Cognitive Aspects of Chronic Illness in Children

COGNITIVE ASPECTS OF CHRONIC ILLNESS IN CHILDREN

Edited by
RONALD T. BROWN

THE GUILFORD PRESS
New York   London

© 1999 The Guilford Press
A Division of Guilford Publications, Inc.
72 Spring Street, New York, NY 10012
http://www.guilford.com

Printed in the United States of America

This book is printed on acid-free paper.

Last digit is print number: 9 8 7 6 5 4 3 2 1

Library of Congress Cataloging-in-Publication Data

Cognitive aspects of chronic illness in children / Ronald T. Brown (editor).
    p.   cm.
   Includes bibliographical references and index.
   ISBN 1-57230-468-5
   1. Chronically ill children—Mental health. 2. Chronically ill children—Psychological aspects. 3. Cognition disorders in children—Health aspects. 4. Chronic diseases in children—Psychological aspects. I. Brown, Ronald T.
RJ380.C64 1999
616'.044'083—dc21   98-56207
                                                CIP

About the Editor

Ronald T. Brown, PhD, ABPP, is Professor of Pediatrics and Director of Program Development in the Department of Pediatrics at the Medical University of South Carolina, Charleston, South Carolina. He also is President-Elect of Section 54 of the American Psychological Association, the Division of the Society of Pediatric Psychology; a Fellow of the American Psychological Association and the American Psychological Society; and a Diplomate of the American Board of Professional Psychology. Dr. Brown serves on the editorial boards of the *Journal of Pediatric Psychology*, the *Journal of Clinical Child Psychology*, *School Psychology Quarterly*, *School Psychology Review*, the *Journal of Learning Disabilities*, and *Children's Services: Social Policy Research and Practice* and has been the recipient of numerous grant awards from the National Institutes of Health. His previous publications include *Medications for School-Age Children: Effects on Learning and Behavior*, coauthored with Michael G. Sawyer (Guilford Press, 1998).

Contributors

Susannah M. Allison, BA, Department of Psychology, George Washington University, Washington, DC

Deborah L. Anderson, PhD, Department of Pediatrics, Medical University of South Carolina, Children's Hospital, Charleston, South Carolina

F. Daniel Armstrong, PhD, Department of Pediatrics, University of Miami School of Medicine, Miami, Florida

Lamia P. Barakat, PhD, Department of Psychology, Sociology, and Anthropology, Drexel University, Philadelphia, Pennsylvania

Douglas R. Bloom, PhD, Division of Developmental Pediatrics, Department of Pediatrics, University of Texas Houston Health Science Center, Houston, Texas

Marc J. Blumberg, PhD, Department of Pediatrics, University of Miami School of Medicine, Miami, Florida

Erika U. Brady, PhD, Department of Pediatrics, University of Miami School of Medicine, Miami, Florida

Pim Brouwers, PhD, Department of Pediatrics, Baylor College of Medicine, Houston, Texas

Ronald T. Brown, PhD, Department of Pediatrics, Medical University of South Carolina, Children's Hospital, Charleston, South Carolina

M. E. Catherine Cant, BA, Department of Psychology, George Washington University, Washington, DC

Alan M. Delamater, PhD, Department of Pediatrics, University of Miami School of Medicine, Miami, Florida

George J. DuPaul, PhD, Department of Education and Human Services, Lehigh University, Bethlehem, Pennsylvania

Linda Ewing-Cobbs, PhD, Division of Developmental Pediatrics, Department of Pediatrics, University of Texas Houston Health Science Center, Houston, Texas

Cheryl Fernandes, BA, Department of Psychology, York University, North York, Ontario, Canada

Natalie C. Frank, PhD, Department of Psychology, George Washington University, Washington, DC

Laura D. Fredrick, PhD, Department of Educational Psychology and Special Education, Georgia State University, Atlanta, Georgia

Marcie Wartel Handler, MEd, Department of Education and Human Services, Lehigh University, Bethlehem, Pennsylvania

Jennifer R. Hiemenz, PhD, Department of Neuropsychology, Kennedy Krieger Institute, Baltimore, Maryland

Catherine Hood, MA, Clinical Child Psychology Program, University of Kansas, Lawrence, Kansas

George W. Hynd, EdD, School of Professional Studies, University of Georgia, Athens, Georgia; Department of Neurology, Medical College of Georgia, Augusta, Georgia

Marta Jimenez, MD, Department of Pediatric Neurology, Instituto Neurológico de Antiquia, Medellin, Colombia

Anne E. Kazak, PhD, Division of Oncology, Children's Hospital of Philadelphia, and Department of Pediatrics, University of Pennsylvania, Philadelphia, Pennsylvania

Betsy D. Kennard, PsyD, Department of Psychiatry, University of Texas Southwestern Medical Center at Dallas, Dallas, Texas

Mary Jo Kupst, PhD, Department of Pediatrics, Medical College of Wisconsin, Milwaukee, Wisconsin

Annette M. La Greca, PhD, Department of Psychology, University of Miami, Coral Gables, Florida

Kathleen L. Lemanek, PhD, Department of Psychology, Children's Hospital, Ohio State University College of Medicine, Columbus, Ohio

Avi Madan-Swain, PhD, Department of Pediatrics, University of Alabama at Birmingham, Birmingham, Alabama

Raymond K. Mulhern, PhD, Division of Behavioral Medicine, St. Jude Children's Research Hospital, Memphis, Tennessee

Lori A. Perez, PhD, HIV and AIDS Malignancy Branch, Cancer Institute and Medical Illness Counseling Center, Bethesda, Maryland

Joanne Rovet, PhD, Department of Psychology, Hospital for Sick Children, and Department of Pediatrics, University of Toronto, Toronto, Ontario, Canada

Wendy B. Schuman, PhD, Department of Psychiatry and Behavioral Sciences, Children's National Medical Center, Washington, DC

Sunita Mahtani Stewart, PhD, Department of Community Medicine, University of Hong Kong, Hong Kong, China

Jan L. Wallander, PhD, Civitan International Research Center and Department of Psychology, University of Alabama at Birmingham, Birmingham, Alabama

Laura Williams, PhD, Department of Psychiatry and Behavioral Sciences, Medical University of South Carolina, Charleston, South Carolina

Mark L. Wolraich, MD, Department of Pediatrics, Division of Child Development, Vanderbilt University, Nashville, Tennessee

Pamela L. Wolters, PhD, HIV and AIDS Malignancy Branch, National Cancer Institute and Medical Illness Counseling Center, Bethesda, Maryland

Preface

This book is intended for clinical child, pediatric, and school psychologists; child psychiatrists; developmental and behavioral pediatricians; and graduate students and trainees in the various disciplines that serve children and adolescents who have chronic diseases, developmental disabilities, and traumatic injuries. The goal of the book is to familiarize the academician, practitioner, and student with the cognitive dysfunctions and learning impairments that are associated with a number of chronic illnesses and developmental disabilities. To some extent, many of these difficulties are rather new, since the prognoses for many diseases have improved markedly over the past several years. In addition, only recently have the cognitive toxicities of specific treatments been realized. Thus, as many of these children and adolescents survive well into their adult years, there is much to learn about their cognitive development. In looking at the excellent contributions of each of the authors, and recalling other articles, book chapters, and books that I have authored or coauthored, I realize that there is more that we need to know than is currently available. To this end, it is anticipated that this book will have some impact on social scientists as they develop programs of research in the field of pediatric psychology. Finally, given the frustration of many pediatric psychologists, health care professionals, and parents of children with chronic illnesses regarding the dearth of services available to children who suffer the adversity of these illnesses, and to their families, it is also anticipated that the book will influence policymakers in the development of much-needed programs. In particular, it is hoped that an even closer alliance will develop between the fields of education, psychology, and pediatrics as we work together to enhance the quality of life for these children and their families.

I wish to express my appreciation to each of the authors who have so willingly given of their time, efforts, and patience to prepare the excellent chapters in this volume. Their tolerance of all of the difficulties associated with preparing an edited book such as this is much appreciated. In addition, I have benefited much from the wisdom of the children and adolescents with whom I have worked at the University of Illinois, Emory University, and the Medical University of South Carolina, as well as the pediatricians with whom I have collaborated at these excellent institutions. Further, all of the editorial guidance from Guilford Publications is very much appreciated, including the wise counsel of Sharon Panulla, the kind assistance of Christopher Jennison, and the meticulous and outstanding editing of Judith Grauman and her associates. No book would be complete without all of the assistance of the staff and faculty with whom I have worked over the years. Martha Hagen's careful typing of the manuscripts as well as Emily Simmerly's excellent editing made the process of writing much more enjoyable. For Kathy and Ryan—for those evenings and weekends away from home and all of the fun things missed, completing this book would not have been possible without your support. Finally, to my many colleagues in the Society of Pediatric Psychology from whom I have learned much about pediatric psychology and scholarship, and who have always provided me with sound advice and counsel, I wish to express my sincere appreciation.

RONALD T. BROWN
Charleston, South Carolina

Contents

III. SPECIAL ISSUES

CHAPTER ONE

Cognition in Chronically Ill Children

A Collaborative Endeavor of Pediatrics and Psychology

RONALD T. BROWN

DEBORAH L. ANDERSON

Tarnowski and Brown (in press) have estimated that 10–15% of children will sustain some type of chronic illness by the age of 18 years. Specifically, a chronic illness refers to a physical condition that may impair health status or psychological functioning. As medical technologies have become increasingly refined and effective, greater numbers of children are surviving diseases that previously carried a more guarded prognosis. Over the past several years, a burgeoning interest in the emotional and behavioral functioning of these children and adolescents has emerged. The psychological community has responded with literature investigating the psychosocial sequelae of various illnesses and their associated treatments.

Four large-scale investigations examining psychological adaptation and associated psychiatric morbidities in children with chronic health conditions are reviewed in Thompson and Gustafson (1996). In the first of these studies, conducted by the United Kingdom National Survey of Health and Development, behavioral questionnaires were administered to children with chronic medical conditions and their parents and teachers. One-fourth of the children had at least two symptoms of behavioral disturbance.

In the second investigation, the Isle of Wight study (Rutter, Tizard, & Whitmore, 1970), parent and teacher reports and psychiatric functioning of children and adolescents with chronic medical conditions were compared to the functioning of their typically developing peers. Findings revealed that nearly 20% of the medically ill sample suffered from psychiatric disorders versus only 7% of their healthy counterparts. The third investigation, the Rochester Child Health Survey (Roghmann & Haggerty, 1970), revealed that children with chronic medical conditions, relative to their healthy peers, had a greater frequency of school, learning, and adjustment difficulties.

The fourth and most comprehensive, rigorous, and methodologically sophisticated investigation of the relationship between psychosocial functioning and chronic illness was completed at McMaster University (Cadman, Boyle, Szatmari, & Offord, 1987). The investigators administered a survey that included items from parent, teacher, and child reports inquiring about symptoms of psychopathology in a sample of over 2,400 children with a chronic illness and their families. The participants were classified by the presence of a disability and compared to healthy peers. The data from this investigation revealed that children with a chronic medical condition comorbid with a disability were 3.4 times more likely than healthy children to have a psychiatric disorder; medically ill children without a disability were only twice as likely to suffer from a psychiatric illness. It is noteworthy that school problems together with social and emotional difficulties were more prevalent in children with both a disability and a medical illness. Clearly, the effects of a chronic medical illness extend beyond the physical domain into the cognitive and psychosocial arenas.

In this book, we conceptualize cognitive functioning as an interplay between the processing of information and affect and how this processing influences mental abilities, attention, memory, language, emotions, and social adaptation. Mounting clinical evidence of learning problems associated with chronic medical illnesses is coupled with the explosion in the literature and widespread clinical interest, resulting in the genesis of a field in pediatric psychology specifically devoted to the identification and management of cognitive and adjustment issues in children with chronic medical conditions. The outcome has been a comprehensive and multidisciplinary approach to the management of disease. Pediatric, clinical, and school psychologists are increasingly well represented on medical school faculties and make viable contributions to research, teaching, and patient care. A great deal of knowledge is required by psychologists and physicians who specialize in this area. Professionals in this field must be equipped with breadth and depth of knowledge in such various disciplines of psychology as physiological bases of behavior, development and psychopathology, principles of learning, and psychological theory as applied to the educational setting. Moreover, all systems that affect the child must be considered, including the family, school, peer group, and health care network.

Neurocognitive assessments are particularly important with this population because cognition may be compromised as a result of the pathophysiology of the disease, the stressors associated in coping with a medical illness, and the iatrogenic effects of medical treatments that affect the cognitive arena. Accordingly, assessments must be comprehensive to include a number of domains of functioning, longitudinal to evaluate for specific disease sequelae, and contextually relevant (e.g., incorporate assessments across settings and informants). This approach requires a vast knowledge of assessment techniques and the ability to communicate recommendations to physicians and school personnel. The competent clinician also must consider secondary prevention issues for children and adolescents at risk for cognitive and adjustment difficulties. Communication of the assessment data to the treating physician allows for informed decision making and permits the identification of the best possible medical treatment while minimizing adverse effects.

SOCIAL–ECOLOGICAL ISSUES ASSOCIATED WITH COGNITIVE ASPECTS OF PEDIATRIC ILLNESS

Children and health care providers are ensconced in a number of systems. These include the school, peer network, family, and health care delivery system. Because these systems affect the adaptation of the child to the illness experience, we review them here.

School

Consultation and liaison with the child's school must be ongoing. In addition to a myriad of neurocognitive deficits that may accompany many pediatric diseases, children also may exhibit associated learning and attention problems that compromise school performance. Frequent school absences related to hospitalizations and outpatient clinic visits only serve to exacerbate an already arduous school reentry experience. The practicing psychologist must be well acquainted with resources offered by the community, the school, and affiliated special education programs. Moreover, educating school personnel regarding various diseases and their associated courses may facilitate the child's reintegration to school and the capacity to cope with classroom expectations. Teachers may require assistance in providing special accommodations for students with limitations. Finally, pediatric psychologists frequently work closely with other allied health professionals to manage medical procedures and to address psychosocial needs of chronically ill children and their families.

Peer Influences

In the chronic illness literature, there has been a recent shift from a focus on psychopathology and risk factors to children's adaptation and protective factors. The interest has been to examine children and adolescents who demonstrate adequate adjustment and adaptation to their chronic illness despite the multitude of stressors that are frequently associated with disease (for review, see Thompson & Gustafson, 1996). The affect of cognitive factors on the emotional arena has been recognized (Tromontana & Hooper, 1997). As a result, children with various brain morphologies and functional deficits also have problems with the regulation and expression of affect. These social-cognitive deficits coupled with restricted peer contact and interaction may diminish the amount of reinforcement that children obtain from the peer group. This may result in decreased social supports and may affect successful disease adaptation detrimentally. Alternatively, social influences and support from peers may positively affect successful adaptation and even enhance disease management and coping (La Greca et al., 1995). In addition, involvement with peers who are able and willing to support chronically ill youngsters in accommodating special needs and dietary restrictions increases adherence and successful disease adaptation.

Family

Social cognition is also influenced by the family system. Family interaction patterns have been demonstrated to mediate successful adaptation to the disease process (Kazak, Segal-Andrews, & Johnson, 1995). The family system not only serves as a vehicle for social support but also models problem solving, coping skills, communication patterns, and mechanisms for seeking social support. Salient variables in this literature include familial cohesion, conflict, expressiveness, and control. In addition, a corpus of research has examined the impact of the disease on the child's family (Rolland, 1987). Family functioning has been found to vary in accordance with the stage of illness and the developmental level of the child. Finally, family functioning influences adjustment of the child to the disease concurrently and prospectively.

Health Care Delivery System

The role of health care providers in children's adaptation to the disease process cannot be underestimated. Implicit within the biopsychosocial model (Engel, 1977) is the notion that the individual's adaptation to an illness is determined both by single systems (i.e., family, school, peers) operating independently and the combined effect of these systems on each other. In essence, the health care delivery system must accommodate the various systems in which the child is involved, just as the child and family must adapt to the medical system. One role of the psychologist is to transverse these systems to assist them in collaborating. In addition, the psychologist may assist the physician in understanding the affect of disease on cognition and adaptation. It is anticipated that this collaborative spirit among clinical, pediatric, and school psychologists will a forge a partnership with our pediatrician colleagues and, ultimately, with the medically ill children whom we serve. We trust that important clinical and research activities will continue to be nurtured as a result of these collaborations and that there will be active liaison among organizations involved with medically ill children.

INTRODUCTION OF THE CHAPTERS

Part I. Basic Issues

There is a clear need for clinical intervention, research, and training for the identification and management of cognitive and learning problems in children and adolescents with chronic illnesses. To address these needs, we have gathered a group of distinguished colleagues to delineate the salient issues in the field; and we review topics that provide the foundation for understanding the basic themes relevant to practice in pediatric psychology. In Chapter 2, Wolraich raises important issues pertaining to the interface of primary care providers and pediatric psychologists and their relationship in a health care setting. The pediatric health care provider is in a seminal position to screen for risk factors or other types of behavioral difficulties. Given that the need for referral is not always readily apparent in the clinical setting, astute medical practitioners who are well versed in issues of child development and adaptation to illness must be vigilant to detect markers that may be indicative of learning or behavioral difficulties. After identification of the problem, practitioners must make a referral to accommodate the patient's needs. Further, the referral question must be posed in a manner that provides the psychologist with the information necessary to assist the patient in the most productive way. Results must be communicated in a manner that the health care provider understands. Finally, this permits the ultimate goal of effective collaboration so that the pediatric patient benefits from the referral process.

Psychometric assessment and interviewing techniques are critical ingredients in pediatric psychologists' provision of services. In a thoughtful chapter related to assessment (Chapter 3), Kupst discusses special issues in the testing of children who are challenged by medical illness. Specifically, attention is devoted to both the neurocognitive assessment process and the behavioral domain. The importance of a developmental perspective is underscored throughout the chapter. The pediatric psychologist must bring to the assessment setting some knowledge of the pathophysiology of various pediatric illnesses and their affect on the cognitive arena. She emphasizes the importance of gathering data across settings so that a comprehensive picture of the child's functioning at home, at school, and with peers is provided. Practical insights are offered that address issues unique to the medical setting and to chronically ill children. Finally, specific information is provided on the available assessment armamentarium.

Part II. Disease-Specific Issues

We have selected disease entities in which pediatric psychologists have made important contributions to research. In fact, in some cases this literature has affected treatment decisions for medically ill children (Tarnowski & Brown, in press). As our empirical knowledge base has increased, we are able to apply these data to clinical practice. In selecting those disease entities to be included in the book, our criteria were that the specific diseases have a rich psychological empirical base and that there has been a history of collaboration with pediatric psychologists.

Armstrong and Mulhern review the research relating to cognitive toxicities associated with prophylactic treatments for acute lymphoblastic leukemia (ALL) and the neurocognitive sequelae of brain tumors (see Chapter 4). In the spirit of our recommendation that psychologists be well grounded in the pathophysiology of diseases in which they are providing services, Armstrong and Mulhern describe aspects of cancer that affect the cognitive arena at baseline, during the course of the disease, and throughout the late-effects period (i.e., at follow-up). An important contribution of the chapter is the lucid review of the many cognitive processes that are affected by various treatments. The data from these studies have been used to guide the development of treatments that minimize neurocognitive toxicities and maximize the quality of life for these children.

To broaden the perspective of the effects of medical illness on cognitive functions, Lemanek and Hood include in their review the influence of cognitive style on children's coping and adaptation to asthma (see Chapter 5). A conceptual framework is provided for specific cognitive processes that affect active coping strategies and adjustment to the disease. Significant implications are raised for the development of self-management programs that promote adherence and quality of life. Finally, a review is provided of the cognitive effects that accompany the pharmacological agents most frequently used to manage children suffering from asthma.

In contrast to asthma, where the pharmacotherapies affect cognitive skills, pediatric HIV infection is a disease that directly exerts deleterious effects on the central nervous system. In Chapter 6, Wolters, Brouwers, and Perez review issues relating to the cognitive assessment of children suffering from this devastating disease. These children and adolescents frequently exhibit global deficits in cognitive functioning as well as in specific areas like attention, memory, and expressive language. The importance of assessing specific areas of functional impairment is highlighted. Although global measures of functioning sometimes yield results indicative of generally normal functioning, more specific neuropsychological testing can identify the exact nature of deficits, thus alerting the physician to further progression of the disease. One must adopt a developmental perspective when evaluating these children, given the importance of age and disease progression. The progressive nature of the disease suggests the need for ongoing evaluation to monitor for exacerbations. Often, adaptation to the disease involves overcoming challenges that are imposed by being disadvantaged as well as coping with a medical condition that is stigmatizing and carries a guarded prognosis. Thus, adaptation may be the result of a complex intertwining of medical and psychosocial factors. With knowledge of cultural sensitivities unique to specific ethnic and social groups, the pediatric psychologist can provide important assistance to children negotiating the hardships imposed by this medical problem.

Insulin-dependent diabetes mellitus is another disease that illustrates the interplay between the family and the patient's understanding of disease, the prescribed treatment regimen, and adherence to treatment demands. Rovet and Fernandes review the affect of diabetes on neurocognitive functioning and then identify associated protective and risk factors (see Chapter 7). In particular, the child must have a threshold of intellectual resources to implement the treatment regimen successfully. Psychologists bring the expertise of developmental disabilities and psychopathology to the medical setting and can assist the health care provider in maximizing adherence in a number of ways. Areas of possible cognitive dysfunction must first be identified by means of careful assessment of mental abilities and learning. Then the psychologist collaborates with the patient, family, and health care provider to develop a treatment program. This will assist the patient in compensating for these deficits so that treatment adherence may be maximized.

A prototype of a disease that requires collaboration between the health care system and pediatric psychologists is sickle cell disease (SCD). Psychologists frequently examine neurocognitive factors and their relationship to disease status and disease management at home and at school. Frank, Allison, and Cant review emerging literature pertaining to neurocognitive and psychosocial functioning of children with SCD (see Chapter 8). Disease severity is discussed as a risk factor for degree of impairment. The chapter highlights the contributions of psychology to the understanding of advances in technology, particularly with neuroimaging techniques (e.g., magnetic resonance imaging).

Development is an important disease parameter in children with cardiac conditions. Chapter 9, by Delamater, Brady, and Blumberg, reviews the literature and suggests that the age of surgical repair for children with congenital heart defects, the type of defect, and the supportive measures used during surgical procedures are important predictors of cognitive outcome. As is evidenced in other childhood chronic illnesses (e.g., leukemia, diabetes), time and process of treatment procedures have critical implications for later cognitive outcome. Again, consistent with the oncology literature, the importance of examining specific components of learning functioning is underscored as essential in providing information needed to design viable intervention programs.

Related to survival, Stewart and Kennard review the clinical and empirical literature on cardiac, kidney, and liver transplantation (see Chapter 10). Salient issues pertaining to outcome include age at onset of the disease and the timing of the transplantation. The authors adapt Wallander's model in predicting risk and resistance factors that interact to determine disease adaptation and psychological adjustment. The chapter highlights the progression in the literature toward theory-driven research and its application to pediatric psychology.

Another patient population in which age at onset is closely associated with later degree of cognitive impairment is children with seizure disorders. Hiemenz, Hynd, and Jimenez review carefully those studies indicating cognitive deficits associated with anticonvulsant medications (see Chapter 11). Fortunately, these effects are transitory, and the skilled pediatric psychologist is an important member of the team in the identification of possible iatrogenic effects of these medications. Children with seizure disorders are best served by a multidisciplinary team that includes the pediatric psychologist, school personnel, and medical staff. The pediatric psychologist plays an essential role in ensuring that the child's psychosocial and academic needs are met while negotiating the stressors of this disease and its associated medical treatment.

Last, assessing and meeting academic and social needs is of prime importance in serving children with traumatic brain injuries (see Chapter 12). Specifically, the cognitive and psychosocial effects of having sustained a traumatic brain injury are reviewed by Ewing-Cobbs and Bloom. Chronological age and type of injury are once again important predictors of extent of cognitive impairment. For psychosocial adjustment, the authors emphasize that premorbid functioning accounts for a greater percentage of the variance in predicting outcome than does the injury itself. This finding underscores the need for practicing psychologists to be well trained in general issues of clinical child psychology. In addition, Ewing-Cobbs and Bloom note that these children frequently are not placed in appropriate classroom settings because their deficits are not always detectable by routine psychological evaluation. Thus, they often must fail academically before appropriate education intervention is recommended. The psychologist can serve these children well by being cognizant of the specific deficits that may result from the injury.

Part III. Special Issues

Working with medically ill children requires the consideration of a multitude of contextual factors, including the family, the peer social network, and the school. These pediatric patients must not only manage the symptoms of their disease but also familial issues and systems, questions from peers, and transition to the classroom. The psychologist may play a pivotal role in facilitating these processes. Further, children with more severe illnesses requiring either aggressive pharmacotherapy or such invasive procedures as transplantation require the full spectrum of services that pediatric psychologists have to offer. Here we may again assist children and their families cope with such stressors and maximize outcome to improve quality of life.

Social cognition and its association with chronic illness is reviewed by Schuman and La Greca in Chapter 13. The authors discuss the affect of chronic illness on social functioning and how the cognitive impairments related to illness couple with the illness itself to impede peer relationships. The authors highlight the essential role that positive peer interactions play in disease management and adaptation. Again, a reciprocal interaction exists in which the illness influences peer relationships and peer support affects disease management. Schuman and La Greca feature innovative treatment programs that promote knowledge of self-management, social skills training, support and coordination among parents, and the reintegration of the child into the classroom.

Madan-Swain, Fredrick, and Wallander discuss the components of successful reintegration to school (see Chapter 14). Chronically ill children face a multitude of adjustment challenges, including academic difficulties and social adjustment issues. This appears to be the case whether the disease is chronic or acute and of short duration. The dearth of research in this area is surprising given the magnitude of the task of school reentry, and the authors emphasize the need for further investigation in this area.

Chapter 15, by Barakat and Kazak, emphasizes the role and affect of family systems on the adaptation of medically ill children to chronic diseases. There is a reciprocal interaction, wherein family functioning affects the child's medical status and the child's illness affects the family system. Again, incorporating a developmental perspective allows the psychologist to formulate hypotheses about specific issues of adjustment during the disease process and to design effective intervention programs for children and adolescents who are at risk. The psychologist must consider non-illness-related factors, including premorbid functioning and external stressors, in developing a plan that will maximally benefit the pediatric patient and the family.

Another important consideration in the management of children with chronic illnesses is the adverse effects of medication on cognition and learning. The cognitive effects of medications used to treat medical disorders are reviewed in Chapter 16 by Handler and DuPaul. They underscore the necessity of assessment and the use of procedures that obtain diagnostic data across settings (i.e., home, school), and informants (teacher, parent, physician) and that establish convergent validity with multiple assessment techniques in the diagnostic process. This is especially important in light of recent advances in medical technology that result in greater numbers of children who survive and return to classrooms.

Finally, we (Anderson, Brown, & Williams, Chapter 17) provide a model by which psychological services are provided to children with chronic illnesses.

SUMMARY

This book provides a framework for reviewing the essential issues associated with the cognitive aspects of chronic medical illness in children. These factors must be considered in accurately assessing and appropriately designing intervention programs for children and adolescents with chronic disease. It is the goal of all disciplines of psychology to enhance adaptation to stressors and to assist in adjustment to the illness. The collaborative nature of our field is mirrored in the flavor and the content of these chapters, each of which focuses on how children receive maximum benefit when there is an integration of divergent sources of information. The best service will come to fruition when psychology forms a strong alliance with pediatrics in this effort to help children affected by chronic illness. We are hopeful that this spirit of collaboration will pervade the research arena by providing the necessary assessment and intervention services to ensure optimal quality of life for these children and their families.

REFERENCES

Cadman, D., Boyle, M., Szatmari, P., & Offord, D. R. (1987). Chronic illness, disability, and mental and social well-being: Findings of the Ontario Child Health Study. *Pediatrics, 79,* 805–813.

Engel, G. L. (1977). The need for a new medical model: A challenge for biomedicine. *Science, 196,* 129–136.

Kazak, A. E., Segal-Andrews, A. M., & Johnson, K. (1995). Pediatric psychology research and practice: A family/systems approach. In M. Roberts (Ed.), *Handbook of pediatric psychology* (2nd ed., pp. 84–104). New York: Guilford Press.

La Greca, A., Auslander, W. F., Greco, P., Spetter, D., Fisher, E. B., & Santiago, J. V. (1995). I get by with a little help from my family and friends: Adolescents' support for diabetes care. *Journal of Pediatric Psychology, 20,* 449–476.

Roghmann, K. J., & Haggerty, R. J. (1970). Rochester Child Health Surveys: I. Objectives, organization and methods. *Medical Care, 8,* 47–59.

Rolland, J. (1987). Chronic illness and the life cycle: A conceptual framework. *Family Process, 26,* 203–221.

Rutter, M., Tizard, J., & Whitmore, K. (1970). *Education, health and behavior*. London: Longmans, Green.

Tarnowski, K. J., & Brown, R. T. (in press). Psychological aspects of pediatric disorders. In M. Hersen & R. T. Ammerman (Eds.), *Advanced abnormal psychology* (2nd ed.). Hillsdale, NJ: Erlbaum.

Thompson, R. J., Jr., & Gustafson, K. E. (1996). *Adaptation to chronic childhood illness*. Washington, DC: American Psychological Association.

Tromontana, M. G., & Hooper, S. R. (1997). Neuropsychology of child psychopathology. In C. R. Reynolds & E. Fletcher-Janzen (Eds.), *Handbook of clinical child neuropsychology* (2nd ed., pp. 120–139). New York: Plenum Press.

PART ONE

BASIC ISSUES

CHAPTER TWO

The Referral Process
The Pediatrician as Gatekeeper

MARK L. WOLRAICH

Recognition and early treatment of psychoeducational and emotional issues in children with chronic illness usually begins with the child's primary care clinician (PCC). This individual is most commonly a general pediatrician, family practitioner, or, in some cases under supervision, a nurse practitioner or physician's assistant. However, in some instances in which a child has a complicated chronic illness, a pediatric subspecialist may also assume the role of PCC. Examples of this would be a pediatric pulmonologist who takes on the primary care responsibilities for children with cystic fibrosis or a pediatric endocrinologist who does so for children with severe cases of diabetes mellitus.

An important characteristic of the PCC–family relationship is that it is usually ongoing. The PCC has the opportunity to interact and observe the children and their families over time and to see them on numerous occasions. When this relationship exists, families feel more comfortable about first seeking help for emotional problems from the PCC whom they know and trust.

In this capacity, PCCs can play an important role in screening their patients for psychosocial and cognitive–developmental problems, and providing them with assistance. Families may be hesitant to admit to or may be unaware of the need for mental health and cognitive–developmental services, particularly if they are caught up in the demands of medical care for their child's chronic illness. In addition, when a PCC provides care to a child with a chronic illness, along with siblings and other family members, he or she is in a position to identify concerns that may develop as a result of the added stress of caring for a child with a chronic illness.

The PCC can also facilitate the family's effort to seek mental health or cognitive–developmental services, frequently a difficult barrier for families to overcome. The presence of a supportive, trusted PCC who can assist caregivers in identifying and obtaining appropriate services may be the difference between receiving and not receiving such services.

Furthermore, the PCC plays an important role in the prevention of greater adjustment or learning difficulties. By identifying problems early, he or she can assist in getting those situations addressed prior to their impact becoming significantly adverse to the child. The PCC can also anticipate problems that are likely to be associated with the developmental level of the child, including language problems during early childhood or compliance issues at adolescence. This anticipatory guidance can help prevent more serious and costly problems by addressing them in their early stages.

The role of the PCC has become even more important with the recent changes in the health care system within the United States and specifically under managed care, where the PCC takes on the additional role of "gatekeeper," reducing health care costs by limiting referrals to those cases where services are appropriate. This concept is not new to health care systems. The British system has traditionally limited subspecialty care to those referred by their general practitioners. This process became more formalized under the government run health care system in the United Kingdom after World War II. The role of gatekeeper, particularly as defined by managed care programs in the United States, can be difficult because the PCC has the competing responsibilities of reducing health costs by restricting the use of specialists, while, at the same time, serving as the advocate for patients and their families.

As gatekeeper for children with psychosocial and cognitive–developmental problems, the PCC has an even more difficult role than when serving as gatekeeper for children's general medical care. In most health care plans, mental health benefits are frequently more limited than the general medical benefits provided to families. There is often a limit, or cap, on the extent of benefits, and the process of obtaining approval from a behavioral health management company prior to receiving services often can be challenging. The company not only determines the appropriateness of the referrals, but also dictates the type of practitioner and in some cases the specific mental health clinician that the families may use. Families and PCCs frequently have to deal with centralized approval procedures (1-800 numbers) and limited services from mental health clinicians who are unknown to them. Cognitive–developmental problems are considered to be under the domain of the education system and are not compensated at all.

Services for psychosocial problems are further complicated because distinctions are not always clear between requirements for mental health services as opposed to educational services or, perhaps, their combination. Cognitive and developmental deficits are mostly relegated to school services. With both educational and mental health programs trying to reduce their expenses, each frequently attempts to shift the gray areas to the other's program. There are no formal mechanisms to easily arbitrate and apportion responsibilities. In sum, even when PCCs identify the need for mental health or cognitive–developmental services and families are in agreement, it is not always possible to obtain adequate services. Further, under the new managed care systems, there is less opportunity for PCCs to work in coordination with their patients' mental health clinicians.

To further understand the role of pediatricians as gatekeepers, it is useful first to review the prevalence of mental illness in children in the primary care settings, the effect of chronic illness on the prevalence of mental illness in children, and what is known about pediatricians' abilities to identify emotional and cognitive problems in children, and then to describe some efforts that can enhance the ability of PCCs to identify and obtain services for emotional and cognitive problems in their patients with chronic illness.

PREVALENCE OF MENTAL ILLNESS IN CHILDREN IN PRIMARY CARE SETTINGS AND IN CHILDREN WITH CHRONIC ILLNESS

No studies were located that have examined the specific issue of psychosocial and cognitive–developmental problems among children with chronic illness seen in a primary care context. However, there is information about the presence of psychosocial and cognitive–developmental issues in primary care and about mental and cognitive–developmental problems in children with chronic illness. A review of both of these areas will help to address indirectly the question of mental and cognitive–developmental disorders in children with chronic illness in a primary care context.

The prevalence of mental disorders in children either in community or primary care settings has been found to range from 18% to 22% (Costello, 1989; Offord et al., 1987). This prevalence rate has increased in the primary care setting from 7% in 1979 (Goldberg, Roghmann, McInerny, & Burke, 1983) to at least 18% in the primary care setting at present (Kelleher et al., 1999). The latter two studies were dependent on physician recognition, so some of the change may reflect better identification by physicians. While there were increases in all diagnostic categories, the greatest absolute increase was in the identification of problems associated with attention and hyperactivity. During this time there also were parallel increases in the number of children living in poverty and in single-parent families (Kelleher et al., 1999). This high prevalence rate in the general population suggests that a high rate of problems is to be expected in the population of children with chronic illnesses. Surprisingly similar prevalence rates were found for mental disorders (Costello, 1989) as were found for the combination of problems and mental disorders (Horwitz, Leaf, Leventhal, Forsyth, & Speechly, 1992; Kelleher et al., 1999). This, again, may reflect the lower disorder recognition rate of PCCs. Many of the children they identified as having problems may actually meet the criteria for a disorder diagnosis.

While a few studies document no increase in the extent of mental illness in children with chronic illness (Cassileth et al., 1984; Drotar et al., 1981), most have found that the prevalence of mental disorders increases with chronic illness. Thus, chronic illnesses pose a specific risk factor for psychiatric disorders, yet are not sufficient conditions for such disorders (Lavigne & Faier-Routman, 1992). There is an associated increase in internalizing conditions, such as anxiety or depression, and in poor self-esteem.

Externalizing conditions (i.e., disruptive behavior disorders including oppositional defiant disorder, conduct disorder, and attention-deficit/hyperactivity disorder), on the other hand, actually appear to be less frequent in children with chronic illness than in the general population. However, the rates are affected by the specific source used to identify children. For example, teachers appear to identify more internalizing conditions than do parents (Lavigne & Faier-Routman, 1992). The risk of psychological adjustment also may vary across different medical conditions, although this remains to be clarified. Conditions involving central nervous system function, such as seizure disorders, increase the risk of psychological and cognitive problems (Lavigne & Faier-Routman, 1992). It is, therefore, important for the PCC to be more vigilant for psychosocial and cognitive–developmental problems in children with chronic illness, and to keep in mind that these problems are more likely to manifest themselves as internalizing conditions that have less outwardly visible symptoms. It is particularly useful to have input from teachers and children themselves to identify these problems.

PEDIATRICIAN IDENTIFICATION

Given the high prevalence rate of mental disorders and psychosocial problems, the next logical step is to determine how well PCCs identify these problems. Little information is available about the identification by PCCs of cognitive and emotional problems in children with chronic illness, but there is some related to the ability of PCCs to identify mental illness in the children in their practices. These results raise a concern that primary care physicians underdiagnose mental disorders in children. Although the prevalence of mental disorders based on epidemiological surveys of children ranges from 10% to 20% (Offord et al., 1987), the prevalence of those actually diagnosed and identified by primary care clinicians has been in the range of 2–5% (Costello, Costello, et al., 1988). The epidemiological studies are based on structured psychiatric interviews with parents and/or patients using the criteria of the third revised edition of the *Diagnostic and Statistical Manual of Mental Disorders* (DSM-III-R; American Psychiatric Association, 1987). Using such rigorous identification methods, Costello, Edelbrock, and colleagues (1988) found that primary care physicians were reasonably specific (.84) but not very sensitive (.17) in classifying mental disorders in children. Results were better in a study examining the specific diagnosis of attention-deficit/hyperactivity disorder, with a specificity of .97 and a sensitivity of .44 (Lindgren et al., 1989). However, it is important to note that both studies suggest that primary care physicians tend to underdiagnose mental disorders in children.

A number of factors contribute to these findings. PCCs receive relatively little training pertaining to mental disorders in children. For example, a review of the Pediatric curriculum in 1978 (Task Force on Pediatric Education, 1978) reported that many residency training programs offered physicians minimal or no training in the psychosocial aspects of pediatrics. Since then most programs have increased developmental–behavioral pediatrics in their curricula, but in most programs it is limited to 1 month, unless the residents themselves elect to pursue the area further during their elective time. The more recent requirements now include the equivalent of 2 months training. However, because the major emphasis of many developmental–behavioral pediatric rotations is on milder behavioral problems, issues of prevention, and developmental disabilities rather than on mental disorders, it is likely that little or no time is spent devoted to diagnostic criteria for mental disorders or, particularly, to DSM nomenclature.

This lack of exposure to mental health diagnostic criteria is reflected in the practice of primary care physicians. In a national survey of pediatricians and family practitioners related to the identification and diagnosis of attention-deficit/hyperactivity disorder (Wolraich et al., 1990), only 24% reported using DSM criteria to make the diagnosis. Most primary care physicians do not use DSM criteria and are therefore not likely to identify many of the children diagnosed on the basis of interviews specifically employing these criteria.

In addition to the lack of information regarding diagnostic criteria, PCCs rarely have sufficient practice time to address psychosocial problems. The average primary care visit is 13 minutes (Bryant & Shimizu, 1988). In that time, it is difficult, if not impossible, to adequately explore psychosocial and cognitive–developmental issues. Consequently, PCCs must deal with issues about which they have relatively little training in too short a period of time. Thus, it is not surprising to find that PCCs are reluctant to address these issues.

The trend of underdiagnosis of mental disorders is further compounded because mothers do not perceive the primary care visit as an appropriate time to raise such issues. In support of this notion, a study by Hickson, Altemeir, and O'Connor (1983) found that 70% of the mothers had psychosocial concerns about their children, but only 28% of them raised them with their physician. The major reason for not doing so was that the mothers were unaware that their pediatricians could help them with these concerns.

A further factor contributing to the low level of identification of mental disorders by PCCs is their reluctance to place a mental disorder label on a child. This is suggested in a study by Starfield and Barkowf (1989). Psychiatric diagnoses still carry social stigma. The negative perceptions are further reinforced by a commonly held belief that many mental disorders imply inadequate child rearing. There also is a belief that, for many disorders, treatment has a limited benefit. All of these beliefs make psychiatric diagnoses upsetting to parents and are likely to make PCCs reluctant to place this added burden on the families.

In addition, psychiatric labeling can have adverse effects on health insurance for the subscriber. There have been instances in which insurance policies have been denied or further restricted in their mental health services coverage because of the diagnosis carried by a family member. Further, as noted earlier, many insurance companies now limit reimbursement for mental disorders and carve out the service system from general medical services so that PCCs do not receive adequate compensation for time taken to address psychosocial issues.

The diagnostic process is further made difficult for PCCs because they are faced with a broad spectrum of psychosocial problems, ranging from normal developmental variations in behaviors dependent on the child's age, to subthreshold conditions or problems, to actual psychiatric disorders. The criteria for diagnosis of psychiatric disorders are not sufficiently clear for the physician to decide if the presenting behaviors are severe enough to meet them. Given the belief that a mental disorder diagnosis is likely to be stigmatizing, the physician is likely to err on the side of underdiagnosing if he or she is unsure of the diagnosis.

The characterization of the spectrum of psychosocial phenomenon is made more difficult by the DSM system, which was developed for psychiatric use. Its emphasis has been on defining disorders so that mental health clinicians can become more precise in their terminology and so that empirical studies of these disorders can be pursued. This system has very effectively increased the empirical knowledge of mental disorders. However, the range of mental problems seen in the primary care setting is much broader than that seen by psychiatrists because children and adolescent patients have not been filtered through a referral system that removes most of the less severely affected children.

RECOMMENDATIONS FOR IMPROVEMENT

To enhance the abilities of PCCs to address psychosocial problems, several recommendations are possible within the constraints faced by these practitioners. It appears that parents' concerns may be a useful way of screening for mental health problems. Parental concern has been shown to be as good as developmental screening tests for identifying developmental delay in children under the age of 5 years (Glascoe, Foster, & Wolraich, 1997). In addition, in a study that examined both physician and parent identification of child mental health disorders, parents' concerns were found to be a useful source of identification, with a sensitivity of .85. However, they were found to overidentify disorders, with a specificity of .55 (Costello, Edelbrock, et al., 1988). It is possible that the children overidentified may be those who do not quite meet the criteria for diagnosis but have significant problems that warrant attention. Utilizing parental concerns as a screening method provides the practical benefit of time- and cost-effectiveness and has the advantage of specifically addressing concerns that caretakers bring to the office setting. PCCs therefore need to make parents aware that they can discuss these issues as part of their physician visits.

Parent rating scales such as the Pediatric Symptom Checklist (Jellinek, Murphy, & Burns, 1986) are another method used to screen children more efficiently. These are not yet used extensively by pediatricians, but do show some promise in helping to identify children in need. They provide the benefit of collecting information from the parent and/or teacher without taking up much physician time. Because the scales have normative data, it is possible to compare a parent's individual rating to a sample of children with a normal distribution.

A practice being instituted as part of family practitioner training also may contribute to the identification of mental health and cognitive–developmental problems in children. Family practitioner training programs have increased their interest in family systems (Doherty & Baird, 1984), resulting in trained family practitioners to address psychosocial and cognitive–developmental issues in their explorations of family dynamics. Use of such procedures as the genogram may help family practitioners to explore family psychosocial and cognitive–developmental issues and to improve their identification of problems in the family that have potentially adverse effects on the children.

Finally, a mental health classification system more suited to the phenomena observed in primary care can assist PCCs in describing what they observe and in documenting their interventions. Horwitz et al. (1992) found that when a classification system designed for primary care is used, PCCs are better able to identify psychosocial problems. In addition, a study of a national sample of general pediatricians and family practitioners found that these physicians identified about 18% of their patients as having psychosocial problems (Kelleher et al., 1999), findings generally consistent with the epidemiological literature (Costello, 1989).

Interest in the development of a broader classification system brought together pediatricians, child psychologists, and child psychiatrists under the auspices of the American Academy of Pediatrics to develop *The Classification of Child and Adolescent Mental Conditions in Primary Care: Diagnostic and Statistical Manual for Primary Care (DSM-PC), Child and Adolescent Version* (Wolraich, 1996). This classification system places environmental situations prominently in the system, defines a spectrum of child manifestations that include normal variations and problems as well as disorders, and provides developmentally based descriptions of the symptoms. It allows the PCC to document the need for preventive interventions prior to a child's situation reaching the point of becoming a diagnosable psychiatric disorder. This classification system, ideally, will better enable researchers to demonstrate the efficacy of preventive interventions to decrease the risk of mental disorders and ultimately to reduce costs of delivering mental health services.

RESEARCH NEEDS

Future research is needed to clarify mental health care for children with chronic illness. First, further delineation of the nature of mental illness in children with chronic illness is needed to distinguish condition-specific from more generic problems that cut across conditions. There is also a need to confirm basic assumptions in the DSM-PC (Wolraich, 1996) where problems as well as disorders are described. It remains to be determined if the distinctions between these levels of severity may be made reliably and to what extent the distinctions between problems and disorders have clinical relevance, issues of considerable import for primary care identification and management.

In this era of cost containment and the need to identify what is efficacious and what is not, research is needed to assess the impact of preventive measures. Will early interventions to address mental health and cognitive–developmental concerns in children with chronic illnesses and their siblings reduce the number of mental disorders or diminish the severity of cognitive–developmental deficits that develop in these children, and, in the long run, are those efforts cost-effective? What is the most efficient and effective method to integrate the physical and mental needs of children with chronic illnesses and their families, and how do you coordinate multiple caregivers to provide family-centered, community-based cost-effective care? These are but two examples of the type of research questions that are required to clarify the need for services, so that intervention can be both effective and efficient.

SUMMARY

PCCs play a central role in the care of children with chronic illness. That role includes identifying, treating, and, if needed, referring children to meet their emotional, cognitive–developmental, and behavioral needs. In the past, PCCs have not been well trained to fill this role and usually do not have adequate time in their practice to do so. Their ability to address psychosocial and cognitive–developmental issues has been further challenged by the development of managed care, which has increased the pressure on PCCs to see more children and refer fewer. The use of techniques such as exploring parental concerns, utilizing parent and teacher rating scales, and employing the classification of mental conditions in primary care (the DSM-PC; Wolraich, 1996) can help note PCCs more effective in addressing psychosocial issues, but more research is needed to evaluate the efficacy of these diagnostic techniques in identifying children who are in need of mental health and developmental services.

REFERENCES

American Psychiatric Association. (1987). *Diagnostic and statistical manual of mental disorders* (3rd ed., rev.). Washington, DC: Author.

Bryant, E., & Shimizu, I. (1988). *Sample design, sampling variance, and estimation procedures for the National Ambulatory Medical Care Survey.* Bethesda, MD: Vital and Health Statistics Public Health Service.

Cassileth, B. R., Lusk, E. J., Strouse, T. B., Miller, D. S., Brown, L. L., Gross, P. A., & Tenaglia, A. N. (1984). Psychosocial status in chronic illness: A comparative analysis of six diagnostic groups. *New England Journal of Medicine, 311,* 506–511.

Costello, E. (1989). Child psychiatric disorders and their correlates: A primary care pediatric sample. *Journal of the American Academy of Child and Adolescent Psychiatry, 28,* 851–855.

Costello, E., Costello, A., Edelbrock, C. Byrns, B. J., Dulcan, M. K., Brent, D., & Janisz-Ewski, S. (1988). Psychiatric disorders in pediatric primary care: Prevalence and risk factors. *Archives of General Psychiatry, 45,* 1107–1116.

Costello, E., Edelbrock C., Costello A., Dulcan, M. K., Byrns, B. J., & Brent, D. (1988). Psychopathology in pediatric primary care: The new hidden morbidity. *Pediatrics, 82,* 415–434.

Doherty, W., & Baird, M. (1984). A protocol for family compliance counseling. *Family and Systemic Medicine, 2,* 333–336.

Drotar, D., Doershuk, C. F., Stein, R. C., Boat, T. F., Boyer, W., & Mathers L. (1981). Psychosocial functioning of children with cystic fibrosis. *Pediatrics, 67,* 338–343.

Glascoe, F., Foster, M., & Wolraich, M. (1997). An economic evaluation of four methods for detecting developmental problems. *Pediatrics, 99,* 830–837.

Goldberg, I. D., Roghmann, K. J., McInerny, T. K., & Burke, J. D. (1983). Mental health problems among children seen in pediatric practice. *Pediatrics, 73*, 278–293.

Hickson, G., Altemeier, W., & O'Connor, S. (1983). Concerns of mothers seeking care in private pediatric offices: Opportunities for expanding services. *Pediatrics, 72*, 619–624.

Horwitz, M., Leaf, J., Leventhal, M., Forsyth, M., & Speechly, N. (1992). Identification and management of psychosocial and developmental problems in community-based primary care pediatric practices. *Pediatrics, 89*, 480–485.

Jellinek, M., Murphy, M., & Burns, J. (1986). Brief psychosocial screening in outpatient pediatric practice. *Journal of Pediatrics, 109*, 371–378.

Kelleher, K. J., McInerny, T. K., Gardner, W. P., Childs, G. E., Wasserman, R. C., & Nutting, P. A. (1999). *Changing prevalence of clinician-identified psychosocial problems among children (1979–1996): A report from ASPN and PROS.* Manuscript submitted for publication.

Lavigne, J. V., & Faier-Routman, J. (1992). Psychosocial adjustment to pediatric physical disorders: A meta-analytic review. *Journal of Pediatric Psychology, 17*, 133–157.

Lindgren, S., Wolraich, M., Stromquist, A., Davis, C., Milich, R., & Watson, D. (1989, November). *Diagnosis of attention deficit hyperactivity disorder by primary care physicians.* Paper presented at Mental Health Services for Children and Adolescents in Primary Care Settings: A Research Conference, New Haven, CT.

Offord, D. R., Boyle, M. H., Szatmari, P., Rae-Grant, N. I., Links, P. S., Cadman, D. T., Byles, J. A., Crawford, J. W., Blum, H. M., Byrne, C., et al. (1987). Ontario Child Health Study: II. Six-month prevalence of disorder and rates of service utilization. *Archives of General Psychiatry, 44*, 832–836.

Starfield, B., & Borkowf, S. (1989). Physicians' recognition of complaints made by parents about their children's health. *Pediatrics, 43*, 168–172.

Task Force on Pediatric Education. (1978). *The future of pediatrics.* Evanston, IL: American Academy of Pediatrics.

Wolraich, M. L. (1996). *The classification of child and adolescent mental conditions in primary care: Diagnostic and statistical manual for primary care (DSM-PC), child and adolescent version.* Elk Grove, IL: American Academy of Pediatrics.

Wolraich, M. L., Lindgren, S., Stromquist, A., Milich, R., Davis, C., & Watson D. (1990). Stimulant medication use by primary care physicians in the treatment of attention deficit hyperactivity disorder. *Pediatrics, 86*, 95–101.

CHAPTER THREE

Assessment of Psychoeducational and Emotional Functioning

MARY JO KUPST

In its many forms, psychological assessment provides an essential contribution to the understanding and care of children with chronic medical conditions. Recommendations based on assessments are influential both in the way medical procedures and treatments are conducted with the individual child and on other facets of the child's life, such as family life and school adjustment. Referrals for assessment may come from medical and nursing staff, social workers, or parents. Alternatively, the psychologist may have reason to conduct an independent evaluation. Reasons for assessment may be similar to those found in general child psychology practice, but pediatric medical conditions, including chronic illnesses, present unique and specific questions that are frequently not encountered in general practice. These situations offer opportunities as well as challenges for the pediatric psychologist.

SPECIFIC ISSUES IN THE ASSESSMENT OF CHILDREN AND ADOLESCENTS

Assessment of children and adolescents requires an understanding of and experience in relevant developmental issues and concerns. Unlike adult assessment, where one or two standardized measures (e.g., Wechsler Adult Intelligence Scale [WAIS-III], Minnesota Multiphasic Personality Inventory [MMPI-2]) may typically be used, the pediatric psychologist must have proficiency and skill in administering and interpreting different measures and modalities depending upon the child's chronological age and developmental level. Thus, in child psychology, the psychologist may administer several different tests of overall cognitive functioning: Bayley Scales of Infant Development, Wechsler Preschool and Primary Scale of Intelligence—Revised (WPPSI-R), Wechsler Intelligence Scale for Children–III (3rd ed., WISC-III), Woodcock–Johnson Tests of Cognitive Abilities, Kaufman Assessment Battery for Children (K-ABC). In cases where serial evaluations are done, the appropriate tests may change as the child grows older.

In contrast to adult assessment, it is frequently necessary to obtain data from several key sources in addition to the child. In a cognitive assessment, direct observation and interaction with the child is the usual mode, but this procedure is often supplemented by reports from teachers and parents. Their information may be elicited through interviews as well as questionnaires and rating scales. In personality, social, and behavioral assessment, there may be multiple sources: parents, teachers, peers, counselors, social workers, and sometimes medical staff, each contributing a unique perspective to the child's functioning. As we know from child psychology, children may exhibit different behaviors in different settings and with different people. The findings of assessments in a clinical setting may be equally valid but conflicting, as in the case of a child who is well behaved at home but very disruptive in school. Different perspectives also may lead to conflicting expectations of the psychologist in terms of recommendations. A parent may view the problem as residing with the school and reject the recommendation for parental involvement in the treatment plan. The teacher, on the other hand, may see the problem as one of lack of behavior management at home. Finally, the child may see the problem as being singled out and picked on by peers at school. In these cases, it is important to obtain as much data as possible, particularly from multiple indicators of the child's behavior across settings and situations to avoid the evaluation of the child within only one setting. A limited assessment in one setting or situation could result in spurious results.

Still another dilemma frequently encountered in assessment of children and adolescents is the diagnostic formulation. While it is sometimes necessary to determine the child's level of functioning, type of problem, direction for intervention and, of course, insurance criteria for reimbursement, there is a risk of creating a diagnostic label that will become a permanent part of a child's hospital, school, or insurance records. For this reason, it is important to note the particular question being asked, to avoid such labels if possible, or to find the least pathological diagnosis that is still valid for this particular child.

In general, the typical assessment in child and adolescent clinical practice involves what Sattler (1988) has labeled the four pillars of assessment: norm-referenced tests, interviews, observations, and "informal" assessment. Most readers will be familiar with the helpful guidelines provided in this text and in a more recent book in which guidelines and techniques of clinical interviewing are presented, including information relevant to specific childhood medical conditions (Sattler, 1997).

ASSESSMENTS CONDUCTED IN PEDIATRIC CHRONIC ILLNESS

As in more general practice, a child or adolescent may be referred for evaluation to determine the existence of a serious mental health problem, such as depression, suicidal ideation, anxiety, or thought disorder. There may also be more formal cognitive and academic evaluations to assist with school placement after a prolonged absence from school due to medical treatment. In addition, assessment of the needs of the child and family and identification of the resources necessary during a time of high stress are also common tasks for the pediatric psychologist.

In addition to the commonalities in traditional psychological practice (i.e., clinical and school psychology), however, many pediatric conditions require more specific expertise from a psychologist trained in health psychology. For example, the psychologist is frequently asked to conduct a pain assessment to assist with the management of specific pediatric conditions, including juvenile rheumatoid arthritis, cancer, or sickle cell anemia. A careful pain assessment will assure that the child receives adequate pain control. Another area is that of adherence to particular medical regimens—for example, diet, medications, exercises—in which the psychologist may perform a behavioral assessment of current adherence problems, where ongoing assessment is employed as an intervention (sticker charts, reward systems) for the purposes of promoting adherence.

For specific medical conditions, children are treated on standard clinical protocols, which are referred to as clinical trials. As part of these clinical trials, psychologists evaluate children to assess differences among treatment arms in neurocognitive toxicities or quality-of-life outcomes. The necessity for these assessments developed out of clinical experiences in practice. Pediatric cancer is an example. About 20 years ago, cranial irradiation was used to prevent leukemia cells from proliferating to the central nervous system (CNS). As more children were treated and these children grew older, it was found that children with leukemia or CNS tumors who endured high doses of cranial irradiation, particularly during early childhood, were at increased risk for lowered mental abilities and basic deficits in memory, attention, processing speed, fine motor control, and mathematical ability (Madan-Swain & Brown, 1991; Mulhern, Hancock, Fairclough, & Kun, 1992). Psychologists frequently work collaboratively, and in the two pediatric clinical trials groups (sponsored by the National Cancer Institute) conduct ongoing assessment studies in order to document the effect of treatment on mental and behavioral abilities, and to develop recommendations to assist in these children's academic progress (Armstrong & Horn, 1995).

In many institutions, psychologists are increasingly called upon to assist in determining the level of understanding of medical information in children and their parents by administering standardized cognitive tests prior to a medical procedure, such as bone marrow transplant. Most importantly, the psychologist may be asked to provide information related to the parent's or patient's capacity to provide consent/assent to such procedures. And, as scientist–practitioner, the psychologist also may provide assessment as part of psychological research in chronic diseases, including coping and adjustment, risk and resistance factors, neuropsychological functioning, and quality of life. Even in clinics and hospitals where routine screening of selected populations is the standard of care, there are usually underlying reasons why screening is conducted, such as to detect children and families at risk for later adjustment problems.

These examples point to the need for the pediatric psychologist to be familiar with the pathophysiology and medical management of various chronic diseases, as they may affect the referral or research question and, subsequently, the choice of assessment tools in addressing the specific referral question. A thorough discussion of behavioral assessment, including interviews, rating scales, and observational procedures, in child and pediatric psychology is provided by Eyberg (1985). In addition, I have surveyed the past 5 years of the *Journal of Pediatric Psychology*, to identify measures common to pediatric research and practice. Table 3.1 presents the most frequently used measures for assessing children with pediatric conditions. Since parents, typically mothers, are also included in many of the reviewed studies, Table 3.2 presents the most frequently used measures for assessing parents of children with pediatric conditions.

Most of these measures are also common to the general clinical child literature, although the practitioner must be judicious in employing these instruments with pediatric chronically ill children. It is common for children with medical conditions to exhibit symptoms of anxiety, depression, anger, denial, and regression, especially when first diagnosed or during the course of difficult treatments, although these are rarely indicators of psychopathology (Sattler, 1997). Coping with these illnesses is a process, and it is important to note the situations under which the behaviors and reactions are observed.

For example, the Child Behavior Checklist (CBCL), the most commonly used rating scale of problem behaviors in articles that have appeared in the past 5 years of the *Journal of Pediatric Psychology*, has several limitations (Perrin, Stein, & Drotar, 1991). Children with physical symptoms may score as having a high frequency of behavior problems due to a subscale associated with somatic complaints as well as a preponderance of items that reflect psychopathology (which may be due to the particular disorder or its treat-

TABLE 3.1. Frequently Used Measures of Child Functioning in Pediatric Psychology

Variable	Title	Type	Respondent
Cognitive functioning	Bayley Scales of Infant Development (Bayley, 1993)	Standardized administration	Infants/ children 0–4
	Wechsler Preschool and Primary Scale of Intelligence (Wechsler, 1989)	Standardized administration	Children 3–6
	McCarthy Scales of Children's Abilities (McCarthy, 1972)	Standardized administration	Children 2–8
	Wechsler Intelligence Scale for Children–III (Wechsler, 1991)	Standardized administration	Children 6–16
	Stanford Binet Intelligence Scale— 4th Edition (Thorndike, Hagen, & Sattler, 1986)	Standardized administration	Children 3– adults
	Kaufman Assessment Battery for Children (Kaufman & Kaufman, 1993)	Standardized administration	Children 2½– 12½
	Woodcock–Johnson Psycho-educational Battery (Cognitive) (Woodcock & Johnson, 1989)	Standardized administration	Children 3– adults
	Wechsler Adult Intelligence Scale–III (Wechsler, 1997)	Standardized administration	Adolescents/ adults
Academic achievement	Wide Range Achievement Test–3 (Wilkinson, 1993)	Paper and pencil; normed	Children 5– adults
	Woodcock–Johnson Tests of Achievement (Woodcock & Johnson, 1989)	Standardized administration	Children 3– adults
Development/ adaptive	Vineland Adaptive Behavior Scales (Sparrow, Balla, & Cicchetti, 1984)	Interview; paper and pencil	Parents, caregivers
	Minnesota Child Development Inventory (Ireton & Thwing, 1974)	Checklist rating scale	Parents, caregivers
Visual–motor	Test of Visual–Motor Integration (Beery, 1989)	Paper-and-pencil drawing	Children 3– adults
Adjustment	Child Behavior Checklist (Achenbach, 1991)	Checklist rating scale	Parents, children, teachers
	Eyberg Child Behavior Inventory (Eyberg & Ross, 1978)	Checklist rating scale	Parents, caregivers
	Conners Parent Rating Scale (Conners, 1989)	Checklist rating scale	Parents, caregivers
	Personal Adjustment and Role Skills Scale–III (Stein & Jessop, 1990)	Checklist rating scale	Parents, adolescents
	Behavior Problems Checklist (Quay & Peterson, 1975)	Checklist rating scale	Parents, caregivers

(*continued*)

TABLE 3.1. *continued*

Variable	Title	Type	Respondent
Depression	Childhood Depression Inventory (Kovacs & Beck, 1977)	Written self-report	Children
Anxiety	State–Trait Anxiety Inventory for Children (Spielberger, Edwards, Lushene, Montuori, &, Platzek, 1973)	Written self-report	Children
	Children's Manifest Anxiety Scale—Revised (Reynolds & Richman, 1978)	Written self-report	Children
Social functioning	Self-Perception Profile for Children (Harter, 1985)	Written self-report	Children
	Social Skills Rating System (Gresham & Elliott, 1990)	Rating scale	Children
Coping	Kidcope (Spirito, Stark, & Williams, 1988)	Interview; written self-report	Children
	Children's Coping Strategies Checklist (Sandler, Tein, & West, 1994)	Checklist	Children
	Ways of Coping Questionnaire (Folkman & Lazarus, 1988)	Checklist	Children 12–adults
Procedural distress	Observational Scale of Behavioral Distress (Elliott, Jay, & Woody, 1987)	Systematic observation	Observers
	Child–Adult Medical Procedure Interaction Scale—Revised (Blount et al., 1997)	Systematic observation	Observers

ment). At the other end of the continuum, the CBCL was designed to identify symptoms associated with psychopathology and is normed on referred clinical populations and nonreferred samples. Thus, it may not be sensitive to these unique behaviors shown in children who are psychologically healthy but who have a physical disorder. Thus, data from rating scales should be supplemented with other assessment techniques, including interviews, observations, and other self-report measures. Similarly, using the example of assessing the neurotoxicities of CNS irradiation, the sole use of a measure of mental abilities such as the Wechsler Full Scale IQ might lead one to conclude that there are no cognitive problems, when the use of additional measures that tap specific memory or processing speed would be more sensitive in identifying the sequelae of this treatment. Indeed, when the referral question pertains to a specific ability associated with a specific medical condition, it is more appropriate and efficient to select measures that are specific and sufficiently sensitive to the issues in question.

Cognitive measures may include neuropsychological tests that tap a

TABLE 3.2. Frequently Used Measures of Parent Functioning
in Pediatric Psychology

Variable	Title	Type
Adjustment	SCL90-R/Brief Symptom Inventory (Derogatis, 1983)	Checklist
	Psychiatric Symptom Index (Ifeld, 1976)	Checklist
	Profile of Mood States (McNair, Lorr, & Droppelman, 1992)	Checklist
Depression	Beck Depression Inventory (Beck, Ward, Mendelson, Mock, & Erbaugh, 1961)	Checklist
Anxiety	State–Trait Anxiety Inventory (Spielberger, Gorsuch, Lushene, Vagg, & Jacobs, 1970)	Checklist
Parenting stress	Parenting Stress Inventory (Abidin, 1986)	Checklist
Family environment	Family Environment Scale (Moos & Moos, 1986)	Checklist
	FACES-III (Olson & Tiesel, 1991)	Checklist
Marital adjustment	Dyadic Adjustment Scale (Spanier, 1976)	Checklist
Coping	Ways of Coping Questionnaire (Folkman & Lazarus, 1988)	Checklist
	Coping–Health Inventory for Parents (McCubbin & Thompson, 1987)	Checklist
Home environment	Home Observation for Measurement of the Environment (HOME) (Caldwell & Bradley, 1984)	Observation

single ability, such as attention (e.g., Conners Continuous Performance Test [Conners, 1995] or Gordon Diagnostic System [Gordon, McClure, & Post, 1983]) or processing speed (e.g., Woodcock–Johnson Visual Matching and Cross Out Tests). Another cognitive variable of interest might be concepts of illness (Bibace & Walsh, 1980) or the level of information about a particular disease or condition (Sattler, 1997). Examples in the recent pediatric literature include structured interviews to assess children's conceptions and understanding of acquired immune deficiency syndrome (AIDS) (Kistner et al., 1996; Walsh & Bibace, 1991; Wells et al., 1995), juvenile rheumatoid arthritis (JRA) (Berry, Hayford, Ross, Pachman, & Lavigne, 1993), and cancer (Claflin & Barbarin, 1991).

In the affective realm, in addition to the standard anxiety and depression scales, one might want to assess anger expression (Hagglund et al., 1994), particularly for the populations for which the scale was developed, that is, those with JRA and diabetes. Another frequently assessed area is that of distress related to medical procedures; assessment employs either one of the well-developed behavioral observation systems (Blount et al., 1997; Elliott, Jay, & Woody, 1987) or patient or parent report (Katz, Kellerman & Siegel, 1980; Kazak, Penati, Waibel, & Blackall, 1996). Some instruments measure both distress and responses to pain. Ideally, a comprehensive pain assessment should include physiological measures as well as observational and self-report measures. The reader is referred to two recent issues of *Children's Health Care* (Fall 1996 and Winter 1997) which were devoted to the issues of theory, assessment, and treatment of pediatric pain.

In many cases, when measures of the constructs of interest have not been available, investigators have either adapted existing measures or created new ones, as was the case in our (M. J. Kupst & J. L. Schulman) program of research on coping and adaptation, when there were few measures of positive adaptation available during the late 1970s and early 1980s (Kupst, 1980). Some examples include measures of adherence (Hanson et al., 1996; Johnson, 1992; Manne, Jacobsen, Gorfinkle, Gerstein, & Redd, 1993), health locus of control (Thompson, Butcher, & Berenson, 1987), impact of illness on the family (Stein & Riessman, 1980), and functional severity (Stein & Jessop, 1990b). Over the past 20 years, there has been increased interest in the area of coping with chronic illness, and several measures have been developed specifically for assessing this construct, such as the Kidcope (Spirito, Stark, & Williams, 1988), the Ways of Coping Questionnaire (Folkman & Lazarus, 1988), and the Coping Health Inventory for Parents (McCubbin & Thompson, 1987). In addition to dispositional scales, there have been recent efforts to observe actual coping behavior, such as one factor of the Child–Adult Medical Procedure Interaction Scale—Revised (CAMPIS-R; Blount et al., 1997). Although the assessment of coping behaviors remains an area of considerable interest, the measurement of coping is fraught with methodological difficulties, such as the frequent discrepancy between dispositional and actual coping, and theoretical differences in coping constructs, process variables, and what constitutes "good" versus "poor coping" (Rudolph, Dennig, & Weisz, 1995; Spirito, 1996).

The wealth of assessment instruments continues to grow in the pediatric psychology literature. However, the selection of constructs of interest and the appropriate assessment and measurement of such constructs is only one part of assessment in chronic illness. Next, practical considerations are offered in conducting such assessments in the pediatric setting.

THE IDEAL AND THE REAL
IN PEDIATRIC ASSESSMENT

Working with children who have chronic medical conditions and their families can be a very exciting and rewarding venture, with the opportunity to be part of a multidisciplinary team in a clinic or hospital, to conduct psychological research, and to work with a generally nonpsychiatric population ("normal" children and families in abnormal situations). As pediatric psychology continues to be a growing and popular choice of practice, there have been proposals regarding the functions of pediatric psychologists. The necessary training and standards are beginning to emerge regarding clinical and research practice. After obtaining experience in this field, following a pediatric psychology internship or fellowship, a realization emerges that, while the field has wonderful opportunities, it also has numerous challenges. There is frequently a disparity between the ideal evaluation (the prototype assessment) and what typically transpires in the pediatric setting (the actual assessment). This is not intended to be discouraging, nor to provide an excuse for sloppy or haphazard assessment, but rather to point out some of the ideal and real situations in pediatric chronic illness assessment, as well as some ways to cope with them. The guidelines for prototype assessments will be presented first, followed by the issues in actual assessments.

Prototype Assessment

The Assessment Questions Should Be Adequately Described (La Greca & Lemanek, 1996)

The referral question is clear: "Is this child's anxiety about procedures higher than one would expect? Based on your assessment, what do you recommend as an intervention?" Or "This child had cranial irradiation 2 years ago. She has been having trouble in school remembering her assignments and following directions. Can you evaluate her memory functioning?" Such referral questions are a pleasure to address due to their specificity regarding the expectations of the evaluation.

Standardized Measures Should Be Used

Most of the measures that are typically administered in pediatric psychology have good psychometric properties, such as reliability, validity, and standardized norms. When the question pertains to overall cognitive functioning, standard tests such as those presented in Table 3.1 (e.g., Wechsler Scales, Bayley Scales) are natural choices. They are universal currency across settings: hospitals, clinics, schools, private practice offices. They have the added benefit of being familiar to insurance carriers. While acceptability to insurance carriers should not be the determinant of the measures to be employed, it does increase one's chances of being authorized to conduct the testing and increases the probability of reimbursement. Fortunately, the cognitive tests most familiar to insurance reviewers and those that are typically used in pediatric psychology generally coincide. In the behavioral realm, the CBCL also is commonly used, and there is a teacher version to assess behavior in the classroom. These instruments also are well recognized by multiple disciplines.

The Assessment Should Be Comprehensive

Ideally, multiple measures and modalities should be used that assess children across situations and with multiple informants. In the cognitive examples presented earlier, one would administer a standardized cognitive test and several of the supplemental scales, depending upon the referral question to be addressed. Similarly, in the case of possible internalizing problems (e.g., anxiety and depression), one might administer a CBCL to parents, but also obtain measures of family functioning, anxiety, depression, and coping strategies. If more diagnostic information is needed, a structured interview, such as the Child Assessment Schedule (Hodges, Kline, Stern, Cytryn, & McKnew, 1982) or a semistructured interview, such as the Semistructured Clinical Interview for Children and Adolescents (SCICA; McConaughy & Achenbach, 1994) could be useful. Several of the structured diagnostic interviews have been well developed, and some have good reliability (for review, see Hodges, 1993, and Sattler, 1997). It may sometimes be necessary, in a comprehensive assessment battery, to extend the evaluation over several sessions, particularly with young children who may not be able to sustain attention and concentration for prolonged periods of time.

Multiple Informants Should Be Obtained

A comprehensive assessment of a child or adolescent should include multiple informants (La Greca & Lemanek, 1966; Thompson & Gustafson, 1996). Typically, sources would include the child, both parents or guardians, and the child's teacher. Additional data on child and family functioning can be gathered from siblings (Sahler et al., 1997), peers (Noll, LeRoy, Bukowski, Rogosch, & Kulkarni, 1991), medical and nursing staff (Manne, et al., 1993), and prior contacts with psychosocial professionals. The choice of informants may depend upon the question of interest. For example, in the assessment of externalizing symptoms (e.g., disruptive behavior disorders), adults (parents, teachers, health care staff) may provide useful information. For internalizing symptoms or pain, children may provide the most useful information. Finally, in the assessment of adherence, parents and children are likely to provide the most useful data, while for peer relationships and social competence, the child and peers (La Greca & Lemanek, 1996) are apt to be the most useful informants. When a child is hospitalized, it is often possible to obtain data from mothers, fathers, and hospital staff.

R., & Pate, J. T. (1997). The Child–Adult Medical Procedure Interaction Scale—Revised: An assessment of validity. *Journal of Pediatric Psychology, 22,* 73–88.

Caldwell, B., & Bradley, R. H. (1984). *Home observation for measurement of the environment.* Little Rock: University of Arkansas at Little Rock.

Claflin, C. J., & Barbarin, O. A. (1991). Does "telling" less protect more?: Relationships among age, information disclosure, and what children with cancer see and feel. *Journal of Pediatric Psychology, 16,* 169–192.

Conners, C. K., (1989). *Conners' rating scales manual.* North Tonawanda, NY: Multi-Health Systems.

Conners, C. K. (1995). *Conners Continuous Performance Test computer program 3.0—User's manual.* Toronto: Multi-Health Systems. Canada.

Dahlquist, L. M., Power, T. G., Cox, C. N., & Fernbach, D. J. (1994). Parenting and child distress during cancer procedures: A multidimensional assessment. *Children's Health Care, 23,* 149–166.

Derogatis, L. R. (1983). *SCL90-R: Administration, scoring and procedures manual II.* Towson, MD: Clinical Psychometric Research.

Eiser, C., Havermans, T., Craft, A., & Kernahan, J. (1995). Development of a measure to assess the perceived illness experience after treatment for cancer. *Archives of Disease in Childhood, 72,* 302–307.

Elliott, C. H., Jay, S. M., & Woody, P. (1987). An observational scale for measuring children's distress during medical procedures. *Journal of Pediatric Psychology, 12,* 543–551.

Eyberg, S. M. (1985). Behavioral assessment advancing methodology in pediatric psychology. *Journal of Pediatric Psychology, 10,* 123–139.

Eyberg, S. M., & Ross, A. W. (1978). Assessment of child behavior problems: Validation of a new inventory. *Journal of Clinical Child Psychology, 7,* 113–116.

Folkman, S., & Lazarus, R. S. (1988) *Ways of Coping Questionnaire.* Palo Alto, CA: Consulting Psychologists Press.

Fritz, G. K., Yeung, A., Wamboldt, M. Z., Spirito, A., McQuaid, E. L., Klein, R., & Seifer, R. (1996). Conceptual and methodologic issues in quantifying perceptual accuracy in childhood asthma. *Journal of Pediatric Psychology, 21,* 153–174.

Gordon, M., McClure, F. D., & Post, E. M. (1983). *The Gordon Diagnostic System.* DeWitt, NY: Gordon Systems.

Gresham, F. M., & Elliott, S. N. (1990). *Social Skills Rating System.* Circle Pines, MN: American Guidance Service.

Haan, H. (1977). *Coping and defending.* New York: Academic Press.

Hagglund, K. J., Clay, D. L., Frank, R. G., Beck, N. C., Kashani, J. H., Hewett, J., Johnson, J., Goldstein, D. E., & Cassidy, J. T. (1994). Assessing anger expression in children and adolescents. *Journal of Pediatric Psychology, 19,* 291–304.

Hanson, C. L., De Guire, M. J., Schinkel, A. M., Kolterman, O. G., Goodman, J. P., & Buckingham, B. A. (1996). Self-care behaviors in insulin-dependent diabetes: Evaluative tools and their associatrions with glycemic control. *Journal of Pediatric Psychology, 21,* 467–482.

Harter, S. (1985). *Manual for the Self-Perception Profile for Children.* Denver, CO: University of Denver.

Hodges, K. (1993). Structured interviews for assessing children. *Journal of Child Psychology and Psychiatry, 34,* 49–68.

Hodges, K., & Kline, J., Stern, L., Cytryn, L., & McKnew, D. (1982). The development of a child assessment schedule for research and clinical use. *Journal of Abnormal Child Psychology, 10*, 173–189.

Hurwitz, J. I., Kaplan, D. M., & Kaiser, E. (1962). Designing an instrument to assess parental coping mechanisms. *Social Care Work, 43*, 527–532.

Ifeld, F. (1976). Further validation of a psychiatric symptom index in a normal population. *Psychological Reports, 39*, 1215–1218.

Ireton, H., & Thwing, E. T. (1974). *Manual for the Minnesota Child Development Inventory*. Minneapolis, MN: Behavior Science Systems.

Johnson, S. B. (1992). Methodological issues in diabetes research: Measuring adherence. *Diabetes Care, 15*, 1658–1667.

Johnson, S. B. (1994). Presidential address: Health behavior and health status: Concepts, methods and applications. *Journal of Pediatric Psychology, 19*, 129–142.

Katz, E. R., Kellerman, J., & Siegel, S. E. (1980). Behavioral distress in children undergoing medical procedures: Developmental considerations. *Journal of Consulting and Clinical Psychology, 52*, 1106–1107.

Kaufman, A. S., & Kaufman, N. L. (1983). *K-ABC administration and scoring manual*. Circle Pines, MN: American Guidance Service.

Kazak, A. E., Penati, B., Waibel, M. K., & Blackall, G. F. (1996). The perception of procedures questionnaire: Psychometric properties of a brief parents report measure of procedural distress. *Journal of Pediatric Psychology, 21*, 195–208.

Kistner, J., Eberstein, I. W., Balthazar, M., Castro, R., Foster, K., Osborne, M., Sly, D., & Quadagno, D. (1996). Assessing children's conceptions of AIDS. *Journal of Pediatric Psychology, 21*(2), 269–282.

Kovacs, M., & Beck, A. T. (1977). An empirical–clinical approach toward a definition of childhood depression. In J. G. Schulterbrandt & A Raskin (Eds.), *Depression in childhood: Diagnosis, treatment, and conceptual models* (pp. 1–25). New York: Raven.

Kupst, M. J. (1980). Family coping with pediatric leukemia: Initial reactions. In J. L. Schulman & M. J. Kupst (Eds.), *The child with cancer* (pp. 111–128). Springfield, IL: Charles C Thomas.

Kupst, M. J., Natta, M. B., Richardson, C. C., Schulman, J. L., Lavigne, J. L., & Das, L. (1995). Family coping with pediatric leukemia: Ten years after treatment. *Journal of Pediatric Psychology, 20*, 601–617.

Kupst, M. J., & Schulman, J. L. (1988). Long-term coping with pediatric leukemia: A six year follow-up study. *Journal of Pediatric Psychology, 13*, 7–22.

La Greca, A. M. (1994). Editorial: Assessment in pediatric psychology: What's a researcher to do? *Journal of Pediatric Psychology, 19*, 283–290.

La Greca, A. M., & Lemanek, K. L. (1996), Editorial: Assessment as a process in pediatric psychology. *Journal of Pediatric Psychology, 21*, 137–152.

Madan-Swain, A., & Brown, R. T. (1991). Cognitive and psychosocial sequelae for children with acute lymphocytic leukemia and their families. *Clinical Psychology Review, 1*, 267–294.

Manne, S. L., Jacobsen, P. B., Gorfinkle, K., Gerstein, F., & Redd, W. H. (1993). Treatment adherence difficulties among children with cancer: The role of parenting style. *Journal of Pediatric Psychology, 18*, 47–62.

McCarthy, D. A. (1972). *Manual for the McCarthy Scales of Children's Abilities*. San Antonio, TX: Psychological Corporation.

McConaughy, S. H., & Achenbach, T. M. (1994). *Manual for the Semistructured*

Clinical Interview for Children and Adolescents. Burlington, VT: University Associates in Psychiatry.

McCubbin, H. I., & Thompson, A. I. (1987). *Family assessment inventories for research and practice.* Madison: University of Wisconsin–Madison.

McNair, D. H., Lorr, M., & Droppleman, L. F. (1992). *Manual for the Profile of Mood States. Revised 1992.* San Diego, CA: Edits Education and Industrial Testing Service.

Moos, R. H., & Moos, B. S. (1986). *Family Environment Scale Manual* (2nd ed.). Palo Alto, CA: Consulting Psychologists Press.

Mulhern, R. K., Hancock, J., Fairclough, D., & Kun, L. (1992). Neuropsychological status of children treated for brain tumors: A critical review and integrative analysis. *Medical and Pediatric Oncology, 20,* 181–191.

Noll, R. B., LeRoy, S., Bukowski, W. M., Rogosch, F. A., & Kulkarni, R. (1991). Peer relationships and adjustment in children with cancer. *Journal of Pediatric Psychology, 16,* 307–326.

Olson, D. H., & Tiesel, J. (1991). *FACES III: Linear scoring and intrepretation.* St. Paul: Family Social Support, University of Minnesota.

Perrin, E. C., Stein, R. E. K., & Drotar, D. (1991). Cautions in using the Child Behavior Checklist: Observations based on research about children with a chronic illness. *Journal of Pediatric Psychology, 16,* 411–422.

Quay, H. C., & Peterson, D. R. (1975). *Manual for the Behavior Problem Checklist.* Coral Gables, FL: University of Miami.

Reynolds, C., & Richmond, B. (1978). What I think and feel: A revised measure of children's manifest anxiety. *Journal of Abnormal Child Psychology, 6,* 271–280.

Rudolph, K. D., Dennig, M. D., & Weisz, J. R. (1995). Determinants and consequences of children's coping in the medical setting: Conceptualization, review, and critique. *Psychological Bulletin, 118,* 328–357.

Sahler, O. J. Z., Roghman, K. J., Mulhern, R. K., Carpenter, P. J., Sargent, J. R., Copeland, D. R., Barbarin, O. A., Zeltzer, L. K., & Dolgin, M. J. (1997). Sibling adaptation to childhood cancer: The association of sibling adaptation with maternal well-being, physical health, and resource use. *Developmental and Behavioral Pediatrics, 18,* 233–243.

Sandler, I. N., Tein, J. Y., & West, S. G. (1994). Coping, stress, and psychological symptoms of children of divorce: A cross-sectional and longitudinal study. *Child Development, 65,* 1744–1763.

Sattler, J. M. (1988). *Assessment of children.* San Diego, CA: Jerome L. Sattler.

Sattler, J. M. (1997). *Clinical and forensic interviewing of children and families.* San Diego, CA: Jerome L. Sattler.

Spanier, G. B. (1976). Measuring dyadic adjustment: New scales for assessing the quality of marriage and similar dyads. *Journal of Marriage and the Family, 38,* 15–28.

Sparrow, S. S., Balla, D. A., & Cicchetti, D. V. (1984). *Vineland Adaptive Behavior Scales—Survey form, classroom, and expanded form manuals.* Circle Pines, MN: American Guidance Service.

Spielberger, C., Edwards, C. D., Lushene, R., Montuori, J., & Platzek, D. (1973). *State–Trait Anxiety Inventory for Children (manual).* Palo Alto, CA: Consulting Psychologists Press.

Spielberger, C., Gorsuch, R. L., Lushene, R., Vagg, P. R., & Jacobs, G. A. (1983).

State–Trait Anxiety Inventory (manual). Palo Alto, CA: Consulting Psychologists Press.

Spieth, L. E., & Harris, C. V. (1996). Assessment of health-related quality of life in children and adolescents: An integrative review. *Journal of Pediatric Psychology, 21*, 175–193.

Spinetta, J. J. (1984). Development of psychometric assessment methods by life cycle stages. *Cancer, 53*, 2222–2225.

Spirito, A. (1996). Pitfalls in the use of brief screening measures of coping. *Journal of Pediatric Psychology, 21*, 573–576.

Spirito, A., Stark, L. J., & Williams, C. (1988). Development of a brief checklist to assess coping in pediatric patients. *Journal of Pediatric Psychology, 13*, 555–574.

Stein, R. E. K., & Jessop, D. J. (1990a). *Manual for Personal Adjustment and Role Skills Scale PARS III*. Bronx, NY: Albert Einstein College of Medicine.

Stein, R. E. K., & Jessop, D. J. (1990b). Functional Status II-R: A measure of child health status. *Medical Care, 28*, 1041–1045.

Stein, R. E. K., & Riessman, C. J. (1980). Development of an impact on family scale: Preliminary findings. *Medical Care, 18*, 465–472.

Thompson, R. J., Butcher, A., & Berenson, G. (1987). Children's beliefs about sources of health: A reliability and validity study. *Measurement and Evaluation in Counseling and Development, 10*, 80–88.

Thompson, R. J., & Gustafson, K. E. (1996). *Adaptation to chronic childhood illness*. Washington, DC: American Psychological Association.

Thompson, R. J., Gustafson, K. E., George, L. K., & Spock, A. (1994). Change over a 12-month period in the psychological adjustment of children and adolescents with cystic fibrosis. *Journal of Pediatric Psychology, 19*, 189–204.

Thorndike, R. L., Hagen, E. P., & Sattler, J. M. (1986). *Guide for administering and scoring the Stanford–Binet Intelligence Scale—Fourth Edition*. Itasca, IL: Riverside.

Walsh, M. E., & Bibace, R. (1991). Children's conceptions of AIDS: A developmental analysis. *Journal of Pediatric Psychology, 16*, 273–286.

Wechsler, D. (1989). *Manual for the Wechsler Preschool and Primary Scale of Intelligence—Revised (WPPSI-R)*. San Antonio, TX: Psychological Corporation.

Wechsler, D. (1991). *Manual for the Wechsler Intelligence Scale for Children—Third edition (WISC-III)*. San Antonio, TX: Psychological Corporation.

Wechsler, D. (1997). *Manual for the Wechsler Adult Intelligence Scale—Third edition (WAIS-III)*. San Antonio, TX: Psychological Corporation.

Wells, E. A., Hoppe, M. J., Simpson, E. E., Gillmore, M. R., Morrison, D. M., & Wilsdon, A. (1995). Misconceptions about AIDS among children who can identify the major routes of HIV transmission. *Journal of Pediatric Psychology, 20* 671–686.

Wilkinson, G. S. (1993). *Manual for the Wide Range Achievement Test 3 (WRAT3)*. San Antonio, TX: Psychological Corporation.

Woodcock, R. W., & Johnson, M. B. (1989). *Manual for the Woodcock–Johnson Psycho-Educational Battery—Revised*. Itasca, IL: Riverside.

PART TWO

DISEASE-SPECIFIC ISSUES

CHAPTER FOUR

Acute Lymphoblastic Leukemia and Brain Tumors

F. DANIEL ARMSTRONG
RAYMOND K. MULHERN

Each year more than 8,000 children under age 15 are diagnosed with cancer in the United States, and recent data suggest that this number has increased over the past 10 years (American Cancer Society, 1997). Of these children, approximately 30% will be diagnosed with acute lymphoblastic leukemia (ALL), and 20% will be diagnosed with some form of malignant brain tumor (Robison, Mertens, & Neglia, 1991). In each of these diagnostic groups, the disease and its treatment can adversely affect the development of the central nervous system, resulting in both short-term and long-term cognitive impairments (Armstrong & Horn, 1995; Mulhern, Armstrong, & Thompson, 1998). Thus, nearly half the children diagnosed with cancer each year in the United States will have at least some degree of risk for learning and/or memory problems, or other difficulties that may impair performance in academic settings. Since current estimates suggest that more than 70% of children are now expected to be cured of their illness (Parker, Tong, Bolden, & Wingo, 1997), the impact of the disease and treatment is likely to involve both performance in school as well as later adaptation and productivity in adulthood. Therefore, it is of critical importance to better understand the nature of the difficulties encountered by children treated for cancer, as well as to begin developing intervention programs to address these issues so that long-term difficulties may be avoided or lessened in severity and intensity.

DISEASE AND TREATMENT ISSUES

Not all types of childhood cancer nor forms of treatment involve the central nervous system or affect its functioning. While there may be significant stress associated with the diagnosis and treatment of any kind of cancer in children, in many cases disabilities that may be evident during treatment will resolve with minimal long-term difficulty. Common factors that may affect school performance for all children include school absences due to hospitalization for treatment, dealing with acute side effects of treatment such as nausea and low blood counts, altered social relationships due to physical changes and emotional stress associated with chemotherapy side effects, and inconsistent or inappropriate educational planning for the child while on treatment. An example of the latter would be having a child whose treatment has minimal side effects receive homebound instruction instead of being reintegrated quickly into a normal school environment (Sexson & Madan-Swain, 1993). Fortunately, these difficulties do not have to be long lasting and may be remediated with careful planning and intervention. However, about 50% of children treated for cancer will be in the situation where either their disease and/or its treatment may adversely affect central nervous system development and functioning. In addition, some children with solid tumors (e.g., neuroblastomas, sarcomas) may require more intensive treatment, such as bone marrow or peripheral stem cell transplantation, when frontline therapy fails (Sanders, 1997). For these children, toxicity associated with high-dose, marrow-ablating chemotherapy or total body radiation may also produce long-term cognitive effects, although the outcome of controlled studies in this area have not yet been reported. The relationships between type of disease, type of treatment, and specific late effects are complex and involve considered evaluation of individual factors, disease factors, acute treatment effects, and long-term developmental changes. Therefore, in the following sections we will attempt to describe disease mechanisms, acute treatment effects associated with specific treatments, and long-term outcomes that are commonly seen in children with specific types of cancer, concluding with a focus on assessment and intervention considerations.

LEUKEMIA

Leukemia is a cancer of the blood that affects nearly 30% of children diagnosed with cancer in the United States each year (Robison et al., 1991). Significant advances have been made in the treatment of leukemia over the last 25 years, resulting in an overall long-term survival rate of nearly 70%, with some types of leukemia even approaching better than 80% survival (Margolin & Poplack, 1997). There are a number of different types of leukemia, some chronic, and some affecting nonlymphoblastic white blood cells, but these types of leukemia are relatively rare in children. The most common form of leukemia is acute lymphoblastic leukemia (ALL), a malignancy most commonly found in children between the ages of 2 and 10. Factors such as the age of the child, white blood cell count at the time of diagnosis, and, recently, chromosomal and DNA abnormalities have been identified as affecting long-term prognosis of children with ALL (Margolin & Poplack, 1997).

Treatment of leukemia usually involves multiagent chemotherapy administered in three distinct phases. The first phase, the induction phase, lasts approximately 28 days, and is designed to eliminate all measurable signs of leukemia, as detected on a bone marrow aspiration. The second phase, the consolidation or intensification phase, involves intensive, higher dose chemotherapy that often requires 3–4 days of hospitalization every 3 weeks for approximately 6 months. The third phase, the maintenance phase, involves oral, subcutaneous, and/or intravenous chemotherapy administered for approximately 1½ years after completion of consolidation. Because leukemia is known to spread into the central nervous system, treatment of leukemia also involves prophylatic administration of chemotherapy directly into the cerebrospinal fluid (intrathecal chemotherapy) using a procedure known as a lumbar puncture or spinal tap. Intrathecal chemotherapy is administered at intervals of 8–12 weeks throughout the first 18 months of treatment. In cases where there is a recurrence (relapse) of the leukemia, children may undergo a bone marrow transplant from a related family member or matched unrelated HLA identical donor, or may receive an umbilical cord blood transplant from an unrelated donor (Margolin & Poplack, 1997).

Prior to the mid-1980s, treatment of the central nervous system in children with ALL involved administration of 1,800–2,400 cGy of whole-brain and spinal radiation therapy, often combined with intrathecal administration of methotrexate, a chemotherapy agent commonly used in the treatment of ALL. This treatment resulted in the identification of growth delays and cognitive impairment in survivors (Kun, 1997; Waber & Tarbell, 1997). In the mid-1980s, the Pediatric Oncology Group began investigating whether a combination of three chemotherapy agents administered by spinal tap could be as effective in preventing the spread of leukemia to the central nervous system as prophylaxis involving craniospinal radiation. This approach, in fact, provided comparable leukemia prophylaxis, without evidence of significant growth and cognitive delays (Margolin & Poplack, 1997). Recently, however, investigators have found that even the use of triple intrathecal chemotherapy may result in subtle brain changes, neuropsychological impairment, and even overt neurological symptoms (Mahoney et al., 1998).

Understanding the components involved in the treatment of ALL is a essential to understanding the behavioral and psychological consequences that may be observed, both during acute care and long-term follow-up. Several of the medications that are administered have acute side effects that may present as behavioral or psychological difficulties. During induction, one of the medications that is commonly used is prednisone, a corticosteroid. Children, particularly young children, may have significantly elevated activity levels accompanied by mood swings and high levels of irritability when receiving this medication. A second medication administered during induction is vincristine. One of the side effects of vincristine is a change in peripheral nervous system functioning, often seen in decreased reflexes and fine motor coordination and speed (Balis, Holcenberg, & Poplack, 1997). Failure to recognize the potential impact of these medications on children's behavioral functioning may lead to inaccurate and inappropriate attribution of mental health or cognitive problems to these children. Copeland and her colleagues (1988) have noted improvements in children's performance on certain fine motor speed and coordination tasks once vincristine is no longer needed in the treatment regimen. Other medications, however, do not present with acute effects on behavior, but have been associated with late physical and cognitive effects. Methotrexate, one of the most common medications used in the treatment of childhood cancer, has been associated with increased risk of calcification and other white matter changes in the brains of children with leukemia (Margolin & Poplack, 1997). Methotrexate is one of the medications included in intrathecal chemotherapy, and it has also been used at increasingly high dosage levels as a systemic medication administered intravenously. Because methotrexate, in higher doses, has been shown to cross the blood–brain barrier, the combination of intrathecal and systemic methotrexate is now being associated with increased risk of neurological damage and neurocognitive impairment in children treated for ALL (Mahoney et al., 1998).

Cognitive and Learning Consequences of ALL

When evaluating cognitive and learning consequences of children treated for ALL, it is important to note the type of treatment that was received. Older adolescents and young adult survivors who were treated in the late 1970s through mid-1980s were likely to have received low (1,800 cGy)- to moderate (2,400 cGy)-dose whole-brain and/or spinal radiation therapy, combined with intrathecal methotrexate. These survivors are at a greater risk of having long-term growth and cognitive consequences than children treated on later protocols.

Radiation-induced central nervous system damage results from oligodendrocyte and endothelial cell damage. The initial endothelial injury within small vessels initiates a cascade of biochemically toxic reactions, including increased formation of oxygen free radicals. These reactions lead to cell swelling, increased vascular permeability, fibrinoid necrosis of the vessel wall, ischemia, edema, and cell death. Late effects of the cascade are evidenced on neuroimaging by diffuse and multifocal white matter hyperintensities, as well as calcifications in the cortical gray matter and basal ganglia. The presence and severity of these imaging changes correlates with cranial radiation therapy (CRT) dose, as do a variety of concurrent neuropsychological syndromes in children treated for cancer, including problems with attention, memory, mental processing speed, and intellectual deterioration. Similar cognitive-processing problems have been noted among other patients with primary white matter pathology, such as those with leukodsytrophy, periventricular leukomalacia, and multiple sclerosis (Mulhern, Armstrong, & Thompson, 1998).

Children treated for ALL in the late 1980s and 1990s are more likely to have received triple intrathecal chemotherapy without radiation therapy, thus reducing their risk of growth delays (Kun, 1997; Margolin & Poplack, 1997). However, recent studies suggest that the risk for cognitive impairment, while not as great as with radiation therapy, still exists for these children (Brown et al., 1992; Brown et al., 1998). A third group is constituted by children who have been treated with systemic and triple intrathecal chemotherapy, suffered a relapse, and then have undergone total body radiation and chemotherapy prior to receiving a bone marrow or umbilical cord blood transplant. Because of these differences in treatment, outcomes may be different and long-term planning may require different approaches.

Late Cognitive Effects Associated with Craniospinal Radiation

Demonstration of the benefits of triple intrathecal chemotherapy without associated growth delays has led to a significant decline in the use of CRT in the treatment of ALL. With the exception of children who present with leukemia present in the central nervous system at the time of diagnosis (<5% of all newly diagnosed ALL), and children who experience a relapse of leukemia in the CNS after beginning treatment (Margolin & Poplack, 1997), most children exposed to CRT will have been treated prior to 1990. Therefore, this population of survivors largely consists of individuals who are of adolescent and young adult age.

Most studies of the effects of CRT and intrathecal methotrexate on the functioning of children with ALL have suggested that there is evidence of changes in the white matter of the brain, particularly in the frontal cortex, that are detected using neuroimaging techniques such as computerized tomography (CT scan) (Fletcher & Copeland, 1988). These changes do not occur for all children treated with CRT and intrathecal methotrexate (Kramer, Norman, Brant-Zawadzki, Ablin, & Moore, 1988), but have been identified on CT (Cap, Foltinová, Szabova, Cinkovska, & Boruta,

1991) or MRI scan (Ciesielski et al., 1994; Kingma, Mooyaart, Kamps, Nieuwenhuizen, & Wilmink, 1993) in nearly half of the children included in several studies. Such changes have not been correlated with CRT dose or age (Kingma et al., 1993). These white matter changes are believed to be associated with an adverse effect on intellectual performance, although not all studies have reported this pattern. (For excellent reviews of these studies, see Mulhern, 1994; Armstrong & Horn, 1995; Butler & Copeland, 1993; and Fletcher & Copeland, 1988.)

A number of factors have been associated with these findings. First, the dose of radiation therapy included in the CNS prophylaxis of children on these various studies has varied. Early treatment typically involved a cranial radiation dose of 2,400 cGy, but more recent protocols that included CRT used a dose of 1,800 cGy. Several studies found that children treated with the higher dose (2,400 cGy) had IQ scores significantly lower than those treated with lower dose (1,800 cGy) radiation therapy (Appleton, Farrell, Zaide, & Rogers, 1990; Halberg et al., 1992; Kingma, et al., 1993; Moore, Kramer, Wara, Halberg, & Albin, 1991). In addition, some studies of the effects of CRT have compared radiation therapy alone with radiation therapy plus intrathecal methotrexate, and an argument has been made that it is the combination of CRT and methotrexate that represents the greatest risk for children treated for ALL (Waber & Tarbell, 1997). In at least one study, no significant deficits were identified for children who received 1,800 cGy of CRT, nor for children who received intrathecal methotrexate alone, but significant deficits were identified in children who received both 1,800 cGy of CRT plus a single high dose of methotrexate (Waber et al., 1995).

Risk Factors

One factor associated with greater risk for cognitive impairment in children treated with CRT plus methotrexate is the age at the time of treatment, with younger children considered at greater risk for problems than older children. Once again, this has not been a consistent finding (Mulhern, 1994), and other factors such as the type and length of exposure to other types chemotherapy (Mulhern, Fairclough, & Ochs, 1991) and interactions between age and gender (Waber, Gioia, et al., 1990; Waber, Urion, et al., 1990) may contribute to these discrepant findings. In one study that compared groups of long-term survivors of ALL (using CNS prophylaxis including intrathecal chemotherapy only, 1,800 cGy, 2,000 cGy, or 2,400 cGy of CRT) to survivors of Wilms' tumor, all diagnosed under the age of 24 months, children with ALL had significantly lower mean IQ scores, poorer performance on measures of visual and auditory memory, lower arithmetic achievement, and greater frequency of special education interventions. Performance within the ALL group was also inversely correlated with total CRT dose, where children who received the highest dose of radiation therapy performed most poorly, while those with no radiation therapy had the highest levels of functioning (Mulhern et al., 1992). Several studies have reported worse performance in younger children even with lower dose CRT (1,800 cGy), particularly when children are under 3 years of age (Appleton et al., 1990; Jankovic et al., 1994; Kingma et al., 1993; Smibert, Anderson, Godber, & Ekert, 1996). In a slightly older cohort (ages 3–6½ years at time of diagnosis), MacLean and his colleagues in the Children's Cancer Group (MacLean et al., 1995) found that children treated with CRT and intrathecal methotrexate scored lower in motor abilities and auditory comprehension than children treated with systemic and intrathecal methotrexate alone. These results were detectable within 9 months of starting treatment. There were no differences in general cognitive abilities, visual–motor integration, or receptive vocabulary.

A second demographic factor associated with cognitive outcome in children treated with CRT has been gender. Mechanisms for differential gender effects have not been identified, but there is at least some evidence that females receiving CRT are a greater risk for cognitive impairment than are males (Mulhern et al., 1991; Schlieper, Esseltine, & Tarshis, 1989; Waber, Urion, et al., 1990; Waber, Tarbell, Kahn, Gelber, & Sallan, 1992). Recent studies suggest the risk of impairment for girls is greater in the verbal area, reflected in both poorer Verbal IQ scores and lower scores on tests of verbal memory (Christie, Leiper, Chessells, Vargha Khadem, 1995). This risk was also found in the area of neuroendocrine functioning (Waber, Urion, et al., 1990), where females were significantly shorter and more overweight for age than were males.

A third factor associated with identification of cognitive deficits in children treated for ALL is the length of time since treatment. As in other areas, contradictory findings have emerged. Early retrospective studies (Schlieper et al., 1989; Said, Waters, Cousens, & Stevens, 1989) failed to find IQ changes associated with increasing time since the treatment, but other investigators (Moore et al., 1991; Mulhern et al., 1992) have identified significant changes in measures of intellectual and neuropsychological functioning with increasing time since treatment. Prospective studies (Rubenstein, Varni, & Katz, 1990; Mulhern et al., 1991) have also reported declines in intellectual functioning over time. In reviewing these studies, Mulhern (1994) noted that when corrections are made for measurement error associated with changing the version of IQ test used because of the child's age at the time of testing or publication of a new version of a test (e.g., WPPSI-R to WISC-III; WISC to WISC-R to WISC-III), the significant decreases in the IQ functioning were no longer detected (see Table 4.1).

Several investigators have also been critical of the emphasis placed on global measures of verbal, nonverbal, and global intellectual functioning as primary outcome variables in studies in this area (Armstrong, 1996;

TABLE 4.1. Risk Factors for Cognitive Impairment in Children Treated for Acute Lymphoblastic Leukemia

Study	Chemo	RT + MTX	TIT	Dose of RT	Age	Gender	Time since treatment	Specific functions affected
Anderson et al. (1994)		Y						Y
Appleton et al. (1990)		Y		Y	Y			
Brown et al. 1992)			Y					Y
Brown et al. (1996)			Y					Y
Brown et al. (1998)			Y			Y		Y
Butler et al. (1994)		Y						Y
Christie et al. (1995)		Y				Y		Y
Ciesielski et al. (1994)		Y						Y
Copeland et al. 1988)	Y							
Copeland et al. (1996)		Y						Y
Cousens et al. (1991)		Y						Y
Giralt et al. (1992)		Y						N
Halberg et al. (1992)		Y		Y				Y
Kingma et al. (1993)		Y		Y	Y			Y
McLean et al. (1995)		Y			Y			
Moore et al. (1991)		Y		Y			Y	
Moore et al. 1992)		Y						Y
Mulhern et al. (1991)		Y				Y	Y	
Mulhern et al. (1992)		Y		Y	Y		Y	
Rodgers et al. (1992)		Y						Y
Rubenstein et al. (1990)		Y					Y	
Said et al. (1989)		Y					N	
Schlieper et al. (1989)		Y				Y	N	
Smibert et al. (1996)		Y			Y			Y
Waber et al. (1990)		Y				Y		Y
Waber et al. (1992)		Y				Y		
Waber, Gioia, et al. (1995)	Y	Y						Y
Williams et al. (1991)			Y					Y

Note. Y, study reported significant finding; N, study included measurement, no significant finding; Chemo, systemic chemotherapy; RT + MTX, cranial radiation therapy plus intrathecal methotrexate; TIT, triple intrathecal chemotherapy (methotrexate, hydrocortisone, cytosine arabinoside [ARA-C]).

Armstrong & Horn, 1995; Butler & Copeland, 1993; Waber & Tarbell, 1997), arguing that the effects of treatment are likely specific and primarily related to hemispheric functions associated with the frontal cortex. Fletcher and Copeland (1988) provided a detailed review both of neuroimaging findings and of cognitive assessments of children receiving CRT for ALL. Neuroradiological findings, primarily based on CT scans of the brain, suggest that the primary structural changes in the brain following CRT and methotrexate are found in the frontal cortex, basal ganglia, and connecting structures. Butler and his colleagues (Butler, Hill, Steinherz, Meyers, & Finlay, 1994) also implicate the posterior section of the dominant hemisphere, associated with auditory language comprehension abilities. When specific tests of neuropsychological functioning were included in assessment batteries, functional deficits were those typically associated with frontal impairment and nondominant hemisphere damage. This review led to a proposal of a model of late effects similar to the nonverbal learning disabilities model proposed by Rourke (1982). A similar theoretical model was proposed by Cousens and her colleagues (Cousens, Ungerer, Crawford, & Stevens, 1991) who suggested that the impact of CRT plus methotrexate resulted primarily in four specific areas of deficit (short-term memory, processing speed, visual–motor coordination, and sequencing ability), all functions associated with the development of the frontal cortex. In a later review, Armstrong and Horn (1995) described an extension of this model that focused on an understanding of developmental emergence of abilities over time. This model suggests that functions associated with structures that develop prior to treatment will remain relatively intact; the effects of CNS prophylaxis are more likely to be seen in abilities that normally emerge in the years after treatment. Thus, the occurrence of a specific deficit and the severity of the deficit are believed to be related to the timing and intensity of treatment. This model also provides a mechanism for understanding discrepant results across studies that failed to control for the age of the child at the time of treatment and the intensity of the treatment delivered. It also leaves open the possibility that not all children will be affected by treatment, or at least not affected to the same degree (Armstrong, 1996). Support for components of each of these models has been obtained in studies conducted over the past 10 years.

Specific Effects

In those studies that have utilized specific measures of neurocognitive functioning, as opposed to global measures of intellectual functioning, support for the specific effects model of neurocognitive outcome in children treated with CRT and methotrexate has emerged. Deficits in children's ability to concentrate and sustain attention have been consistently found (Anderson, Smibert, Ekert, & Godber, 1994; Butler et al., 1994; Cousens et al., 1991; Christie et al., 1995), as have problems with visual motor integration (Butler et al., 1994; Ciesielski et al., 1994; Kingma et al., 1993). Measures of nonverbal abilities, such as coding from the Wechsler tests (Waber et al., 1995), tests of processing speed (Cousens et al., 1991; Moore, Copeland, Ried, & Levy, 1992), and measures of fine motor speed and accuracy (Butler et al., 1994; Christie et al., 1995; Kingma et al., 1993) have also represented areas of difficulty for children treated for ALL, providing additional support for some of the components of the specific effects model proposed by Cousens and her colleagues (1991).

Empirical data contributing to this model for other functions are not as clear. Several studies have pointed to difficulties with memory when children with ALL are compared to siblings and other children with cancers that do not affect the CNS (Mulhern, Wasserman, Fairclough, & Ochs, 1988; Rodgers, Britton, Morris, Kernahan, & Craft, 1992), and in children treated under the age of 4 years treated with CRT and methotrexate (Christie et al., 1995). There are, however, many different measures of different types of memory. When studies have assessed specific types of memory, findings have not been as clear. Kingma and her colleagues (1993) found significant deficits in verbal memory in a cohort of children treated with CRT and methotrexate, but Giralt and his colleagues found no deficits in this area, nor in verbal learning abilities (Giralt et al., 1992). Children treated with CRT and methotrexate, compared with children treated with intrathecal methotrexate only, have also been found to function more poorly on measures of verbal memory (Waber et al., 1995). A similar pattern has been found when figural memory, or memory for visual material, has been assessed (Ciesielski et al., 1994). While the number of studies in this area is still relatively small, the data point to a potential impact of treatment on memory functioning, but with the caveat that age, type, and dose of treatment and type of memory may be critical variables to further explore before this effect is fully understood.

While the relationship between specific deficits and functional outcome has not been clearly established, there is a growing literature to suggest that children treated with CRT and intrathecal methotrexate are at significant risk for learning problems. Global deficits in academic achievement (Halberg et al., 1992), as well as specific deficits in spelling, reading (Anderson et al., 1994; Copeland, Moore, Francis, Jaffe, & Culbert, 1996; Smibert et al., 1996), and arithmetic (Cousens et al., 1991) have been reported. A large number of children treated with CRT and methotrexate are identified as in need of special education services, with 40–50% ultimately placed in programs providing assistance with learning disabilities (Kingma et al., 1993; Rubenstein et al., 1990).

Despite some inconsistencies, the studies to date clearly point to a significant risk for children who received CRT and intrathecal methotrexate as part of their CNS prophylaxis. There is evidence for global impairment, and factors such as the child's gender; age, both at the time of treatment and at the time of assessment; and the dose of radiation therapy are emerging as important determinants of the severity of the outcome. Recent studies using more precise measurement approaches provide additional support for models that suggest more specific cognitive outcomes following this treatment, although the number of studies completed and lack of similarity of measures across studies limit interpretation. It is important to note, however, that there is inconsistency in the findings across studies, and not all children treated for ALL with these modalities experience adverse effects. While all children treated in this manner are at potential risk for cognitive deficits, some children seem at greater risk while others are protected, although the factors increasing risk or protection have not yet been identified.

Intrathecal Chemotherapy

As delays in cognitive development and physical growth were noted following CRT, changes were made in cancer treatment protocols to determine whether eliminating CRT would decrease toxicity while maintaining good CNS prophylaxis. Initially, studies relied on the administration of intrathecal methotrexate for CNS prophylaxis. Over time, two additional drugs, cytosine arabinoside (ARA-C) and hydrocortisone, were added to methotrexate to develop what became known as triple intrathecal CNS prophylaxis. The operating assumption for this change was that utilizing chemotherapy would reduce toxicity and eliminate many of the cognitive and growth problems encountered with the use of CRT. This strategy proved to be as effective in preventing CNS leukemia as the combination of CRT and methotrexate (Margolin & Poplack, 1997), and preliminary studies suggested that children treated with intrathecal chemotherapy prophylaxis had significantly higher global intellectual functioning compared to children treated with CRT (Schlieper et al., 1989).

Unfortunately, this advancement in treatment may not have been completely benign. Transient changes in white matter of the brain were detected within a year of the initiation of treatment (Nitschke, Wilson, Bowman, Chaffin, & Sexauer, 1990; Ochs et al., 1991). In a study of parent report of their children's academic performance, Williams and his colleagues (Williams, Ochs, Williams, & Mulhern, 1991) found that parents of children with ALL reported their children doing more poorly on everyday cognitive and academic tasks than children who had no illnesses, although better than children with diagnosed learning disabilities. In a study that evaluated a group of children with ALL at diagnosis, after 1 year of treatment, and at the completion of treatment, Brown and his colleagues (1992) found that children who had completed treatment performed significantly poorer than children with less than 1 year of treatment in the areas of delayed recall, general nonverbal abilities, attention, motor speed, and visual motor integration. These were the same areas of deficit that had been identified for children treated with CRT and methotrexate, suggesting that even though the severity of toxicity, particularly for physical growth, was reduced with the triple intrathecal chemotherapy, the risk for later learning problems was not eliminated. Likewise, a cohort of children with ALL from Australia, all using only intrathecal methotrexate for CNS prophylaxis, performed significantly more poorly than a comparison group of children with solid tumors on all measures of academic achievement, with declines greater than one standard deviation noted over a 3-year period (Brown et al., 1996). A concurrent study by Copeland and her colleagues

(1996) detected no differences on measures of neuropsychological functioning between children with ALL treated with intrathecal methotrexate and those treated for other solid tumors. There were declines for both groups in academic achievement, but all other functions remained stable or improved across time.

In a recent multisite study of children with ALL treated on a Pediatric Oncology Group protocol (Protocol No. 8602), 47 children who had received triple intrathecal chemotherapy CNS prophylaxis were evaluated between 2 and 7 years after completing treatment (Brown et al., 1998). While there were no significant deficits identified in global and verbal areas of functioning, these survivors had significantly lower performance, compared to age-adjusted test norms, on measures of nonverbal performance, perceptual organizational skills, and freedom from distractability/attention measures. Performance on nonverbal measures was significantly lower than performance on verbal measures, and mild impairments were noted in visual–motor integration for the group of survivors. Gender differences were evident. Females scored significantly lower than males and test norms on measures of Performance IQ, perceptual organization, and visual–motor integration, but there was no difference in the performance of males compared to the test norms. Thus, while these data are not fully representative of the ALL population, they point to gender (female) as a significant risk factor for cognitive deficits in the face of triple intrathecal chemotherapy. An additional finding of the study was that 37% of the sample was receiving part-time special education assistance, and 7% were in a full-time special education program (all females), figures that were consistent with those for children treated with CRT and methotrexate (Kingma et al., 1993; Rubenstein et al., 1990).

The number of studies examining the role of intrathecal chemotherapy alone on children's neurocognitive functioning remains rather small, and, as in the case of CRT and methotrexate, results are varied. There is inadequate evidence at this point to make a definitive statement that children treated with either intrathecal methotrexate or triple intrathecal chemotherapy in addition to other systemic chemotherapy will have adverse cognitive late effects. However, there are adequate data to suggest that at least a subset of these children are at risk for neurocognitive difficulties, most likely presenting in the form of academic and school-related problems. As treatment protocols continue to include intrathecal chemotherapy for CNS prophylaxis, while at the same time increasing the intensity of systemic chemotherapy with escalating doses of methotrexate and 6-mercaptopurine, the possibility of neurocognitive deficits significant enough to interfere with a child's performance in the classroom continues to exist. Fortunately, it appears that not every child treated in this manner will experience deficits. It is critical for research to continue, not only to document areas of deficits, but to identify risk and preventive factors associated with this outcome.

effect of the tumor is increased intracranial pressure, resulting in symptoms of headache, vomiting, visual impairment, and sometimes hydrocephalus. Less frequent, but occurring nonetheless, are seizures, changes in behavior such as depressive or suicidal thinking, irritability, obsessive behaviors, and endocrine changes (van Eys, 1991). Other symptoms specific to the involved structure of the brain may be seen, with one of the more common patterns in young children being a diencephalic syndrome characterized by significant failure to thrive, leading to emaciation. Since many of these presenting signs are associated with other medical problems, as well as to mental health concerns, it is critical that all health professionals be aware of the possibility of a brain tumor as part of a differential diagnosis, since it has been our experience that some behavioral referrals (e.g., sudden onset depression in a previously well-adjusted child; weight loss, food refusal, and early morning vomiting patterns presented as an eating behavior problem) have ultimately resulted in the diagnosis of a childhood brain tumor.

Treatment

Treatment of brain tumors in children is complex, and difficulties associated with treatment may be highly specific to the type of tumor. The type of treatment selected may also depend upon the behavior of the specific tumor. Some brain tumors are highly malignant, meaning that they tend to be invasive to brain tissue and have the potential to spread to other parts of the brain, spinal column, and even other parts of the body. These tumors are considered high grade, and are often highly responsive to radiation therapy and chemotherapy treatment. Other tumors are much more slow in their growth and tend to remain localized. These tumors are considered low grade, or sometimes termed benign. Unfortunately, the low-grade tumors are largely unresponsive to radiation and chemotherapy, and if their location limits the use of surgery, even a low-grade tumor may prove to be fatal. Because of the complexity involved with each specific tumor, we will provide a brief description of the components of treatment of childhood brain tumors as an overview, but will reserve specific comments as outcome data for specific tumor types are discussed.

Neurosurgery

The most frequent component of brain tumor treatment is neurosurgery, whether used to extract tissue for a definitive diagnosis or to completely resect all identifiable tumor tissue. Because the location (e.g., brainstem) or type of tumor cell may be associated with significant morbidity (e.g., loss of vision, sight, cognitive functioning, physiological regulation), complete resection is not a possibility in a number of pediatric tumors. In fact, for some, even surgical biopsy is not possible. In other cases, neurosurgery may be used to resect a portion of the tumor, resulting in residual disease remaining after surgery. Finally, some pediatric tumors have clearly defined margins separating them from normal brain tissue and are located in sites that are surgically accessible, thus frequently presenting the opportunity for a complete resection. Depending upon the aggressiveness and skill of the surgeon, many tumors can be surgically removed while leaving functional abilities intact. There are, however, complications of surgery that can and do occur, including intracranial bleeding that results in permanent disability. Neurosurgery is also used to provide assistance with complications of a tumor, as in the case of placement of a ventriculo-peritoneal (VP) shunt to aid in reduction of intracranial pressure. An acute complication of any surgery on the brain is edema, a situation frequently managed by the use of high-dose steroids such as decadron. Side effects of this medication may result in short-term irritability and behavioral changes, although these typically subside once the medication is discontinued (Balis et al., 1997; van Eys, 1991).

Radiation Therapy

Radiation therapy has been a stalwart of treatment of brain tumors for a number of years. It is most effective with high-grade tumors, since its course of action is to destroy tumor cells at the time of cell division. Radiation therapy is typically delivered in a series of fractions over multiple days up to a cumulative total dose in an effort to provide maximal exposure to the tumor while minimizing acute morbidity. The doses of radiation therapy administered to children with brain tumors vastly exceed those used in CNS prophylaxis for leukemia, so concerns about cognitive and endocrine late effects are significant. In addition to these late effects, radiation therapy may result in a somnolence syndrome, characterized by significant fatigue, increased sleep, and, in some cases, significant interference with appetite and adequate food intake. In some of these cases, nutrition by nasogastric or gasterointestinal feeding may be necessary. This somnolence syndrome may be of short duration, but in some cases may persist for months after radiation treatment is discontinued (Kun, 1997).

Chemotherapy

For many years, chemotherapy was considered an unknown adjunct to the primary therapies of surgery and radiation. However, the discovery that some chemotherapy can penetrate the CNS when administered systemically, and that this chemotherapy resulted in tumor reduction, has led to its increased use for a variety of pediatric tumors. The most common drugs used include cyclophosphamide, cisplatin or carboplatin, VP-16, and vincristine. These medications all have acute side effects, although cisplatin is of greatest concern from a late effects perspective. Cisplatin is one of the more active agents used in treating brain tumors, but it is known to result in ototoxicity, or hearing loss, particularly when used in children who are also treated with whole-brain radiation therapy. Other side effects of chemotherapy used in the treatment of children with brain tumors are similar to those confronted by children treated for other types of cancer (Balis et al., 1997; van Eys, 1991).

Factors Affecting Neuropsychological Outcome

For a few types of childhood brain tumors, studies have been conducted with homogeneous samples of children with tumors treated in similar ways. These studies will be summarized within the descriptions of the specific tumors. However, because childhood brain tumors are relatively rare, and the frequency of any given type of tumor at a single institution is small, many of the reports on neurocognitive outcomes are based on histologically different tumors, grouped by tumor location, age of the child at the time of diagnosis, or treatment with or without radiation therapy. Before describing outcomes for specific tumors, findings from mixed sets of tumors will be reviewed in an effort to identify factors associated with neurocognitive outcome (see Table 4.2).

Tumors in Young Children

Children under age 3 at the time of diagnosis are considered to have significantly greater risk for severe cognitive impairment than older children. Several studies have found a significant incidence of mental retardation in children under 3 years of age at diagnosis (Danoff, Cowchock, Marquette, Mulgrew, & Kramer, 1982; Spunberg, Change, Goldman, Auricchio, & Bell, 1981), and a number of studies have found younger age statistically related to significantly poorer outcome (Cohen et al., 1993; Dennis, Spiegler, Hetherington, & Greenberg, 1996; Ellenberg, Mccomb, Siegel, & Stowe, 1987; Lannering, Marky, Lundberg, & Olsson, 1990; Mulhern & Kun, 1985; Packer et al., 1989). In addition to significant neurocognitive deficits, these children also have a high incidence of neurological problems, with one study identifying blindness or severe visual impairment in 36% of long-term survivors (Cohen et al., 1993). Careful interpretation of these findings is important, since several studies have suggested that a factor interacting with age of treatment is the length of time since treatment, with longer time since treatment associated with poorer intellectual functioning (Dennis et al., 1996; Kun & Mulhern, 1983; Packer et al., 1989) and psychological adjustment (Seaver et al., 1994).

In these studies, children were treated with surgery and whole-brain radiation therapy, with at least one study reporting significantly lower Full Scale IQ scores in a large percentage of children with mixed supratentorial

TABLE 4.2. Risk Factors for Cognitive Impairment in Children with Brain Tumors

Study	Tumor type	Surgery	RT	Chemo	RT dose	Age at diagnosis	Global function	Specific function
Cohen et al. (1993)	Mixed		Y			Y		
Danoff et al. (1982)	Mixed		Y			Y		
Dennis et al. (1991)	Medullo		Y				Y	Y
Dennis et al. (1996)	Mixed		Y			Y	Y	Y
DeVos et al. (1995)	Cerebral low grade						N	
Duffner et al. (1993)	Mixed			N		N	N	
Ellenberg et al. (1987)	Mixed		Y			Y		
Hirsch et al. (1989)	Cerebral low grade	Y					Y	
Johnson et al. (1994)	Medullo		Y			Y	Y	Y
Lannering et al. (1990)	Mixed		Y			Y		
LeBaron et al. (1988)	Medullo		Y				Y	Y
Mulhern, Kovnar, et al. (1988)	Astrocytoma	Y	Y			Y	Y	Y
Mulhern & Kun (1985)	Mixed		Y			Y		
Mulhern et al. (1998)	Medullo		Y		Y	Y	Y	
Packer et al. (1987)	Medullo		N			Y	N	Y
Packer et al. (1989)	Mixed		Y			Y		
Seaver et al. (1994)	Medullo			Y		Y	Y	Y
Spunberg et al. (1981)	Mixed		Y			Y	Y	

Note. Y, study reported significant finding; N, study included measurement, no significant finding; Medullo, medulloblastoma; Mixed, heterogeneous sample of brain tumors; RT, whole-brain radiation therapy; Chemo, systemic chemotherapy.

and infratentorial tumors treated with whole-brain radiation therapy (68%), compared to children treated with surgery alone (18%) (Lannering et al., 1990). In an effort to reduce the long-term neurotoxicity associated with radiation therapy in very young children, the Pediatric Oncology Group conducted a study using postoperative chemotherapy to delay radiation in children diagnosed prior to 36 months of age. There appeared to be no significant difference in tumor progression in the children who did not receive radiation therapy, and evaluation of neurodevelopmental functioning at 1-year after diagnosis revealed no evidence of deterioration in cognitive ability (Duffner et al., 1993). Long-term follow-up data on these children are not yet available, but the early data suggest a protective factor associated with delayed radiation therapy.

Types of Tumors

As noted earlier, brain tumors in children may arise in any part of the brain. However, there are groups of tumors that are much more common in children. In the following sections, we will describe the more common types of childhood brain tumors, discussing studies that had examined the neuropsychological functioning of these children following appropriate treatment.

Primitive Neuroepithelial Tumors (PNETs) or Medulloblastomas. PNETs are a class of primitive tumors of the brain that can occur at either a supratentorial or infratentorial level of the brain. The most common type of PNET is the medulloblastoma, which is also the most common tumor of the CNS of childhood. Eighty percent of children diagnosed with medulloblastoma will present before the age of 15, and boys are more likely to have this tumor than girls in a 4:1 ratio. Medulloblastoma typically presents in the posterior fossa adjacent to the cerebellum, and may involve the ventricular system. Identification of risk factors has led to the classification of medulloblastomas as either high risk or low risk, depending primarily upon the degree of involvement and whether the tumor can be completely resected. There are significant survival differences based on the risk classification, with low-risk patients experiencing survival of 70% or greater. Treatment of a medulloblastoma involves as complete a surgical resection as possible, followed by an approximately 1-year course of chemotherapy. Whole-brain radiation therapy, involving a fractionated dose in the range of 3,500 cGy with an additional boost to the posterior fossa for a total dose near 5,500 cGy (van Eys, 1991), is administered after one to two cycles of chemotherapy in older children, or delayed, as long as there is no evidence of tumor recurrence, in younger children (Duffner et al., 1993).

Studies of survivors of medulloblastoma have produced mixed results related to neuropsychological late effects. In a study of 43 children with PNETs in the posterior fossa, Packer and his colleagues (1987) found 97% to have intellectual functioning in the normal range. All other studies have found significantly higher rates of cognitive impairment, with Full Scale IQ scores more than 1 standard deviation below the normative mean in 75–100% of patients studied (Dennis et al., 1996; Johnson et al., 1994; LeBaron, Zeltzer, Zeltzer, Scott, & Marlin, 1988; Seaver et al., 1994). More importantly, each of the studies identified significant impairment (performance > 1 standard deviation below normative means) in specific areas of functioning. Deficits in memory have been identified in 53% (Dennis, Spiegler, Hoffman, et al., 1991) to 72% (Packer et al., 1987) of patients studied, with serial memory most affected (Dennis, Spiegler, Fitz, et al., 1991). A number of studies have identified significant impairment in motor abilities, dexterity, and speed (Packer et al., 1987; Johnson et al.,

1994; LeBaron et al., 1988; Mulhern, Kovnar, Kun, Crisco, & Williams, 1988), visual–motor and perceptual–motor abilities (Johnson et al., 1994; LeBaron et al., 1988; Mulhern et al., 1988; Packer et al., 1987), and academic achievement, with difficulties noted in 67–80% of survivors (LeBaron et al., 1988; Packer et al., 1987; Seaver et al., 1994). Academic achievement difficulties were associated with younger age at diagnosis (Seaver et al., 1994) and placement of a shunt, with children with shunts performing better than children without shunts (Johnson et al., 1994). One study also reported significant deficits in cognitive flexibility, tactile perception, and motor planning (LeBaron et al., 1988).

Several factors were associated with these results. Younger children performed worse on measures of intellectual functioning and academic achievement than older children (Dennis et al., 1996; Johnson et al., 1994), and performance on nonverbal tasks was worse than on verbal tasks (Dennis et al., 1996), with performance deficits significantly related to younger age at diagnosis. Age differences in Verbal IQ were not related to age and diagnosis, but instead related to length of time since treatment (Dennis et al., 1996). In the area of academic achievement, reading scores were better than math scores by more than 10 points (Packer et al., 1987).

A recent Pediatric Oncology Group study examined the neuropsychological functioning of 22 long-term survivors of low-risk medulloblastoma treated with standard dose or reduced dose CRT (Mulhern, Kepner, et al., 1998). Stratification by treatment group and by age at diagnosis found that children treated with reduced-dose (2,340 cGy) as opposed to standard-dose (3,600cGy) CRT had significantly higher IQ scores, and younger children benefited more from the reduced cranial radiation dose than did older children. This prospective study suggests an interaction between dose of treatment and age at diagnosis.

Astrocytomas. Astrocytomas are glial tumors that represent 50% of tumors in the cerebral hemispheres of children. They are typically low grade, and most often located in the parietal region of the brain. The high-grade form of astrocytoma (glioblastoma multiforme) is an aggressive and highly malignant form of this tumor. Treatment of astrocytomas typically involves surgical resection of as much of the tumor as possible. Whole-brain radiation therapy may be indicated, and chemotherapy has been used in clinical trials but outcome results are not yet available (van Eys, 1991). In one report following seven children with temporal lobe astrocytomas treated with surgical resection and CRT, a postoperative neuropsychological evaluation found one of the children to be functioning in the mentally retarded range and four to have significant learning disabilities and academic problems. The reason for these impairments were not clear, since they were also associated with inadequate seizure control, tumor recurrence, and younger age at diagnosis (Mulhern, Kovnar, et al., 1988).

Ependymomas. Ependymomas are another type of glial tumor, representing 9% of intracranial brain tumors in children. These tumors often arise from the fourth ventricle, and present with obstructive hydrocephalus. They are typically low-grade tumors that can be controlled but not cured by surgery alone. Postoperative radiation therapy is often included as part of treatment, with attempts made to provide local as opposed to whole-brain radiation in many cases. The efficacy of chemotherapy has not yet been demonstrated in this tumor (van Eys, 1991). There are no reports of studies specifically assessing neurocognitive outcome in children with ependymomas; instead, children with this tumor are included in heterogeneous samples of children with many different types of tumor (Lannering et al., 1990; Dennis, Speigler, Hoffman, et al., 1991).

Optic Pathway Tumors. A group of low-grade glial tumors arising from the optic pathway, most frequently the optic chiasm, represent a fairly common type of brain tumor in children under 5 years of age. These children often present with defects of vision, and sometimes may present with a diencephalic syndrome. Because these tumors are low grade, surgery represents the best treatment option, and maybe repeated if necessary. Survival beyond 5 years in these children is very good (approximately 80%), but tumor progression may suggest the addition of chemotherapy and radiation therapy if necessary (van Eys, 1991). As in the case of ependymomas, there are no reports of specific neurocognitive outcome in children with optic pathway tumors, although clinical trials are currently underway in a cooperative effort between the Pediatric Oncology Group and a Children's Cancer Group. Children with optic pathway tumors often experience long-term visual impairment, requiring careful assessment and services for the visually impaired.

High-Grade Gliomas. Approximately 10–15% of childhood brain tumors will present as glial tumors arising from the brainstem. These tumors typically develop slowly, but present with significant symptoms that may acutely compromise the life of the child. Tissue diagnosis is very difficult because of the location of the tumor, so diagnosis is usually based upon neuroradiological imaging. Surgical resection is not an option, so the treatment of choice is typically high-dose whole-brain radiation therapy. Chemotherapy has not proven to be effective in managing this tumor (van Eys, 1991). Survival following diagnosis of a brainstem glioma is time limited, often less than 1-year from diagnosis, so studies of neurocognitive outcome have not been conducted.

Other Rare Low-Grade Tumors. Children with other rare low-grade tumors of the cerebral hemispheres and choroid plexus may occasionally be referred for neuropsychological assessment. The choroid plexus carcinoma is a rare tumor representing 2–3% of childhood brain tumors. It typically presents with increased intracranial pressure, and is a very low-grade, slow-growing tumor. Surgery is the only current treatment option, and survival outcome is good (van Eys, 1991). However, this tumor is associated with significant cognitive morbidity, including at least one case that we have seen resulting in autistic characteristics. Another rare, low-grade tumor is the craniopharyngioma, a tumor of developmental origin. This tumor is also low grade, but surgical treatment sometimes followed by radiation therapy presents an excellent survival outlook (van Eys, 1991). In each of these cases, the location of the tumor represents a potential high risk for cognitive morbidity. In one study of low-grade tumors of the cerebral hemisphere, 30% of children treated with surgery alone had Full Scale IQs less than 80 and experienced significant academic problems (Hirsch, Rose, Pierre-Kahn, Pfister, & Hoppe-Hirsch, 1989). Despite this risk, surgical removal of tumors in the cerebral hemisphere near the language centers has been associated with an average 12-point improvement in postoperative language functioning (DeVos, Wyllie, Geckler, Kotagal, & Comair, 1995). Careful consultation with neurosurgeons and neurologists and review of neuroimaging studies will be necessary in designing assessment studies and clinical evaluations of children with these types of tumors.

Summary

In summary, children with brain tumors are at significant risk for long-term cognitive impairment. Factors such as the type and location of the tumor, use of radiation therapy and dose of radiation therapy, and time since treatment constitute substantial risks for these children. The greatest risk factor appears to be the age of the child at the time of diagnosis and treatment, but efforts to delay radiation therapy suggest a more positive outlook in terms of cognitive functioning. As more protocols are developed that rely heavily on chemotherapy, in addition to or in place of radiation therapy, careful attention must be paid to the late cognitive effects associated with this treatment change.

SOCIAL AND PSYCHOLOGICAL ADJUSTMENT

Functioning on tests of neuropsychological ability is not the only area of a child's existence that may be affected by treatment for leukemia or a brain tumor. Fortunately, aside from some acute problems associated with parental distress during treatment (Dahlquist, Czyzewski & Jones,1993; Kazak & Barakat, 1997; Manne et al., 1995), or in acute stress reactions to treatment or preparation for bone marrow transplantation (Butler, Rizzi, & Handwerger, 1996), children with acute leukemia appear to have minimal problems with social functioning (Noll, Bukowski, Davies, Koontz, &

Kulkarni, 1993) or long-term psychological adjustment or coping (Kupst et al., 1995). Similar family factors, along with reactions to disfigurement and functional impairment have been reported for children recently diagnosed (Mulhern, Carpentieri, Shema, Stone, & Fairclough, 1993), with minimal problems noted 2–5 years off treatment for brain tumors (Radcliffe, Bennett, Kazak, Foley, & Phillips, 1996). However, a recent study of 110 children, treated with CRT and methotrexate, but off treatment for ALL an average of 15 years, suggest that this treatment combination is associated with significant long-term problems in academic achievement, poorer self-image related to physical appearance, and greater general psychological distress (Hill et al., 1998). As this is the only study that has examined this issue in a cohort of children treated for the same disease using the same treatment protocol for a period of greater than 10 years, it raises significant concerns about the long-term implications of this treatment.

CONCLUSIONS

In this chapter, we have focused on neurocognitive outcomes in children with acute lymphoblastic leukemia or brain tumors, relying largely on description of impairments and identification of different aspects of disease and treatment that place children at increased risk. Unfortunately, these neurocognitive impairments can have a significant impact on a child's success in school, self-esteem, social relationships, and long-term quality of life. It appears that we have made significant progress in identifying children at risk and the specific patterns of cognitive deficits likely to result. However, simply acknowledging that a deficit exists is inadequate in addressing these other noncognitive needs.

What approaches can be taken to avoid, minimize, or remediate neurocognitive deficits resulting from cancer and its treatment? First, the results of neuropsychological testing of survivors are increasingly used to guide pediatric oncologists in the development of new, less neurotoxic, treatment protocols. Such testing is logistically difficult because of the involvement of multiple institutions and variable reimbursement from third-party payers (Armstrong & Drotar, in press). However, the ultimate value of treatment that includes consideration of neuropsychological impact leading to sparing children unnecessarily aggressive therapy can no longer be disputed. Second, an appropriate standard of care dictates that children at risk receive routine surveillance of their cognitive abilities and academic progress using instruments of proven validity in indentifying cognitive deficits associated with their disease and treatment (Mulhern, Armstrong, & Thompson, 1998). Third, early intervention for identified deficits must be provided, including education of parents, teachers, and children about etiology and the scope of affected functions.

Unfortunately, there are no published studies that systematically evaluate the effectiveness of either pharmacological, behavioral, and/or educational interventions for these children, although social skills intervention as part of a school integration program has been shown to be effective in increasing children's perceptions of classmate and teacher social support (Varni, Katz, Colegrove, & Dolgin, 1993). One report suggests that methylphenidate may be beneficial in alleviating some of the attentional problems experienced by children with ALL and brain tumors (Delong, Friedman, Friedman, Gustafson, & Oakes, 1992), but this was a noncontrolled series of cases involving children treated clinically with the drug. Butler and his colleagues (Butler & Rizzi, 1995) have reported on preliminary work using a cognitive rehabilitation program that addresses specific deficits associated with CRT, but controlled trials with adequate samples have not been conducted nor reported. We have suggested a model utilizing technological support (e.g., audiotaping of notes and lectures, use of a calculator, oral as opposed to written evaluation, and untimed testing) as strategies to assist children in reintegrating to an academic environment (Armstrong & Horn, 1995), but these interventions have also been proposed in the absence of empirical support.

There is perhaps no more pressing issue in the psychological management of children with ALL and brain tumors than the development and empirical demonstration of effectiveness of interventions targeting the neurocognitive, social, and behavioral deficits associated with treatment of these diseases. It is critical that psychological and educational treatment keep pace with advances in the medical care and cure of these childhood cancers.

ACKNOWLEDGMENTS

Partial support for this chapter was provided to Raymond K. Mulhern by the American Lebanese Syrian Associated Charities (ALSAC) and Cancer Center Support (CORE) Grant No. P30-CA21765 from the National Cancer Institute. Partial support for F. Daniel Armstrong for the preparation of this chapter was provided by the Division of Pediatric Hematology/Oncology, University of Miami School of Medicine.

REFERENCES

American Cancer Society. (1997). *Cancer facts and figures*. Atlanta: Author.

Anderson, V., Smibert, E., Ekert, H., & Godber, T. (1994). Intellectual, educational, and behavioural sequelae after cranial irradiation and chemotherapy. *Archives of Diseases in Childhood, 70*, 476–483.

Appleton, R. E., Farrell, K., Zaide, J., & Rogers, P. (1990). Decline in head growth and cognitive impairment in survivors of acute lymphoblastic leukaemia. *Archives of Diseases in Childhood, 65*, 530–534.

Armstrong, F. D. (1996). Commentary: Childhood cancer. *Journal of Pediatric Psychology, 20*, 417–421.

Armstrong, F. D., & Drotar, D. (in press). Multi-institutional and multi-disciplinary research collaboration: Strategies and lessons from cooperative trials. In D. Drotar (Ed.), *Handbook on pediatric and clinical psychology*. New York: Plenum Press.

Armstrong, F. D., & Horn, M. (1995). Educational issues in childhood cancer. *School Psychology Quarterly, 10*, 292–304.

Balis, F. M., Holcenberg, J. S., & Poplack, D. G. (1997). In P. A. Pizzo & D. G. Poplack (Eds.), *Principles and practice of pediatric oncology* (3rd ed., pp. 215–272), Philadelphia: Lippincott-Raven.

Brown, R. T., Madan-Swain, A., Pais, R., Lambert, R. G., Sexson, S., & Ragab, A. (1992). Chemotherapy for acute lymphocytic leukemia: Cognitive and academic sequelae. *Journal of Pediatrics, 121*, 885–889.

Brown, R. T., Madan-Swain, A., Walco, G. A., Cherrick, I., Ievers, C. E., Conte, P. M., Vega, R., Bell, B., & Lauer, S. J. (1998). Cognitive academic late effects among children previously treated for acute lymphocytic leukemia receiving chemotherapy as CNS prophylaxis. *Journal of Pediatric Psychology, 23*, 219–228.

Brown, R. T., Sawyer, M. B., Antoniou, G., Toogood, I., Rice, M., Thompson, N., & Madan-Swain, A. (1996). A 3-year follow-up of the intellectual and academic functioning of children receiving central nervous system prophylactic chemotherapy for leukemia. *Journal of Developmental and Behavioral Pediatrics, 17*, 392–398.

Butler, R. W., & Copeland, D. R. (1993). Neuropsychological effects of central nervous system prophylactic treatment in childhood leukemia: Methodological considerations. *Journal of Pediatric Psychology, 18*, 319–338.

Butler, R. W., Hill, J. M., Steinherz, P. G., Meyers, P. A., & Finlay, J. L. (1994). Neuropsychologic effects of cranial irradiation, intrathecal methotrexate, and systemic methotrexate in childhood cancer. *Journal of Clinical Oncology, 12*, 2621–2629.

Butler, R. W., & Rizzi, L. P. (1995). The remediation of attentional deficits secondary to treatment for childhood cancer. *Progress Notes, Society of Pediatric Psychology, 19*, 5, 13.

Butler, R. W., Rizzi, L. P., & Handwerger, B. A. (1996). Brief report: The assessment of posttraumatic stress disorder in pediatric cancer patients and survivors. *Journal of Pediatric Psychology, 21*, 499–504.

Cap, A., Foltinová, A., Szabova, I., Cinkovska, S., & Boruta, P. (1991). Disorders in neuropsychological development and their relation to computed tomography brain scan in children with acute lymphoblastic leukemia in long-term remission. *Neoplasma, 38*, 351–356.

Christie, D., Leiper, A. D., Chessells, J. M., & Vargha Khadem, F. (1995). Intellectual performance after presymptomatic cranial radiotherapy for leukaemia: Effects of age and sex. *Archives of Diseases in Childhood, 73*, 136–140.

Ciesielski, K. T., Yanofsky, R., Ludwig, R. N., Hill, D. E., Hart, B. L., Astur, R. S., & Snyder, T. (1994). Hypoplasia of the cerebellar vermis and cognitive deficits in survivors of childhood leukemia. *Archives of Neurology, 51*, 985–993.

Cohen, B. H., Packer, R. J., Siegel, K. R., Rorke, L. B., D'Angio, G., Sutton, L. N., Bruce, D. A., & Schut, L. (1993). *Pediatric Neurosurgery, 19,* 171–179.

Copeland, D. R., Dowell, R. E., Fletcher, J. M., Sullivan, M. P., Jaffee, N., Cangir, A., Frankel, L. S., & Judd, B. W. (1988). Neuropsychological test performance of pediatric cancer patients at diagnosis and one year later. *Journal of Pediatric Psychology, 13,* 183–196.

Copeland, D. R., Moore, B. D., III, Francis, D. J., Jafffe, N., & Culbert, S. J. (1996). Neuropsychologic effects of chemotherapy on children with cancer: A longitudinal study. *Journal of Clinical Oncology, 14,* 2826–2835.

Cousens, P., Ungerer, J. A., Crawford, J. A., & Stevens, M. M. (1991). Cognitive effects of childhood leukemia therapy: A case for four specific deficits. *Journal of Pediatric Psychology, 16,* 475–488.

Dahlquist, L. M., Czyzewski, D. I., & Jones, C. L. (1996). Parents of children with cancer: A longitudinal study of emotional distress, coping style, and marital adjustment two and twenty months after diagnosis. *Journal of Pediatric Psychology, 21,* 541–554.

Danoff, B. F., Cowehock, F. S., Marquette, C., Mulgrew, L., & Kramer, S. (1982). Assessment of the long-term effects of primary radiation therapy for brain tumors in children. *Cancer, 49,* 1580–1586.

Delong, R., Friedman, H., Friedman, N., Gustafson, K., & Oakes, J. (1992). Methylphenidate in neuropsychological sequelae of radiotherapy and chemotherapy of childhood brain tumors and leukemia. *Journal of Child Neurology, 7,* 462–463.

Dennis, M., Spiegler, B. J., Fitz, C. R., Hoffman, H. J., Hendrick, E. B., Humphreys, R. P., & Chuang, S. (1991). Brain tumors in children and adolescents: II. The neuroanatomy of deficits in working, associative, and serial-order memory. *Neuropsychologia, 29,* 829–847.

Dennis, M., Spiegler, B. J., Hetherington, C. R., & Greenberg, M. L. (1996). Neuropsychological sequelae of the treatment of children with medulloblastoma. *Journal of Neuro-Oncology, 29,* 91–101.

Dennis, M., Spiegler, B. J., Hoffman, H. J., Hendrick, E. B., Humphreys, R. P., & Becker, L. E. (1991). Brain tumors in children and adolescents: I. Effects on working, associative, and serial-order memory of IQ, age at tumor onset and age of tumor. *Neuropsychologia, 29,* 813–827.

DeVos, K. J., Wyllie, E., Geckler, C., Kotagal, P., & Comair, Y. (1995). Language dominance in patients with early childhood tumors near left hemisphere language areas. *Neurology, 45,* 349–356.

Duffner, P. K., Horowitz, M. E., Krischer, J. P., Friedman, H. S., Burger, P. C., Cohen, M. E., Sanford, R. A., Mulhern, R. K., James, H. E., Freeman, C. R., Seidel, F. G., & Kun, L. E. (1993). *New England Journal of Medicine, 328,* 1725–1731.

Ellenberg, L., Mccomb, J. G., Siegel, S. E., & Stowe, S. (1987). Factors affecting intellectual outcome in pediatric brain tumor patients. *Neurosurgery, 21,* 638–644.

Finlay, J. L. (1996). The role of high-dose chemotherapy and stem cell rescue in the treatment of malignant brain tumors. *Bone Marrow Transplantation, 18,* S51–55.

Fletcher, J. M, & Copeland, D. R. (1988). Neurobehavioral effects of central nervous system prophylactic treatment of cancer in children. *Journal of Clinical and Experimental Neuropsychology, 10,* 495–538.

Giralt, J., Ortega, J. J., Olive, T., Verges, R., Forio, I., & Salvador, L. (1992). Long-term neuropsychologic sequelae of childhood leukemia: Comparison of two CNS prophylactic regimens. *International Journal of Radiation Oncology and Biologic Physics, 24*, 49–53.

Glauser, T. A., & Packer, R. J. (1991). Cognitive deficits in long-term survivors of childhood brain tumors. *Children's Nervous System, 7*, 2–12.

Halberg, F. E., Kramer, J. H., Moore, I. M., Wara, W. M., Matthay, K. K., & Ablin, A. R. (1992). Prophylactic cranial irradiation dose effects on late cognitive function in children treated for acute lymphoblastic leukemia. *International Journal of Radiation Oncology and Biologic Physics, 22*, 13–16.

Hill, J. M., Kornblith, A. B., Jones, D., Freeman, A., Holland, J. F., Glicksman, A. S., Boyett, J. M., Lenherr, B., Brecher, M. L., Dubowy, R., Kung, F., Mauer, H., & Holland, J. C. (1998). A comparative study of the long term psychosocial functioning of childhood acute lymphoblastic leukemia survivors treated by intrathecal methotrexate with or without cranial radiation. *Cancer, 82*, 208–218.

Hirsch, J. F., Rose, C. S., Pierre-Kahn, A., Pfister, A., & Hoppe-Hirsch, E. (1989). Benign astrocytic and oligodendritic tumors of the cerebral hemispheres in children. *Journal of Neurosurgery, 70*, 568–572.

Jankovic, M., Brouwers, P., Valsecchi, M. G., VanVEldhuizen, A., Huisman, J., Kamphuis, R., Kingma, A., Mor, W., Van Dongen-Melman, J., Ferronato, L., Mancini, M. A., Spinetta, J. J., & Masera, G. for the International Study Group on Psychosocial Aspects of Childhood Cancer. (1994). Association of 1800 cGy cranial irradiation with intellectual function in children with acute lymphoblastic leukaemia. *Lancet, 344*, 224–227.

Johnson, D. L., McCabe, M. A., Nicholson, H. S., Joseph, A. L., Getson, P. R., Byrne, J., Brasseux, C., Packer, R. J., & Reaman, G. (1994). Quality of long-term survival in young children with medulloblastoma. *Journal of Neurosurgery, 80*, 1004–1010.

Kazak, A. E., & Barakat, L. P. (1997). Brief report: Parenting stress and quality of life during treatment for childhood leukemia predicts child and parent adjustment after treatment ends. *Journal of Pediatric Psychology, 22*, 749–758.

Kingma, A., Mooyaart, E. L., Kamps, W. A., Nieuwenhuizen, P., & Wilmink, J. T. (1993). Magnetic resonance imaging of the brain and neuropsychological evaluation in children treated for acute lymphoblastic leukemia at a young age. *American Journal of Pediatric Hematology/Oncology, 15*, 231–238.

Kramer, J. H., Norman, D., Brant-Zawadski, M., Ablin, A., & Moore, I. M. (1988). Absence of white matter changes on magnetic resonance imaging in children treated with CNS prophylaxis therapy for leukemia. *Cancer, 61*, 928–930.

Kun, L. E. (1997). General principles of radiation therapy. In P. A. Pizzo & D. G. Poplack (Eds.), *Principles and practice of pediatric oncology* (3rd ed., pp. 289–321). Philadelphia: Lippincott-Raven.

Kun, L. E., Camitta, B. M., Mulhern, R., Lauer, S., Kline, R., Caspter, J., Kamen, B., Kaplan, B., & Barber, S. (1984). Treatment of meningeal relapse in childhood acute lymphoblastic leukemia: I. Results of craniospinal irradiation. *Journal of Clinical Oncology, 6*, 359–364.

Kun, L. E., & Mulhern, R. K. (1983). Neuropsychologic function in children with brain tumors: II. Serial studies of intellect and time after treatment. *American Journal of Clinical Oncology, 6*, 651–665.

Kupst, M. J., Natta, M. B., Richardson, C. C., Schulman, J. L., Lavigne, J. V., & Das, L. (1995). Family coping with pediatric leukemia: Ten years after treatment. *Journal of Pediatric Psychology, 20,* 601–617.

Lannering, B., Marky, I., Lundberg, A., & Olsson, E. (1990). Long-term sequelae after pediatric brain tumors: Their effect on disability and quality of life. *Medical and Pediatric Oncology, 18,* 304–310.

LeBaron, S., Zeltzer, P. M., Zeltzer, L. K., Scott, S. E., & Marlin, A. E. (1988). Assessment of quality of survival in children with medulloblastoma and cerebellar astrocytoma. *Cancer, 62,* 1215–1222.

Longeway, K. L., Mulhern, R., Crisco, J., Kun, L. E., Lauer, S., Casper, J., Camitta, B., & Hoffman, R. G. (1990). Treatment of meningeal relapse in childhood acute lymphoblastic leukemia: II. A prospective study of intellectual loss specific to CNS relapse and therapy. *American Journal of Pediatric Hematology/Oncology, 12,* 45–50.

MacLean, W. E., Noll, R. B., Stehbens, J. A., Kaleita, T. A., Schwartz, E., Whitt, J. K., Cantor, N., Waskerwitz, M., Ruymann, F., Novak, L. J., Woodard, A., Hammonds, G. D., for the Children's Cancer Group. (1995). Neuropsychological effects of cranial irradiation in young children with acute lymphoblastic leukemia 9 months after diagnosis. *Archives of Neurology, 52,* 156–160.

Mahoney, D. H., Jr., Shuster J. J., Nitschke, R., Lauer, S. J., Steuber, C. P., Winick, N., & Camitta, B. (1998). Acute neurotoxicity in children with B-precursor acute lymphoid leukemia: An association with intermediate dose intravenous methotrexate and intrathecal tripe therapy: A Pediatric Oncology Group study. *Journal of Clinical Oncology, 16,* 1712–1722.

Manne, S. L., Lesanics, D., Meyers, P., Wollner, N., Steinherz, P., & Redd, W. (1995). Predictors of depressive symptomatology among parents of newly diagnosed children with cancer. *Journal of Pediatric Psychology, 20,* 491–510.

Margolin, J. F., & Poplack, D. G. (1997). Acute lymphoblastic leukemia. In P. A. Pizzo & D. G. Poplack (Eds.), *Principles and practice of pediatric oncology* (3rd ed., pp. 409–462), Philadelphia: Lippincott-Raven.

Moore, B. D., III, Copeland, D. R., Reid, H., & Levy, B. (1992). Neuropsychological basis of cognitive deficits in long-term survivors of childhood cancer. *Archives of Neurology, 49,* 809–817.

Moore, I. M., Kramer, J. H., Wara, W., Halberg, F., & Ablin, A. R. (1991). Cognitive function in children with leukemia: Effect of radiation dose and time since irradiation. *Cancer, 68,* 1913–1917.

Mulhern, R. K. (1994). Neuropsychological late effects. In D. J. Bearison & R. K. Mulhern (Eds.), *Pediatric psychooncology: Psychological perspectives on children with cancer* (pp. 99–121). New York: Oxford Press.

Mulhern, R. K., Armstrong, F. D., & Thompson, S. J. (1998). Function-specific neuropsychological assessment. *Medical and Pediatric Oncology Supplement, 1,* 34–40.

Mulhern, R. K., Carpentieri, S., Shema, S., Stone, P., & Fairclough, D. (1993). Factors associated with social and behavioral problems among children recently diagnosed with brain tumor. *Journal of Pediatric Psychology, 18,* 339–350.

Mulhern, R. K., Crisco, J. J., & Kun, L. E. (1983). Neuropsychological sequelae of childhood brain tumors: A review. *Journal of Clinical Child Psychology, 12,* 66–73.

Mulhern, R. K., Fairclough, D., & Ochs, J. (1991). A prospective comparison of neuropsychologic performance of children surviving leukemia who received 18-Gy, 24-Gy or no cranial irradiation. *Journal of Clinical Oncology, 9,* 1348–1356.

Mulhern, R. K., Kepner, J., Thomas, P. R. M., Armstrong, F. D., Friedman, H., & Kun, L. (1998). Neuropsychological functioning of survivors of childhood medulloblastoma randomized to receive conventional (3,600 cGy/20) or reduced (2,340 cGy/13) dose cranospinal irradiation: A Pediatric Oncology Group study. *Journal of Clinical Oncology, 16,* 1723–1728.

Mulhern, R. K., Kovnar, E. H., Kun, L. E., Crisco, J. J., & Williams, J. M. (1988). Psychologic and neurologic function following treatment for childhood temporal lobe astrocytoma. *Journal of Child Neurology, 3,* 47–52.

Mulhern, R. K., Kovnar, E. H., Langston, J., Carter, M., Fairclough, D., Leigh, L., & Kun, L. E. (1992). Longterm survivors of leukemia treated in infancy: Factors associated with neuropsychological status. *Journal of Clinical Oncology, 10,* 1095–1102.

Mulhern, R. K., & Kun, L. E. (1985). Neuropsychologic function in children with brain tumors: III. Interval changes in the six months following treatment. *Medical and Pediatric Oncology, 13,* 318–324.

Mulhern, R. K., Ochs, J., Fairclough, D., Wasserman, A., Davis, K., & Williams, J. M. (1987). Intellectual and academic achievement status after CNS relapse: A retrospective analysis of 40 children treated for ALL. *Journal of Clinical Oncology, 5,* 933–940.

Mulhern, R. K., Wasserman, A. L., Fairclough, D., & Ochs, J. (1988). Memory function in disease-free survivors of childhood acute lymphocytic leukemia given CNS prophylaxis with or without 1800 cGy cranial irradiation. *Journal of Clinical Oncology, 6,* 315–320.

Nitschke, R., Wilson, D., Bowman, M., Chaffin, M., & Sexauer, C. (1990, September). *MRI detection of transient leukoencephalopathy and neuropsychological findings in children treated for acute lymphoblastic leukemia.* Paper presented at the third annual meeting of the American Society of Pediatric Hematology/Oncology, Chicago.

Noll, R. B., Bukowski, W. M., Davies, W. H., Koontz, K., & Kulkarni, R. (1993). Adjustment in the peer system of adolescents with cancer: A two-year study. *Journal of Pediatric Psychology, 18,* 351–364.

Ochs, J., Mulhern, R. K., Fairclough, D., Parvey, L., Whitaker, J., Chien, L., Mauer, A., & Simone, J. (1991). Comparison of neuropsychologic functioning and clinical indicators of neurotoxicity in long-term survivors of childhood leukemia given cranial radiation or parenteral methotrexate: A prospective study. *Journal of Clinical Oncology, 9,* 145–151.

Ochs, J., Rivera, G., Aur, R. J. A., Hustu, H. O., Berg, R., & Simone, J. (1985). Central nervous system morbidity following an initial isolated central nervous system relapse and its subsequent therapy in childhood acute lymphoblastic leukemia. *Journal of Clinical Oncology, 3,* 622–625.

Packer, R. J., Sposto, R., Atkins, T. E., Sutton, L. N., Bruce, D. A., Siegel, K. R., Rorke, L. B., Littman, P. A., & Schut, L. (1987). Quality of life in children with primitive neuroectodermal tumors (medulloblastoma) of the posterior fossa. *Pediatric Neuroscience, 13,* 169–175.

Packer, R. J., Sutton, L. N., Atkins, T. E., Radcliffe, J., Bunnin, G. R., D—Angio, G., Siegel, K. R., & Schut, L. (1989). A prospective study of cognitive function in children receiving whole brain radiotherapy and chemotherapy: Two year results. *Journal of Neurosurgery, 70,* 707–713.

Parker, S. L., Tong, T., Bolden, S., & Wingo, P. A. (1997). Cancer statistics. *CA-A Cancer Journal for Clinicians, 47,* 5–27.

Radcliffe, J., Bennett, D., Kazak, A. E., Foley, B., & Phillips, P. C. (1996). Adjustment in childhood brain tumor survival: Child, mother, and teacher report. *Journal of Pediatric Psychology, 21,* 529–539.

Robison, L. L., Mertens, A., & Neglia, J. P. (1991). Epidemiology and etiology of childhood cancer. In D. J. Fernbach & T. J. Vietti (Eds.), *Clinical pediatric oncology* (pp. 11–28). St. Louis: Mosby Year Book.

Rodgers, J., Britton, P. G., Morris, R. G., Kernahan, J., & Craft, A. W. (1992). Memory after treatment for acute lymphoblastic leukaemia. *Archives of Diseases in Childhood, 67,* 266–268.

Rourke, B. P. (1982). Central processing deficiencies in children: Toward a developmental neuropsychological model. *Journal of Clinical Neuropsychology, 4,* 1–18.

Rubenstein, C. L., Varni, J. W., & Katz, E. R. (1990). Cognitive functioning in long-term survivors of childhood leukemia: A prospective analysis. *Journal of Developmental and Behavioral Pediatrics, 11,* 301–305.

Said, J. A., Waters, B. G. H., Cousens, P., & Stevens, M. M. (1989). Neuropsychological sequelae of central nervous system prophylaxis in survivors of childhood acute lymphoblastic leukemia. *Journal of Consulting and Clinical Psychology, 57,* 251–256.

Sanders, J. E. (1997). Bone marrow transplantation in pediatric oncology. In P. A. Pizzo & D. G. Poplack (Eds.), *Principles and practice of pediatric oncology* (3rd ed., pp. 357–373), Philadelphia: Lippincott-Raven.

Schlieper, A. E., Esseltine, D. W., & Tarshis, E. (1989). Cognitive function in long survivors of childhood acute lymphoblastic leukemia. *Pediatric Hematology Oncology, 6,* 1–9.

Seaver, E., Geyer, R., Sulzbacher, S., Warner, M., Batzel, L., Milstein, J., & Berger, M. (1994). Psychosocial adjustment of long-term survivors of childhood medulloblastoma and ependymoma treated with craniospinal irradiation. *Pediatric Neurosurgery, 20,* 248–253.

Sexson, S. B., & Madan-Swain, A. (1993). School reentry for the child with chronic illness. *Journal of Learning Disabilities, 26,* 115–125.

Smibert, E., Anderson, V., Godber, T., & Ekert, H. (1996). Risk factors for intellectual and educational sequelae of cranial irradiation in childhood acute lymphoblastic leukaemia. *British Journal of Cancer, 73,* 825–830.

Spunberg, J. J., Change, C. H., Goldman, M., Auricchio, E., & Bell, J. J. (1981). Quality of long-term survival following irradiation for intracranial tumors in children under the age of two. *International Journal of Radiation Oncology and Biological Physics, 7,* 727–736.

van Eys, J. (1991) Malignant tumors of the central nervous system. In D. J. Fernbach & T. J. Vietti (Eds.), *Clinical pediatric oncology* (pp. 409–426). St. Louis: Mosby Year Book.

Varni, J. W., Katz, E. R., Colegrove, R., Jr., & Dolgin, M. (1993). The impact of social skills training on the adjustment of children with newly diagnosed cancer. *Journal of Pediatric Psychology, 18*, 751–767.

Waber, D. P., Gioia, G., Paccia, J., Sherman, B., Dinklage, D., Sollee, N., Urion, D. K., Tarbell, N. J., & Sallan, S. E. (1990). Sex differences in cognitive processing in children treated with CNS prophylaxis for acute lymphoblastic leukemia. *Journal of Pediatric Psychology, 15*, 105–122.

Waber, D. P., & Tarbell, N. J. (1997). Toxicity of CNS prophylaxis for childhood leukemia. *Oncology, 11*, 259–265.

Waber, D. P., Tarbell, N. J., Fairclough, D., Atmore, K., Castro, R., Isquith, P., Lussier, F., Romero, I., Carpenter, P. J., & Schiller, M. (1995). Cognitive sequelae of treatment in childhood acute lymphoblastic leukemia: Cranial radiation requires an accomplice. *Journal of Clinical Oncology, 13*, 2490–2496.

Waber, D. P., Tarbell, N. J., Kahn, C. M., Gelber, R. D., & Sallan, S. E. (1992). The relationship of sex and treatment modality to neuropsychologic outcome in childhood acute lymphoblastic leukemia. *Journal of Clinical Oncology, 10*, 810–817.

Waber, D. P., Urion, D. K., Tarbell, N. J., Niemeyer, C., Gelber, R., & Sallan, S. E. (1990). Late effects of central nervous system treatment of acute lymphoblastic leukemia in childhood are sex-dependent. *Developmental Medicine and Child Neurology, 32*, 238–248.

Williams, K. S., Ochs, J., Williams, J. M., & Mulhern, R. K. (1991). Parental report of everyday cognitive abilities among children treated for acute lymphoblastic leukemia. *Journal of Pediatric Psychology, 16*, 13–26.

CHAPTER FIVE

Asthma

KATHLEEN L. LEMANEK
CATHERINE HOOD

Children's and adolescent's adaptation to chronic illnesses, including asthma, has been a research and clinical focus in pediatric psychology. As with other chronic illnesses, wide variability in adaptation to asthma exists in children. Some children have adapted well to their illness, seeming to have few academic, social, emotional, and behavioral problems. On the other hand, children with asthma do present twice as often with behaviors considered to be indicative of a poor adaptation to their illness, especially if they are receiving inpatient treatment (Furrow, Hambley, & Brazil, 1989; MacLean, Perrin, Gortmaker, & Pierre, 1992). Poor adaptation to asthma may be displayed in the form of internalizing behavior problems (e.g., anxiety, depression), externalizing behavior problems (e.g., disruptive behaviors), deficient social interactions, academic difficulties, and inadequate illness management. To understand such differential responses to any chronic illness, investigators have stressed the importance of delineating factors that foster or hinder adaptation (Creer, Stein, Rappaport, & Lewis, 1992; Drotar, 1997; Varni & Wallander, 1988). One set of protective factors identified in most chronic illnesses can be characterized as cognitions. In general, cognitions, such as attributions and coping style, influence children's and adolescents' adaptation to positive and negative events, including events related to a chronic illness. This chapter will present the literature that highlights the role cognitions have in adaptation to asthma by examining various domains of biological and psychological functioning. First, a brief description of the clinical features and medical management of asthma will be provided followed by a conceptual framework defining the term cognition and describing certain cognitive processes.

CLINICAL FEATURES
AND MEDICAL MANAGEMENT

Asthma is a common childhood chronic illness, occurring in approximately 6% of children less than 18 years old (Taggart & Fulwood, 1993). In 1988, this figure corresponded to an estimated 2.7 million children (Taylor & Newacheck, 1992). In the most recent report by the National Institutes of Health (NIH; 1997), asthma is defined as a chronic inflammation disorder that causes airflow obstruction (narrowing/blocking), which is often reversible either spontaneously or with treatment, and bronchial hyperresponsiveness to a variety of stimuli. In general, this obstruction, hyperreactivity of airways, and inflammation lead to the most common clinical feature of asthma—breathing difficulties, which are manifested as coughing, wheezing, or shortness of breath.

In order to understand how asthma affects children and adolescents clinically, certain of the terms in the preceding definition require clarification. Airway hyperresponsiveness or "bronchoconstriction" involves narrowing of the small airways due to muscle spasm, mucosa edema, mucosa inflammation, and excessive mucus secretion (Creer & Bender, 1995). Airway inflammation refers to swelling and excess mucus secretion. Stimuli to which the hyperresponsiveness and inflammation may arise include both environmental and internal agents, such as allergens (e.g., dust mites, animal dander), irritants (e.g., cigarette smoke, perfumes, cold air), drugs (e.g., aspirin), respiratory infections, exercise, changes in air temperature, and emotional reactions (e.g., laughing, crying) (Creer & Bender, 1995; Young, 1994). This range of stimuli then contributes to the wide variability in the frequency and the severity of asthma attacks within and across children and adolescents (Creer & Bender, 1995).

The specific clinical symptoms of asthma are also variable and can range from mild to severe (Lemanek, Trane, & Weiner, 1999). Children and adolescents may experience such mild symptoms as coughing with laughing, crying, or running, or when exposed to cold air; feelings of chest tightness; and diminished stamina for vigorous exercise. These symptoms may progress to wheezing (i.e., squeaking or whistling noises as air moves through narrowed airways) or labored breathing (i.e., increased respiratory rate and use of accessory muscles to assist in breathing). In severe cases, cyanosis (i.e., blue skin color due to lack of oxygen) may occur.

As with most chronic illnesses, both heredity and the environment are implicated in the etiology of asthma. For example, the risk of inheriting an atopic disease, such as asthma or hay fever/allergic rhinitis, is 50% when at least one parent has the disease. The NIH report (1997) suggests that hyperresponsiveness is attributable to multiple factors: airway inflammation, deficiencies in bronchial epithelial integrity, changes in autonomic neural control of airways, modifications in intrinsic smooth muscle function, and baseline airway obstruction (cited in Creer & Bender, 1995). Inflammation in the airways is also due to an interaction among cellular processes, such as inflammatory cells, mediators (e.g., mast cells, macrophages, histamines, platelet-activating factors), and airway cells and tissues. With respect to the environment, factors associated with a higher prevalence of asthma include living in an urban setting, residing in certain countries (e.g., 20% in New Zealand vs. 3% in Japan), exposure to indoor allergens (e.g., dust mites, animal dander), and smoking (Lemanek et al., 1999).

The mortality and morbidity of asthma can be significant. During the 1980s, deaths in children due to asthma increased by 6.2% per year in the United States, with greater increases in children ages 5–14 years compared to individuals ages 15–34 years (Weiss & Wagener, 1990). The most common variables contributing to these deaths appear to be poor communication between patients, their parents, and the physician, as well as reactions of anger and hopelessness regarding their illness (Lemanek et al., 1999). In addition to these psychological factors, physiological variables (e.g., seizures, respiratory failure) are considered risk factors for death in children and adolescents (Fritz, Rubinstein, & Lewiston, 1987). In terms of morbidity, asthma can have both health and economic consequences for children, their families, and society. For example, asthma is a leading contributor to school absenteeism and can restrict participation in school-related activities (Lemanek, 1990; Taggart & Fulwood, 1993; Taylor & Newacheck, 1992). Children with asthma also have more contacts with physicians and a greater frequency of hospitalizations than children without asthma. With respect to inpatient hospitalizations and emergency room visits, millions of dollars are spent on health care for asthma (Weiss, Gergen, & Hodgson, 1992). Furthermore, 2–30% of a family's income may be spent on the medical management of asthma (Creer, Renee, & Chai, 1982).

Despite the development of more efficacious treatment regimens, the prevalence and the severity of asthma have increased in the United States over the past two decades (Creer & Bender, 1993). Ultimately, the goals of treatment regimens for asthma include controlling symptoms with minimal medication, maximizing pulmonary function, optimizing functional status (e.g., ability to attend school or participate in activities), and educating children and their families in self-management strategies (Cockcroft & Hargreave, 1990; Lemanek, 1990). To achieve these goals, three treatment approaches are recommended and pertain to environmental control, pharmacological intervention, and immunotherapy (Lemanek et al., 1999; NIH, 1997; Young, 1994). In terms of environmental control, instructions are given on how to reduce exposure to known triggers of asthma attacks, such as by eliminating tobacco smoke and avoiding animals, and controlling dust mites and mold allergies through the use of air conditioners and humidifiers. Immunotherapy is frequently recommended if allergens are constant or cannot be avoided. Finally, medications are prescribed to prevent and manage asthma attacks, whether these attacks are episodic, recurrent, or exercise-induced. In general, two classes of medications are used to control asthma symptoms: bronchodilators and anti-inflammatory drugs. Bronchodilators (e.g., albuterol, metaproterenol) are adrenaline-like drugs that relax the constriction of smooth muscles surrounding the airways. Anti-inflammatory medications (e.g., cromolyn sodium, nedocromil) lessen airway hyperreactivity and the swelling and mucus secretions of airway membranes. These medications can be administered on a daily (usually anti-inflammatory medications) or intermittent basis, and can be taken orally or inhaled; the latter route is preferred because the frequency of symptoms are lessened, thereby avoiding the necessity of recurrent administration of bronchodilators. Oral steroids (e.g., prednisone) may also be given during exacerbations of asthma that do not resolve with inhaled medications (e.g., viral infections or chest colds). Management of status asthmaticus usually requires administration of oxygen and varying combinations of medications, including injections of epinephrine or terbutaline, inhaled beta$_2$-adrenergic agonists, or intravenous theophylline (Cockcroft & Hargreave, 1990). Encompassing all three treatment approaches is an emphasis on educating children and families about the rationale for medication, potential side effects, correct use of inhalers and peak flow meters, the importance of adherence, and adequate home care and collaboration with health care professionals (Lemanek et al., 1999).

CONCEPTUAL FRAMEWORK

The role of cognition in learning was introduced by Albert Bandura when he proposed that individuals can acquire and perform behaviors through imitation (Bandura, 1977, 1982). Cognitions also play a prominent role in cognitive-behavioral approaches to the assessment and treatment of various psychological disorders. Psychologists following this approach theorize that an individual's behavior is a product of the environment's contingencies *and* the mediating thoughts and information-processing style of the person (Kendall et al., 1992). Within this approach, the concept "cognition" can be described in terms of cognitive structures, content, processes, and products. Cognitive structures represent the memory of information and the template through which new experiences in social contexts are perceived (Kendall et al., 1992). Children with asthma, for instance, have the memory capability for prior experiences with asthma attacks. As will be elucidated later, these memories may trigger feelings of anxiety and depression, thus altering their perception of future attacks. Cognitive content comprises the events or information in the memory of a person (Kendall et al., 1992). Adolescents with asthma may remember their response to past asthma attacks as well as those of family members, especially if emergency room services were required. Cognitive processes refer to the cognitions that emerge from the perception and interpretation of the content (Kendall et al., 1992). Depression and anxiety are examples of cognitive processes resulting from the adolescent's experience with an asthma attack. Cognitive products include, for example, attributions and self-efficacy, and are examined in the following sections (Kendall et al., 1992).

Attributions

Researchers have identified attributional style, also known as explanatory style, as consisting of people's explanations of reasons for the occurrence of uncontrollable events in their lives (Abramson, Seligman, & Teasdale, 1978; Palmer & Rhodes, 1989). Explanatory style emerged as a way to identify individual differences in cognitions and describe the manner in which the cognitions influence emotions and behavior. The belief or attribution, in theory, results in specific behaviors, emotions, and cognitions. Borrowing from the learned helplessness theory of depression (Seligman, 1975), three dimensions theoretically determine a person's future response to similar stimuli. An internal versus external dimension concerns the extent to which a person subscribes to an internal explanation ("It's me") versus an external explanation ("It's someone else"). This notion represents what is more commonly referred to as "locus of control." If a person believes that a bad event was caused by something internal to him, the person will feel less competent in his behavior. The stability dimension refers to how stable a person views things in the environment ("It's short lived" vs. "It's permanent"). A more stable attribution for a bad event will lead a person to think bad events will occur again under similar circumstances. The final dimension of explanatory style is a global versus a specific dimension. A statement such as "Everything will be affected" is an example of the global dimension, while "Only this will be affected" represents a specific dimension. The belief that a bad event will affect numerous domains of functioning will cause negative experiences to permeate multiple areas. Upon examining cognitive features associated with asthma, this concept of attribution or explanatory style will be the focus in the discussion of intrapersonal functioning of children and adolescents with asthma.

Self-Efficacy

The concept of self-efficacy is intimately related to attributional style and coping strategies. Self-efficacy refers to children's confidence in their ability to perform certain activities in their lives, usually to achieve a desired outcome (Bandura, 1977, 1982). Bandura (1982, 1986) expands the concept of self-efficacy by stating that people's judgment of their self-efficacy will determine their persistence in reaching their specified goal when presented with difficult or aversive situations. This notion of self-efficacy influencing a person's motivation to perform certain behaviors is evident in the discussion of anxiety and illness management in children with asthma. Three other sources of self-efficacy have been highlighted as important in determining one's perceived ability to perform desired behaviors. First, observation of people's success at tasks may bolster a person's confidence that similar success can occur in one's own, similar situation. Second, encouragement from others may reinforce individuals' belief that they are capable of performing a desired behavior. For example, one goal of asthma management programs is to encourage children that adequate adherence to treatment regimens alleviates many complications from asthma symptoms (Evans & Mellins, 1991; Perrin, MacLean, Gortmaker, & Asher, 1992). This goal is based on findings that self-efficacy is an important predictor of adherence to treatment recommendations (Clark et al., 1988). Third, physiological signals may lead an individual to believe that future efforts will not produce a desired outcome. Depression and uncontrolled asthma symptoms may cause a person to feel less effective in his or her actions, and, therefore, alter future behavior in similar circumstances. Overall, along with other attributions, positive evaluations of self-efficacy are considered essential for children's adaptation to a chronic illness and have been incorporated into various models of adaptation (e.g., Thompson, Gustafson, Hamlett, & Spock, 1992; Varni & Wallander, 1988); these models will be reviewed below.

Coping

Coping is defined as cognitive or behavioral responses that individuals use to handle problematic situations or events (Lazarus & Launier, 1978). The correlation found between stressful events and childhood psychopathology suggests that individuals' own coping style may account for individual differences in psychopathology by possibly shielding the relationship between stress and disorders. Lazarus and Folkman (1984) have outlined six components of coping, including health, positive beliefs, problem-solving skills, social skills, social support, and material resources. Two general coping styles have also been identified by various investigators: emotion-focused/ avoidance coping and problem-focused/approach coping (e.g., Lazarus & Folkman, 1984; Spirito, Stark, & Williams, 1988). The emotion-focused coping style is characterized by distraction, blaming others, wishful thinking, resignation, and negative emotional regulation. The problem focused coping style is portrayed by cognitive restructuring, problem-solving, social support, and positive emotional regulation. In general, the use of problem-focused coping strategies in children is related to fewer adjustment problems based on self-report or parent report (Compas, 1987; Compas, Malcarne, & Fondacaro, 1988). Unfortunately, few researchers have investigated coping in such a systematic method using populations of children and adolescents with chronic illnesses (Frank, Blount, & Brown, 1997). Stimulating such research efforts may be the fact that coping has been included as a protective factor in models of psychosocial adaptation to chronic illnesses.

Models of Psychosocial Adaptation

Models of psychosocial adaptation have been proposed in recent years to delineate factors that place children and adolescents with a chronic illness and their families at increased risk for the development of social, emotional, and behavioral difficulties. Two of these models are the disability–stress–coping model proposed by Wallander and Varni (Varni & Wallander, 1988; Wallander, Varni, Babani, Banis, & Wilcox, 1989) and the transactional stress and coping model devised by Thompson and his colleagues (Thompson, 1985; Thompson et al., 1992). Both of these models depict sets of risk and protective factors that interact to affect adaptation, directly and indirectly, and typically include child characteristics (e.g., coping style), family functioning (e.g., cohesion), social–ecological variables (e.g., external support), and illness/disability variables (e.g., severity). Both models also assign a critical role to cognitive processes of children and parents with respect to influences on psychosocial adaptation. In Wallander and Varni's model, coping strategies and cognitive appraisal of disease-related and disease-unrelated events are considered stress-processing factors that may enhance a parent's resistance to stress. In Thompson's model, the following three processes act as mediators to adjustment above and beyond the influence of children's illness and family demographic variables: (1) cognitive processes in children and parents, such as appraisal of daily hassles and illness tasks, efficacy expectations, and self-esteem; (2) family functioning, emphasizing support or conflict; and (3) coping strategies (i.e., emotion-focused vs. problem-focused) used by children and parents.

Although there are no published reports on the application of these models to children and adolescents with asthma, the focus on risk and protective factors is consistent with a transactional or biopsychosocial model advanced by investigators in the area of asthma (e.g., Creer et al., 1992). The following sections explore how cognitions influence adaptation to asthma, particularly how children function emotionally and behaviorally, interact with peers, manage their illness, and achieve academically.

INTRAPERSONAL FUNCTIONING

Children and adolescents are more vulnerable to internalizing behavior problems, such as depression and anxiety, than to externalizing behavior problems. Since attributional style has been linked to the presence of these internalizing problems, the following sections focus on depression and anxiety as aspects of intrapersonal functioning.

Depression

Attributional style was formulated from research investigating the etiology of depression (Seligman, 1975). Seligman et al. (1984) refer to an individual's attributional style of negative events as a depressogenic style when the person believes the negative events are a result of an internal, stable, and global origin. Supporting the role of attributional style in the manifestation of depressive symptoms is a study by Kaslow, Rehm, and Siegel (1984). In this study, children in grades 1, 4, and 8 who reported greater symptoms of depression made significantly more internal, stable, and global attributions for negative events. With respect to asthma, depressive symptomatology is one of the most common problems identified in children and adolescents who do experience difficulties in emotional and behavioral functioning (e.g., Bennett, 1994; MacLean et al., 1992). Unfortunately, the attributional style of children and adolescents with asthma and its influence on adaptation has received minimal attention in the literature.

In an unpublished investigation, Trane (1995) examined the attributional style, coping strategies, psychosocial adaptation, and parent–child relationships in school-age children with mild to moderate asthma. The KASTAN–Revised Children's Attributional Style Questionnaire (Kaslow, Tanenbaum, & Seligman, 1978) was administered to assess attribution for causation for positive and negative events in children's lives regardless of their medical condition. Results showed no association between girls' attributional style and parent-reported functional status or adaptation. However, in boys a less depressive attributional style correlated with more internalizing behavior problems. Specifically, internalizing behaviors were associated with a belief that negative events were caused by something external, unstable, and specific to the situation. These results suggest that boys with asthma may perceive their ability to control their symptoms as limited, especially if symptoms are unpredictable and triggered by external agents. A related study examined the extent of irrational beliefs in adolescents (ages 12–18 years) with asthma (Silverglade, Tosi, Wise, & D'Costa, 1994). Irrational beliefs were defined as the emphasis the adolescents placed on the importance of the past, importance of approval from others, and control of emotions. The results supported the authors' hypothesis that many adolescents with asthma have a strong dependency on others (a finding yielded from the endorsement of the importance of approval from others). The adolescents also exhibited symptoms of helplessness, depression, and anxiety, as measured by a self-report adjective checklist. These studies provide some evidence of disease-specific cognitive processes in children and adolescents with asthma.

Anxiety

Anxiety is another psychological factor identified in children and adolescents with asthma (Bussing, Burket, & Kelleher, 1996; Butz & Alexander, 1993; Park, Sawyer, & De Glaun, 1996). In fact, Bussing et al. (1996) found that children with asthma, ages 7–17 years old, exhibited two times the rate of anxiety disorders (e.g., separation anxiety, overanxious, obsessive–compulsive disorder) compared with a healthy control group. The severity of asthma was not, however, related to the presence or severity of an anxiety disorder. This latter finding is interesting in that emotional factors, such as heightened arousal and anxiety, can create airway obstruction in individuals with asthma, thus triggering an asthma attack (Isenberg, Lehrer, & Hochron, 1992). Studies have, in fact, revealed that children who demonstrate more chronic anxiety visit the emergency room and are hospitalized more often than children who present with milder forms of anxiety (Staudenmayer, 1982).

These findings have led researchers to examine individuals' perceptions of asthma symptoms in an effort to understand exactly how anxiety exacerbates asthmatic symptoms. Researchers have found that anxiety interferes with adults' accurate perception of symptoms and stalls one's motivation to seek appropriate treatment (cited in Park et al., 1996). Baron et al. (1986) obtained similar results with children, where those with more severe asthma and a longer time since diagnosis were more likely to underestimate obstruction in their airway passages. However, Fritz et al. (1996) noted the difficulty in using various objective and subjective methods of physiological functioning, especially in those individuals who cannot accurately identify documented physiological changes. According to Fritz et al. (1996), it is, therefore, critical to standardize methodological approaches in the perception of physiological symptoms of asthma.

Two other studies focus on attributional style in explaining the occurrence of anxiety in children and adolescents with asthma. Carpenter (1992) elaborated on the learned helplessness theory of depression by examining the internality or locus of control dimension in children (4–18 years of age) undergoing an invasive medical procedure. Carpenter (1992) hypothesized and found that those children and adolescents who did not perceive an internal source of control for successfully coping with an acute medical procedure had higher levels of anxiety, as assessed by self-report, parent report, and independent observation. Park et al. (1996) suggested that a similar process may occur with preadolescents with asthma. This retrospective study examined children, 10–12 years of age, and documented precipitating events that led to an asthma attack; the dimension of control or its specific impact on asthma symptoms was not evaluated. Similar research analyzing these three dimensions in asthma may provide a clearer understanding of the development of anxiety and depression in children and adolescents with asthma.

Self-Esteem and Self-Concept

Researchers have examined self-esteem and self-concept in children with asthma, as these constructs often are related to depression (Kazdin, 1988). The literature on self-esteem in children and adolescents is inconsistent. Some studies have shown low self-esteem among girls with moderate to severe asthma (Hambley, Brazil, Furrow, & Chua, 1989; Price, 1996). The majority of the research, however, suggests that children with asthma and healthy control groups have comparable levels of self-esteem and self-concept, despite disease severity (Kashani, König, Shepperd, Wilfley, & Morris, 1988; Panides, 1984; Vázquez, Fontan-Bueso, & Buceta, 1992).

A review article by Price (1994) on the explanations and reasons for nonadherence to asthma treatments suggests that one aspect of children's self-concept concerns their perceived body image. Price (1994) compared the altered body image that adolescents have with anorexia nervosa and bulimia and suggested that a similar phenomenon may occur with children and adolescents with asthma. For example, he stated that the symptoms of asthma, such as dyspnea and co-occurring anxiety, may lead individuals to view their body, especially their lungs, as less than adequate compared to others'. This particular area of self-concept remains a fruitful area for research, as positive findings of an altered body image may suggest the need for cognitive-behavioral interventions to change these perceptions.

Social Competence

Children and adolescent interpersonal relationships have been an important area of research, especially with respect to children who have chronic illnesses (La Greca, 1990). One reason for this emphasis is the concern that any illness-related interference in developmentally appropriate activities will impede the development of adequate peer interactions and relationships (La Greca, 1990). Girls with asthma or diabetes do, in fact, report lower levels of athletic competence and physical appearance than boys with these illnesses (Holden, Chmielewski, Nelson, Kager, & Foltz, 1997). Adequate peer interactions and relationships are partly based on the level of children's social competence, which is conceptualized as entailing social adjustment, social performance, and social skills (Cavell, 1990; Gresham & Elliott, 1990). This last component of social competence is identical to one component of coping as outlined by Lazarus and Folkman (1984), serving to link the cognitive and behavioral facets of children's peer interactions.

Overall, little research exists assessing the social competence of children and adolescents with asthma. The available research suggests little difference in the number of friends or ratings of popularity and rejection between school-age children with asthma and healthy controls (Graetz & Shute, 1995), but those children who have more hospitalizations may be preferred less as playmates and experience more feelings of loneliness (Graetz & Shute, 1995). Nassau and Drotar (1995) compared the social competence of 8- to 10-year-old children with asthma to children with diabetes, and their healthy peers. No differences in social adjustment, social performance, or social skills were found between any group of children. Children in this study may have represented a limited sample in that they maintained regular contact with their health care providers and were from middle-level socioeconomic status families. Given the finding that asthma appears to be increasing in prevalence among families of lower socioeconomic status (NIH, 1997), future research is needed to evaluate if such children are at increased risk of experiencing inadequate peer interactions and relationships. In addition, research should clarify the conceptual nature of social skills as a component of social competence versus coping in adaptation to asthma.

Coping

Developmental and situationally specific factors appear to play a role in children's coping style and its relation to adaptation to chronic illnesses. Brown, O'Keeffe, Sanders, and Baker (1986) concluded that adolescents coped better, used more positive self-talk, and employed a greater variety of coping strategies compared to younger children. However, other studies have shown that coping strategies may decrease when the adolescent is faced with a chronic illness, and that the developmental trajectory found by Brown et al. (1986) may not apply to children with chronic illnesses (as discussed in Friedrich & Jaworski, 1995). Similarly, a study looking at children with different chronic illnesses, including asthma, revealed the use of more adaptive coping strategies when the children were faced with procedures and events that were specific to their illness management (Olson, Johansen, Powers, Pope, & Klein, 1993). However, the coping strategies employed by these children did not generalize to stressful situations with which they may have had limited experience. The relationship between coping style and psychosocial adaptation has been examined in one unpublished study (Trane, 1995). In this study, girls with asthma (ages 8–13 years) who used a more problem-focused coping style were less likely to have adjustment problems, as measured by parent reports of internalizing and externalizing behavior; this pattern was not found for the boys in the study. However, when the status of daily functioning was taken into consideration, coping style was not predictive of adjustment to their illness. The coping measure used in this study (KANCOPE; Danovsky, 1994) was a general measure of coping and did not include disease-specific stressors. As such, these findings and those of Olson et al. (1993) support the assertion by Compas et al. (1988) that the relationship between coping and adjustment may depend on the type of stress experienced. Future research is needed to elucidate the relationship between coping style and adjustment in children and adolescents with asthma for both general and disease-specific stressors as well as successful disease management.

ILLNESS MANAGEMENT

Evans and Mellins (1991) have delineated obstacles to successful disease management, including children and parents lacking crucial information, techniques, and decisional skills on home management (e.g., when emergency care is necessary; symptoms of asthma attack). In addition to acquisition of knowledge and skills, successful management of asthma requires adherence to the treatment regimen. These factors (i.e., inadequate education and understanding of asthma and its treatment, poor self-management skills, nonadherence) also contribute directly to treatment failure (Ashkenazi, Amir, Volovitz, & Varsano, 1993; Donnelly, Donnelly, & Thong, 1989).

In most investigations, adherence is defined as "the extent to which a person's behavior (in terms of medications, following diets, or executing lifestyle changes) coincides with medical or health advice" (Haynes, 1979, pp. 2–3). The utility of this definition is high in that it not only delineates a range of adherent behaviors (e.g., taking medications, following diets) but also includes whether adherence agrees with medical recommendations (Rapoff & Barnard, 1991). There is also an underlying assumption in this literature that adherence to medical recommendations will affect mortality, morbidity, and health promotion; an assumption that may or may not be accurate (La Greca & Schuman, 1995; Rapoff & Barnard, 1991).

Nonadherence rates for pediatric asthma have ranged from 34% (Wood, Casey, Kolski, & McCormick, 1985) to 98% (Sublett, Pollard, Kadlec, & Karibo, 1979) when examining serum assays for therapeutic levels of theophylline. Fewer studies and, therefore, estimates of nonadherence are available on the use of medications that are administered through metered-dose inhalers. Two published studies reported a nonadherence rate of between 40% and 55% in children and adolescents who were prescribed prophylactic cortiocosteroids based on either canister weighing (Zora, Lutz, & Tinkelman, 1989) or a Nebulizer Chronolog (the Chronolog is an electronic device that counts and times each actuation of a metered-dose inhaler)(Coutts, Gibson, & Paton, 1992). Both studies also found adherence rates to decrease over a period of 2 weeks, 4 weeks, and 3 months.

Reports of negative consequences following nonadherence to medical regimens for asthma include increased morbidity, such as exacerbation of symptoms, medical complications, and school absences, as well as greater mortality (Lemanek, 1990; Rapoff & Barnard, 1991). Nonadherence is also related to escalated health care utilization rates (e.g., physician visits, hospitalizations) and expenses from unused medications and unnecessary laboratory tests (Ashkenazi et al., 1993; Lemanek, 1990; Weinstein, 1995). In addition, these expenses may subsequently raise insurance premiums and taxes to families of youth with chronic illnesses and to society at large (Rapoff & Barnard, 1991). If such negative consequences follow nonadherence, why is the rate of nonadherence so high?

The majority of research on nonadherence is correlational in nature, where factors related to nonadherence to medical regimens are identified. These factors can be identified with the regimen itself, the disease, or to patient–family characteristics (Creer & Levstek, 1996; La Greca & Schuman, 1995; Rapoff & Barnard, 1991). Examples of regimen characteristics correlated with nonadherence include longer duration of the medical regimen, complexity of the regimen (e.g., taking multiple medications at different times throughout the day; changes in lifestyle), presence of negative side effects of the medication or the regimen (e.g., weight gain with repeated use of corticosteroids; restrictions placed on physical activity), and unstable efficacy of the regimen, especially when the medication is costly (Creer & Levstek, 1996; Lemanek, 1990; Voyles & Menendez, 1983).

Disease characteristics associated with nonadherence in asthma consist of asymptomatic periods, younger age at illness onset, and illness severity as perceived by the family. This third characteristic may be related to the degree of parental supervision and vigilance about following the regimen components, since increased supervision by parents and physicians has been shown to improve adherence (Rapoff & Barnard, 1991). In contrast, physician and patient estimates of severity and duration of asthma are not consistently associated with adherence compared to such illnesses as diabetes (Smith, Seale, Ley, Shaw, & Bracs, 1986; Weinstein & Cuskey, 1985). The intermittent nature of asthma attacks in children and adolescents (i.e., number of attacks within and across patients) and the reversibility of airway obstruction with or without treatment is likely to influence patient perception of severity, and, consequently, adherence (Creer & Levstek, 1996). Specifically, these two features of asthma increase the possibility that memory decay, lack of practice using the inhaler or nebulizer, and problems transferring skills across time and settings will occur, thereby, negatively impacting adherence (Creer & Levstek, 1996). Such events may be particularly evident with those medications that are used on an as-needed basis, as is typically the case with bronchodilators (Creer & Levstek, 1996).

Patient and family variables involve youth characteristics and family interaction patterns rather than demographic variables, such as gender and ethnicity (Lemanek, 1990). Premorbid behavioral and emotional problems (e.g., oppositional behaviors), family dysfunction (e.g., disharmony, poor problem solving), and lack of social support are related to nonadherence to medical regimens in asthma (Christiaanse, Lavigne, & Lerner, 1989;

Spector, 1985; Wamboldt, Wamboldt, Gavin, Roesler, & Brugman, 1995). However, extensive data do not exist in this area, nor is there a consistent relationship between individual and family disturbance and nonadherence. For example, in the study by Christiaanse et al. (1989), parents' perceptions of asthma severity and family environment (i.e., cohesion vs. conflict) were not correlated with adherence in children (ages 7–17), as measured by either mean theophylline levels or percentage nonadherence theophylline levels. But, the best predictors of nonadherence were a combination of high levels of behavior problems *and* family conflict. How do cognitive variables, such as attitudes and beliefs, mediate relationships between regimen, disease, and patient–family characteristics and nonadherence?

A patient's attitude toward the illness, confidence in his or her ability to manage the illness, and knowledge about the illness all contribute to whether or not a medical regimen is successful (Wigal et al., 1993). With respect to attitudes, data suggest that children with asthma hold positive attitudes toward the illness and health care professionals and settings, compared to children with acute illnesses (Koontz, Bachanas, & Rae, 1995). However, in comparison to children with other chronic illnesses, such as hemophilia and sickle cell disease, children with asthma hold neutral attitudes about treatment and its effects (Van Sciver, D'Angelo, Rappaport, & Woolf, 1995). In addition, they possess limited confidence in the ability of treatment to control symptoms and to achieve a healthy outcome. Children's confidence in their own ability to successfully manage their asthma constitutes self-efficacy, as defined by Bandura (1982). In the area of pediatric asthma, the examination of the influence of self-efficacy on self-management and adherence is only beginning. Investigators (e.g., Tobin, Wigal, Winder, Holroyd, & Creer, 1987; Wigal et al., 1993) propose that self-efficacy influences outcome (i.e., favorable or unfavorable, depending on level of efficacy) and whether one can perform the actual behaviors required to produce the outcome. Furthermore, self-efficacy affects whether knowledge of asthma and its treatment will be employed to manage asthma successfully. Available studies indicate that older children perceive themselves to be more competent in managing their asthma than do younger children (Miles, Sawyer, & Kennedy, 1995; Schlosser & Havermans, 1992). In addition, parental knowledge about asthma and its treatment is associated with children's perceived competence to manage their asthma. However, studies thus far have not investigated whether or not higher levels of self-efficacy actually lead to greater adherence to the medical regimen. A related study by Deaton (1985), in fact, suggests that parental adaptiveness about adherence decisions and accuracy of predictions of task performance correlated with better outcomes, but actual degree of adherence did not. Research in this area deserves attention, especially in terms of the correspondence between self-efficacy, management behaviors, and therapeutic outcome, as well as adherence.

Asthma education and self-management programs have been developed to provide children and/or their parents with information and skills about asthma and its treatment. Topics covered within these programs typically include physiological mechanisms of asthma, identifying symptoms and triggers, managing symptoms and attacks, and living with asthma. Positive outcomes following participation in self-management programs consist of decreases in the number of emergency room visits, hospitalizations, and days spent in the hospital; fewer school days missed; and improved asthma-management behaviors (e.g., symptom discrimination). However, the support for increases in asthma knowledge is mixed. Perrin et al. (1992) found a linear relationship between knowledge and daily activities, but Rubin, Bauman, and Lauby (1989) found a nonlinear relationship between knowledge and management behaviors. Their data suggest that once a patient reaches a level of knowledge, further knowledge does not have an effect on behavior. Studies by Deaton (1985) and Miles et al. (1995) would support the inclusion of parents in all management programs due to the association between parent knowledge and children's competence as well as adherence. Controlled studies also need to be conducted to evaluate the effectiveness of asthma self-management programs with respect to analyzing management behaviors and determining whether skill acquisition leads to actual task performance at home and in school (Creer, Wigal, Kotses, & Lewis, 1990; Lemanek, 1990).

Intervention strategies directly targeting adherence can be grouped into one of three categories: (1) educational, (2) organizational, and (3) behavioral (La Greca & Schuman, 1995; Lemanek, 1990; Weinstein, 1995). In general, educational strategies alone are necessary but not sufficient in improving adherence in pediatric asthma (Bender & Milgrom, 1996; Lemanek, 1990; Weinstein, 1995). Studies have usually found an increase in knowledge following educational programs but not a corresponding increase in adherence (e.g., Selner & Staudenmayer, 1979). The majority of studies in this area have implemented a multicomponent treatment program consisting of educational, organizational, and behavioral strategies to increase adherence rates and optimize functioning (e.g., da Costa, Rapoff, Lemanek, & Goldstein, 1997; Lemanek, Rapoff, Carr, & Hope, 1996; Smith et al., 1986; Smith, Seale, Ley, Mellis, & Shaw, 1996; Weinstein, 1995). The educational component usually entails written information (e.g., leaflets, program handouts) given to parents and children about asthma, the medical regimen, and the importance of adherence. Organizational strategies most often address tailoring the medication regimen and expanding the supervision of adherence by the physician. The behavioral strategies emphasize either self-regulatory procedures, such as self-monitoring of pulmonary functioning and asthma management (e.g., Smith et al., 1996) or reinforcement-based procedures, such as contracting (e.g., Weinstein, 1995) and token systems (e.g., da

Costa et al., 1997). These studies result in general improvement in adherence and other outcome measures (e.g, peak flow rates, emergency room visits), as well as treatment acceptability. However, future studies will need to incorporate both short- and long-term follow-up periods to examine the directional relationship over time between attitudes and expectations, and adherence.

ACADEMIC ACHIEVEMENT

Asthma has been hypothesized to impact children's and adolescents' academic achievement either directly through neurocognitive alterations associated with the disease or its treatment, or indirectly through school absence or psychological changes related to the disease (Bender, 1995). The literature on academic achievement in children with asthma has emphasized school absentee rates or the possible effects of theophylline on learning and behavior (Fowler, Davenport, & Garg, 1992). An increasing number of studies (e.g., Bender, Lerner, & Kollasch, 1988; Gutstadt et al., 1989) have been examining academic performance and effects of other medications used in the management of asthma (e.g., corticosteroids). Unfortunately, differences in methodology, such as various assessment measures and duration of past and current therapy, have resulted in conflicting results (Celano & Geller, 1993; Weinberger, Lindgren, Bender, Lerner, & Szefler, 1987).

Academic Performance

The available data indicate that children and adolescents with asthma do not evidence deficiencies in academic performance when compared to children in a control group (McLoughlin et al., 1983) or standardized tests of intelligence and achievement (Bender, Belleau, Fukuhara, Mrazek, & Strunk, 1987; Gutstadt et al., 1989). For example, Gutstadt and colleagues found that intelligence test scores and standardized achievement scores in reading and mathematics were average to above average in a large group of hospitalized children (ages 9–17 years) with moderately severe to severe asthma. In contrast, data from the 1988 U.S. National Health Interview Survey on Child Health revealed that children with asthma were at moderate risk of academic problems in terms of learning disabilities, compared to children without asthma (Fowler et al., 1992). Low income, rather than a diagnosis of asthma, has been consistently related to poor academic performance in these studies. In addition, the influence of poor health status or history of respiratory arrest on academic performance has been demonstrated in some studies (i.e., Dunleavy, 1981; Gutstadt et al., 1989) but not in others (i.e., Bender et al., 1987; Fowler et al., 1992).

Theophylline

Numerous studies have been published on the effects of theophylline on the central nervous system and on the behavior of children and adolescents with asthma. Subjective reports from parents and teachers have suggested considerable changes in learning and behavior, but objective reports from double-blind studies have indicated few adverse side effects (Bender, 1995). For example, notable changes in such areas as attention, activity level, and behavior problems have been reported by parents and teachers (e.g., Furukawa et al., 1984; Rachelefsky et al., 1986). However, statistically significant differences have not been obtained on neuropsychological tests or questionnaires in more methodologically rigorous studies (i.e., Rappaport et al., 1989; Schlieper, Alcock, Beaudry, Feldman, & Leikin, 1991). For example, Schlieper et al. (1991) assessed the effects of theophylline on behavior, cognitive processing, and mood in 31 children (ages 8–12 years) with moderate asthma. A double-blind, randomized, crossover design was employed where theophylline/placebo or placebo/theophylline was administered for 10 days with a 2-day wash-out period. Strengths of this study were the restrictions placed on xanthine-containing foods and beverages and the monitoring of therapeutic levels of theophylline. No significant effects on parent-reported attention or activity level, self-reported mood (i.e., depression, anxiety), or cognitive processing (i.e., memory, attention) were revealed. A study by Bender and associates (Bender, Lerner, Ikle, Comer, & Szefler, 1991) is perhaps the only evaluation of theophylline on cognitive processing, behavior, and mood over a 6-month period of time. Comparisons were made among three groups of children: children without asthma, children with mild to moderate asthma who were taking theophylline, and children with asthma who were not receiving theophylline. Improved scores on laboratory measures of attention were obtained, as well as slightly increased behavior problems according to parent report (e.g., hyperactivity). Results from these studies suggest that the effects of theophylline on learning and behavior are ambiguous and contradictory (Bender, 1995; Weinberger et al., 1987). However, two general statements can be made: Subtle changes in learning and behavior may occur, and there is a wide variability and susceptibility to theophylline in children (Bender, 1995; Schlieper et al., 1991).

Corticosteroids

A history of continuous oral steroid use has been examined in relationship to cognitive skills (Bender, Lerner, & Poland, 1991; Suess, Stump, Cahi, & Kalisker, 1986), academic performance (e.g., Gutstadt et al., 1989), and mood (e.g., Bender et al., 1988; Bender, Lerner, & Poland, 1991). For example, Suess et al. (1986) compared the performance of 120 hospitalized children (ages 9–18 years) within three groups: those with asthma who were receiving theophylline, those with asthma who were on both theophylline and steroids, and those without asthma. Impaired performance on tests of visual and verbal retention were found in those children who received both theophylline and steroids, but only when tested 6–8 hours postmedication. No group differences were obtained when testing occurred 22–24 hours or 46–48 hours postmedication. Bender et al. (1988) investigated both cognitive and affective processes in 27 inpatients with severe asthma (ages 8–16 years) at high steroid levels (i.e., 61.5 mg/day) and at low steroid levels (i.e., 3.33 mg/day). A variety of responses were examined, such as attention, impulsivity, hyperactivity, verbal learning, mood, and behavior problems. Problems with symptoms related to depression, anxiety, and long-term recall of information were associated with high doses of steroids compared to low doses. However, no relationship was shown between the psychological variables and asthma severity or theophylline level. Overall, subtle effects on memory and mood seem to be evident with the use of oral steroids, but in a dose-dependent way (Bender, 1995; Celano & Geller, 1993). With respect to aerosolized steroids, the development of behavior problems (e.g., hyperactivity, aggression, opposition) primarily in preschool-age children have been described in a few case reports (e.g., Connett & Lenney, 1991; Lewis & Cochran, 1983). Based on these findings, Bender (1995) recommends the inclusion of preschool-age children in future controlled studies of the side effects of oral and inhaled steroids on learning and behavior.

Beta-Agonists, Cromolyn Sodium, and Antihistamines

A limited number of studies have examined the effects of beta-agonists, cromolyn sodium, and antihistamines on learning and behavior. These studies have been reviewed in detail by Bender (1995). Regarding beta-agonists (e.g., albuterol), no impairments have been identified in such cognitive abilities as attention, visual perception, visual–motor coordination, and speed and dexterity (e.g., Mazer, Figueroa-Rosario, & Bender, 1990). However, use of these inhaled medications has been related to short-lived, muscular-skeletal tremors (Bender, 1995). In three studies (i.e., Furukawa et al., 1984, 1988; Springer, Goldenberg, Ben Dov, & Godfrey, 1985), the effects of cromolyn sodium on learning and behavior have been compared to theophylline in blind comparisons. In general, slightly favorable responses were obtained on tests of memory, concentration, and visual–spatial planning when the children were on cromolyn sodium compared to theophylline. In addition, greater behavioral difficulties at home and in school (e.g., nervousness) were reported when theophylline was administered in comparison to cromolyn sodium. Bender (1995) concludes from these studies that cromolyn sodium produces fewer behavioral toxicities, but inclusion of untreated control groups is necessary in future research to verify this conclusion. In terms of antihistamines, too few studies are available to draw definitive conclusions regarding the effects of either traditional or nonsedating antihistamines on learning and behavior (Bender, 1995). However, the occurrence of aberrant behaviors (e.g., hallucinations) following the administration of traditional antihistamines in preschool-age children have been reported in the literature (e.g., Sankey, Nunn, & Sills, 1984). Bender (1995) suggests that controlled research is clearly needed on the side effects of these medications, especially nonsedating types, due to the popular use of antihistamines in children and adolescents.

RESEARCH AND CLINICAL IMPLICATIONS

Research on the role of cognitions in pediatric asthma is in its early stage of growth. Most of the research to date has addressed neurocognitive changes related to asthma or its treatment. Multiple avenues of research are available to pursue in the future. Investigators should first systematically examine whether cognitions serve as mediators or moderators of adaptation, which includes not only psychological and social functioning but also disease management and adherence. Research has not yet established if psychological variables precede asthma or coincide with and exacerbate its symptoms (Kashani et al., 1988). In this area, a recommendation for future research involves the goals of self-management programs, such as training children how to accurately perceive their symptoms in order to implement the most effective treatment strategy (e.g., rescue dose of medication; seek emergency room services). The question can be raised whether differences in attitudes about the illness and its treatment and in self-efficacy expectations should be taken into account during such training. Furthermore, what is the relationship between attitudes and self-efficacy on actual implementation of management strategies versus discussion of these strategies in a group setting? In short, does generalization and transfer of knowledge and skills occur from a training setting to daily functioning?

Another area to address is differentiating the role of cognitions with respect to events applicable to all children and adolescents versus those specific to asthma and its management. The study by Trane (1995) implies an inverse relationship between internalizing behavior, depressive cognitive style, and, perhaps, disease management. Perhaps a depressive style serves a different function in children with asthma, in that they would then believe themselves to be more in control of their symptoms and management. In addition, the studies on body image and physical appearance in adolescents (i.e., Holden, Chmielewski, Nelson, Kager, & Foltz, 1997; Price, 1994) suggest the usefulness of narrowing the focus of future research efforts by investigating not only general constructs (e.g., self-concept) but specific aspects of these constructs, when applicable.

This recommendation for greater specificity also applies to examination of coping strategies in children and adolescents with asthma. Future research should delineate what strategies (i.e., problem-focused versus emotion-focused) are typically used by these youth and whether they differ over time. Perhaps more importantly, do these strategies differ by type of stressor—general or disease-specific?

A final area of research is controlled investigations of the effects, especially long-term, of various asthma medications on both learning and behavior. While this area provides the most data at this time, the methodological weaknesses of many studies limit the clinical and practical application of the results. Important in all of these areas is a greater emphasis on examining chronological and mental age differences and cultural variables on how cognitions influence adaptation. Influences of age on medication adverse effects have already been determined in pediatric asthma, but the extent of age and cultural variables on intrapersonal functioning and disease management needs to be explored.

While there appear to be more questions than answers regarding cognitions and pediatric asthma, the answers will have direct relevance to clinical practice. The current health care system is requiring psychologists to document the effectiveness of assessment and treatment practices. However, there is also a need to more fully understand the directional relationship between cognitions and behavior in children and adolescents with asthma in order to identify critical variables for assessment and treatment. Ultimately, the health and welfare of youth with asthma will be enhanced through these research initiatives.

REFERENCES

Abramson, L. Y., Seligman, M. E. P., & Teasdale, J. D. (1978). Learned helplessness in humans: Critique and reformulation. *Journal of Abnormal Psychology, 87,* 49–74.

Ashkenazi, S., Amir, J., Volovitz, B., & Varsano, I. (1993). Why do asthmatic children need referral to an emergency room? *Pediatric Allergy and Immunology, 4,* 93–96.

Bandura, A. (1977). *Social learning theory.* Englewood Cliffs, NJ: Prentice-Hall.

Bandura, A. (1982). Self-efficacy mechanism in human agency. *American Psychologist, 37,* 122–147.

Bandura, A. (1986). *Social foundations of thought and action: A social cognitive theory.* Englewood Cliffs, NJ: Prentice-Hall.

Baron, C., Lamarre, A., Veilleux, P., Ducharme, G., Spier, S., & Lapierre, J. G. (1986). Psychomaintenance of childhood asthma: A study of 34 children. *Journal of Asthma, 23,* 69–79.

Bender, B. G. (1995). Are asthmatic children educationally handicapped? *School Psychology Quarterly, 10,* 274–291.

Bender, B. G., Belleau, L., Fukuhara, J. T., Mrazek, D. A., & Strunk, R. C. (1987). Psychomotor adaptation in children with severe chronic asthma. *Pediatrics, 79,* 723–727.

Bender, B. G., Lerner, J. A., Ikle, D., Comer, C., & Szefler, S. (1991). Psychological change associated with theophylline treatment of asthmatic children: A 6-month study. *Pediatric Pulmonology, 11,* 233–242.

Bender, B. G., Lerner, J. A., & Kollasch, E. (1988). Mood and memory changes in asthmatic children receiving corticosteroids. *Journal of the American Academy of Child and Adolescent Psychiatry, 27,* 720–725.

Bender, B. G., Lerner, J. A., & Poland, J. E. (1991). Association between corticosteroids and psychologic change in hospitalized asthmatic children. *Annals of Allergy, 66,* 414–419.

Bender, B., & Milgrom, H. (1996). Compliance with asthma therapy: A case for shared responsibility. *Journal of Asthma, 33,* 199–202.

Bennett, D. S. (1994). Depression among children with chronic medical problems: A meta-analysis. *Journal of Pediatric Psychology, 19,* 149–169.

Brown, J. M., O'Keeffe, J., Sanders, S. H., & Baker, B. (1986). Developmental changes in children's cognition to stressful and painful situations. *Journal of Pediatric Psychology, 11,* 343–357.

Bussing, R., Burket, R. C., & Kelleher, E. T. (1996). Prevalence of anxiety disorders in a clinic-based sample of pediatric asthma patients. *Psychosomatics, 37,* 108–115.

Butz, A. M., & Alexander, C. (1993). Anxiety in children with asthma. *Journal of Asthma, 30,* 199–209.

Carpenter, P. J. (1992). Perceived control as a predictor of distress in children undergoing invasive medical procedures. *Journal of Pediatric Psychology, 17,* 757–773.

Cavell, T. A. (1990). Social adjustment, social performance, and social skills: A tri-component model of social competence. *Journal of Clinical Child Psychology, 19,* 111–122.

Celano, M. P., & Geller, R. J. (1993). Learning, school performance, and children with asthma: How much at risk? *Journal of Learning Disabilities, 26,* 23–32.

Christiaanse, M. E., Lavigne, J. V., & Lerner, C. V. (1989). Psychosocial aspects of compliance in children and adolescents with asthma. *Journal of Developmental and Behavioral Pediatrics, 10,* 75–80.

Clark, N. M., Rosentstock, I. M., Hassan, H., Evans, D., Wasilewski, Y., Feldman, C., & Mellins, R. B. (1988). The effect of health beliefs and feelings of self-efficacy on self management behavior of children with chronic disease. *Patient Education and Counseling, 11,* 131–150.

Cockcroft, D. W., & Hargreave, F. E. (1990). Outpatient management of bronchial asthma. *Medical Clinics of North America, 74,* 797–808.

Compas, B. E. (1987). Coping with stress during childhood and adolescence. *Psychological Bulletin, 101,* 393–403.

Compas, B. E., Malcarne, V. L., & Fondacaro, K. M. (1988). Coping with stressful events in older children and young adolescents. *Journal of Consulting and Clinical Psychology, 56,* 405–411.

Connett, G., & Lenney, W. (1991). Inhaled budensonids and behavioral disturbances. *Lancet, 338,* 634–635.

Coutts, J. P., Gibson, N. A., & Paton, J. Y. (1992). Measuring compliance with inhaled medication in asthma. *Archives of Diseases in Childhood, 67*, 332–333.

Creer, T. L., & Bender, B. G. (1993). Asthma. In R. J. Gatchel & E. B. Blanchard (Eds.), *Psychophysiological disorders* (pp. 151–203). Washington, DC: American Psychological Association.

Creer, T. L., & Bender, B. G. (1995). Pediatric asthma. In M. C. Roberts (Ed.), *Handbook of pediatric psychology* (2nd ed., pp. 219–240). New York: Guilford Press.

Creer, T. L., & Levstek, D. (1996). Medication compliance and asthma: Overlooking the trees because of the forest. *Journal of Asthma, 33*, 203–211.

Creer, T. L., Renne, C. M., & Chai, H. (1982). The application of behavioral techniques to childhood asthma. In D. C. Russo & J. W. Varni (Eds.), *Behavioral pediatrics* (pp. 27–67). New York: Plenum Press.

Creer, T. L., Stein, R. E., Rappaport, L., & Lewis, C. (1992). Behavioral consequences of illness: Childhood asthma as a model. *Pediatrics, 90*, 808–815.

Creer, T. L., Wigal, J. K., Kotses, H., & Lewis, P. (1990). A critique of 19 self-management programs for childhood asthma: Part II. Comments regarding the scientific merit of the programs. *Pediatric Asthma, Allergy, and Immunology, 4*, 41–55.

da Costa, I. G., Rapoff, M. A., Lemanek, K. L., & Goldstein, G. L. (1997). Improving adherence to medication regimens for children with asthma and its effect on clinical outcome. *Journal of Applied Behavior Analysis, 30*, 687–691.

Danovsky, M. (1994). *Development of a coping measure for children: The KANCOPE.* Unpublished doctoral dissertation, University of Kansas, Lawrence.

Deaton, A. V. (1985). Adaptive noncompliance in pediatric asthma: The parent as expert. *Journal of Pediatric Psychology, 10*, 1–14.

Donnelly, J.E., Donnelly, W.J., & Thong, Y.H. (1989). Inadequate parental understanding of asthma medications. *Annals of Allergy, 62*, 337–341.

Drotar, D. (1997). Relating parent and family functioning to the psychological adjustment of children with chronic health conditions: What have we learned? What do we need to know? *Journal of Pediatric Psychology, 22*, 149–165.

Dunleavy, R. A. (1981). Neuropsychological correlates of asthma: Effect of hypoxia or drugs? *Journal of Consulting and Clinical Psychology, 49*, 137.

Evans, D., & Mellins, R. B. (1991). Educational programs for children with asthma. *Pediatrician, 18*, 317–323.

Fowler, M. G., Davenport, M. G., & Garg, R. (1992). School functioning of US children with asthma. *Pediatrics, 90*, 939–944.

Frank, N. C., Blount, R. L., & Brown, R. T. (1997). Attributions, coping, and adjustment in children with cancer. *Journal of Pediatric Psychology, 22*, 563–576.

Friedrich, W. N., & Jaworski, T. M. (1995). Pediatric abdominal disorders: Inflammatory bowel disease, rumination/vomiting, and recurrent abdominal pain. In M. C. Roberts (Ed.), *Handbook of pediatric psychology* (2nd ed., pp. 479–497). New York: Guilford Press.

Fritz, G. K., Rubinstein, S., & Lewiston, N. J. (1987). Psychological factors in fatal childhood asthma. *American Journal of Orthopsychiatry, 57*, 253–257.

Fritz, G. K., Yeung, A., Wamboldt, M. Z., Spirito, A., McQuaid, E. L., Klein, R., & Seifer, R. (1996). Conceptual and methodologic issues in quantifying perceptual accuracy in childhood asthma. *Journal of Pediatric Psychology, 21*, 153–173.

Furrow, D., Hambley, J., & Brazil, K. (1989). Behavior problems in children requiring inpatient rehabilitation treatment for asthma. *Journal of Asthma, 26*, 123–132.

Furukawa, C. T., DuHamel, T. R., Weimer, L., Shapiro, G. G., Pierson, W. E., & Bierman, C. W. (1988). Cognitive and behavioral findings in children taking theophylline. *Journal of Allergy and Clinical Immunology, 81,* 83–88.

Furukawa, C. T., Shapiro, G. G., Bierman, C. W., Kraemer, M. J., Ward, D. J., & Pierson, W. E. (1984). A double-blind study comparing the effectiveness of cromolyn sodium and sustained-release theophylline in childhood asthma. *Pediatrics, 74,* 453–459.

Graetz, B., & Shute, R. (1995). Assessment of peer relationships in children with asthma. *Journal of Pediatric Psychology, 20,* 205–216.

Gresham, F. M., & Elliott, S. N. (1990). *Social Skills Rating System.* Circle Pines, MN: American Guidance Service.

Gutstadt, L. B., Gillette, J. W., Mrazek, D. A., Fukuhara, J. T., LaBrecque, J. F., & Strunk, R. C. (1989). Determinants of school performance in children with chronic asthma. *American Journal of Diseases of Children, 143,* 471–475.

Hambley, J., Brazil, K., Furrow, D., & Chua, Y. Y. (1989). Demographic and psychosocial characteristics of asthmatic children in a Canadian rehabilitation setting. *Journal of Asthma, 26,* 167–175.

Haynes, R. B. (1979). Introduction. In R. B. Haynes, D. W. Taylor, & D. L. Sackett (Eds.), *Compliance in health care* (pp. 1–7). Baltimore: Johns Hopkins University Press.

Holden, E. W., Chmielewski, D., Nelson, C. C., Kager, V. A., & Foltz, L. (1997). Controlling for general and disease-specific effects in child and family adjustment to chronic childhood illness. *Journal of Pediatric Psychology, 22,* 15–27.

Isenberg, S. A., Lehrer, P. M., & Hochron, S. (1992). The effects of suggestion and emotional arousal on pulmonary function in asthma: A review and a hypothesis regarding vagal mediation. *Psychosomatic Medicine, 54,* 192–216.

Kashani, J. H., König, P., Shepperd, J. A., Wilfley, D., & Morris, D. A. (1988). Psychopathology and self-concept in asthmatic children. *Journal of Pediatric Psychology, 13,* 509–520.

Kaslow, N. J., Rehm, L. P., & Siegel, A. W. (1984). Social-cognitive and cognitive correlates of depression in children. *Journal of Abnormal Child Psychology, 12,* 605–620.

Kaslow, N. J., Tanenbaum, R. L., & Seligman, M. E. P. (1978). *The KASTAN-R: A children's attributional style questionnaire (KASTAN-R-CASQ).* Unpublished manuscript, University of Pennsylvania.

Kazdin, A. E. (1988). Childhood depression. In E. J. Mash & L. G. Terdal (Eds.), *Behavioral assessment of childhood disorders* (2nd ed., pp. 157–195). New York: Guilford Press.

Kendall, P. C., Chansky, T. E., Kane, M. T., Kim, R. S., Kortlander, E., Ronan, K. R., Sessa, F. M., & Siqueland, L. (1992). The cognitive-behavioral perspective. In A. P. Goldstein, L. Krasner, & S. L. Garfield (Eds.), *Anxiety disorders in youth: Cognitive-behavioral interventions* (pp. 12–29). Boston: Allyn & Bacon.

Koontz, A. D., Bachanas, P. J., & Rae, W. A. (1995, April). *Children's attitudes toward health care and adherence to medical regimens: A comparison of acutely ill and chronically ill pediatric patients.* Poster session presented at the Fifth Annual Florida Conference on Child Health Psychology, Gainesville.

La Greca, A. M. (1990). Social consequences of pediatric conditions: Fertile area for future investigation and intervention? *Journal of Pediatric Psychology, 15,* 285–307.

La Greca, A. M., & Schuman, W. B. (1995). Adherence to prescribed medical regimens. In M. C. Roberts (Ed.), *Handbook of pediatric psychology* (2nd ed., pp. 55–83). New York: Guilford Press.

Lazarus, R. S., & Folkman, S. (1984). *Stress, appraisal and coping.* New York: Springer.

Lazarus, R. S., & Launier, R. (1978). Stress-related transactions between persons and environment. In L. A. Pervin & M. Lewis (Eds.), *Perspectives in interactional psychology* (pp. 287–327). New York: Plenum.

Lemanek, K. L. (1990). Adherence issues in the medical management of asthma. *Journal of Pediatric Psychology, 15,* 437–458.

Lemanek, K. L., Rapoff, M., Carr, T., & Hope, T. (1996, April). *Improving adherence regimens in children with asthma.* Paper presented at the meeting of the Southwest/Gulf Coast Regional Pediatric Psychology Conference, Fort Worth, TX.

Lemanek, K. L., Trane, S. T., & Weiner, R. E. (1999). Asthma. In A. Goreczny & M. Hersen (Eds.), *Handbook of pediatric and adolescent health psychology* (pp. 141–158). Needham Heights, MA: Allyn & Bacon.

Lewis, L. D., & Cochran, G. M. (1983). Psychosis in a child inhaling budesonide. *Lancet, 2,* 634.

MacLean, W. E., Perrin, J. M., Gortmaker, S., & Pierre, C. B. (1992). Psychological adjustment of children with asthma: Effects of illness severity and recent stressful life events. *Journal of Pediatric Psychology, 17,* 159–171.

Mazer, B., Figueroa-Rosario, W., & Bender, B. (1990). The effect of albuterol aerosol on fine-motor performance in children with chronic asthma. *Journal of Allergy and Clinical Immunology, 86,* 243–248.

McLoughlin, J., Nall, M., Isaacs, B., Petrosko, J., Karibo, J., & Lindsey, B. (1983). The relationship of allergies and allergy treatment to school performance and student behavior. *Annals of Allergy, 51,* 506–510.

Miles, A., Sawyer, M., & Kennedy, D. (1995). A preliminary study of factors that influence children's sense of competence to manage their asthma. *Journal of Asthma, 32,* 437–444.

Nassau, J. H., & Drotar, D. (1995). Social competence in children with IDDM and asthma: Child, teacher, and parent reports of children's social adjustment, social performance, and social skills. *Journal of Pediatric Psychology, 20,* 187–204.

National Institutes of Health. (1997). *Guidelines for the diagnosis and management of asthma: Highlights of the expert panel report II* (NIH National Heart, Lung, and Blood Institute Publication No. 4857). Bethesda, MD: U.S. Government Printing Office.

Olson, A. L., Johansen, S. G., Powers, L. E., Pope, J. B., & Klein, R. B. (1993). Cognitive coping strategies of children with chronic illness. *Developmental and Behavioral Pediatrics, 14,* 217–223.

Palmer, D. J., & Rhodes, W. S. (1989). Conceptual and methodological issues of the assessment of children's attributions. In J. N. Hughes & R. J. Hall (Eds.), *Cognitive-behavioral psychology in the schools: A comprehensive handbook* (pp. 166–205). New York: Guilford Press.

Panides, W. (1984). The perception of the past, present, and future in preadolescent asthmatic children: An exploratory study. *Sex Roles, 11,* 1141–1152.

Park, S. J., Sawyer, S. M., & De Glaun (1996). Childhood asthma complicated by anxiety: An application of cognitive behavioural therapy. *Journal of Paediatrics and Child Health, 32,* 183–187.

Perrin, J. M., MacLean, W. E., Gortmaker, S. L., & Asher, K. N. (1992). Improving the psychological status of children with asthma: A randomized controlled trial. *Developmental and Behavioral Pediatrics, 13,* 241–247.

Price, B. (1994). The asthma experience: Altered body image and non-compliance. *Journal of Clinical Nursing, 3,* 139–145.

Price, J. F. (1996). Issues in adolescent asthma: What are the needs? *Thorax, 51*(Suppl. 1), S13–S17.

Rachelefsky, G. S., Wo, J., Adelson, J., Mickey, M. R., Spector, S. L., Katz, R. M., Siegel, S. C., & Rohr, A. S. (1986). Behavior abnormalities and poor school performance due to oral theophylline use. *Pediatrics, 78,* 1133–1138.

Rapoff, M. A., & Barnard, M. U. (1991). Compliance with pediatric medical regimens. In J. A. Cramer & B. Spiker (Eds.), *Patient compliance in medical practice and clinical trials* (pp. 73–98). New York: Raven Press.

Rappaport, L., Coffman, H., Guare, R., Fenton, T., DeGraw, C., & Twarog, F. (1989). Effects of theophylline on behavior and learning in children with asthma. *American Journal of Diseases of Children, 143,* 368–372.

Rubin, D. H., Bauman, L. J., & Lauby, J. L. (1989). The relationship between knowledge and reported behavior in childhood asthma. *Journal of Developmental and Behavioral Pediatrics, 10,* 307–312.

Sankey, R. J., Nunn, A. J., & Sills, J. A. (1984). Visual hallucinations in children receiving decongestants. *British Medical Journal, 288,* 1369.

Schlieper, A., Alcock, D., Beaudry, P., Feldman, W., & Leikin, L. (1991). Effect of therapeutic plasma concentrations of theophylline on behavior, cognitive processing, and affect in children with asthma. *Journal of Pediatrics, 118,* 449–455.

Schlosser, M., & Havermans, G. (1992). A self-efficacy scale for children and adolescents with asthma: Construction and validation. *Journal of Asthma, 29,* 99–108.

Seligman, M. E. P. (1975). *Helplessness: On depression, development, and death.* San Francisco: Freeman.

Seligman, M. E. P., Peterson, C., Kaslow, N. J., Tanenbaum, R. L., Alloy, L. B., & Abramson, L. Y. (1984). Attributional style and depressive symptoms among children. *Journal of Abnormal Psychology, 93,* 235–238.

Selner, J. C., & Staudenmayer, H. (1979). Parents' subjective evaluation of a self-help education-exercise program for asthmatic children and their parents. *Journal of Asthma Research, 17,* 13–22.

Silverglade, L., Tosi, D. J., Wise, P. S., & D'Costa, A. (1994). Irrational beliefs and emotionality in adolescents with and without bronchial asthma. *Journal of General Psychology, 121,* 199–207.

Smith, N. A., Seale, J. P., Ley, P., Mellis, & Shaw, J. (1996). Better medication compliance is associated with improved control of childhood asthma. *Archives of Chest Diseases, 49,* 470–474.

Smith, N. A., Seale, J. P., Ley, P., Shaw, J., & Bracs, P. U. (1986). Effects of intervention on medication compliance in children with asthma. *Medical Journal of Australia, 144,* 119–122.

Spector, S. (1985). Is your asthmatic patient really complying? *Annals of Allergy, 55,* 552–556.

Spirito, A., Stark, L. J., & Williams, C. (1988). Development of a brief coping checklist for use with pediatric populations. *Journal of Pediatric Psychology, 13,* 555–574.

Springer, C., Goldenberg, B., Ben Dov, I., & Godfrey, S. (1985). Clinical, physiologic, and psychologic comparison of treatment by cromolyn or theophylline in childhood asthma. *Journal of Allergy and Clinical Immunology, 76,* 64–69.

Staudenmayer, H. (1982). Medical manageability and psychosocial factors in childhood asthma. *Journal of Chronic Diseases, 35,* 183–198.

Sublett, J. L., Pollard, S. J., Kadlec, G. J., & Karibo, J. M. (1979). Noncompliance in asthmatic children: A study of theophylline levels in a pediatric emergency room population. *Annals of Allergy, 43,* 95–97.

Suess, W. M., Stump, N., Chai, H., & Kalisker, A. (1986). Mnemonic effects of asthma medication in children. *Journal of Asthma, 23,* 291–296.

Taggart, V. S., & Fulwood, R. (1993). Youth health report card: Asthma. *Preventive Medicine, 22,* 579–584.

Taylor, W. R., & Newacheck, P. W. (1992). Impact of childhood asthma on health. *Pediatrics, 90,* 657–662.

Thompson, R. J., Jr. (1985). Coping with the stress of chronic childhood illness. In A. N. O'Quinn (Ed.), *Management of chronic disorders of childhood* (pp. 11–41). Boston: G. K. Hall.

Thompson, R. J., Jr., Gustafson, K. E., Hamlett, K. W., & Spock, A. (1992). Psychological adjustment of children with cystic fibrosis: The role of child cognitive processes and maternal adjustment. *Journal of Pediatric Psychology, 17,* 741–755.

Tobin, D. L., Wigal, J. K., Winder, J. A., Holroyd, K. A., & Creer, T. L. (1987). The asthma self-efficacy scale. *Annals of Allergy, 59,* 273–277.

Trane, S. T. (1995). *Adaptational processes among children with asthma.* Unpublished master's thesis, University of Kansas, Lawrence.

Van Sciver, M. M., D'Angelo, E. J., Rappaport, L., & Woolf, A. D. (1995). Pediatric compliance and the roles of distinct treatment characteristics, treatment attitudes, and family stress: A preliminary report. *Journal of Developmental and Behavioral Pediatrics, 16,* 350–358.

Varni, J. W., & Wallander, J. L. (1988). Pediatric chronic disabilities: Hemophilia and spina bifida as examples. In D. K. Routh (Ed.), *Handbook of pediatric psychology* (pp. 190–221). New York: Guilford Press.

Vázquez, M. I., Fontan-Bueso, J., & Buceta, J. M. (1992). Self-perception of asthmatic children and modification through self-management programmes. *Psychological Reports, 71,* 903–913.

Voyles, J. B., & Menendez, R. (1983). Role of patient compliance in the management of asthma. *Journal of Asthma, 20,* 411–418.

Wallander, J. L., Varni, J. W., Babani, L. V., Banis, H. T., & Wilcox, K. T. (1989). Family resources as resistance factors for psychological maladjustment in chronically ill and handicapped children. *Journal of Pediatric Psychology, 14,* 157–173.

Wamboldt, F. S., Wamboldt, M. Z., Gavin, L. A., Roesler, T. A., & Brugman, S. M. (1995). Parental criticism and treatment outcome in adolescents hospitalized for severe, chronic asthma. *Journal of Psychosomatic Research, 39,* 995–1005.

Weinberger, M., Lindgren, S., Bender, B., Lerner, J. A., & Szefler, S. (1987). Effects of theophylline on learning and behavior: Reason for concern or concern without reason? *Journal of Pediatrics, 111,* 471–474.

Weinstein, A. G. (1995). Correspondence: Behavioral strategies and theophylline compliance in asthmatic children. *Annals of Allergy, 55,* 16–21.

Weinstein, A. G., & Cuskey, W. (1985). Theophylline compliance in asthmatic children. *Annals of Allergy, 54,* 19–24.

Weiss, B., & Wagener, D. K. (1990). Changing patterns of asthma mortality: Identifying target populations at risk. *Journal of the American Medical Association, 264,* 1683–1687.

Weiss, K. B., Gergen, P. J., & Hodgson, T. A. (1992). An economic evaluation of asthma in the United States. *New England Journal of Medicine, 326,* 862–866.

Wigal, J. K., Stout, C., Brandon, M., Winder, J. A., McConnaughy, K., Creer, T. L., & Kotses, H. (1993). The knowledge, attitude, and self-efficacy asthma questionnaire. *Chest, 104,* 1144–1148.

Wood, P. R., Casey, R., Kolski, G. B., & McCormick, M. C. (1985). Compliance with oral theophylline therapy in asthmatic children. *Annals of Allergy, 54,* 400–404.

Young, G. A. (1994). Asthma: Medical issues. In R. A. Olson, L. L. Mullins, J. B. Gillman, & J. M. Chaney (Eds.), *The sourcebook of pediatric psychology* (pp. 57–69). Boston: Allyn & Bacon.

Zora, J. A., Lutz, C. N., & Tinkelman, D. G. (1989). Assessment of compliance in children using inhaled beta adrenergic agonists. *Annals of Allergy, 62,* 406–409.

CHAPTER SIX

Pediatric HIV Infection

PAMELA L. WOLTERS
PIM BROUWERS
LORI A. PEREZ

Children infected with human immunodeficiency virus (HIV) are at risk for developing impairments in cognitive, language, motor, and behavioral functions, primarily associated with the effects of HIV on the central nervous system (CNS). The onset of HIV-related CNS disease, rate of deterioration in functioning, severity of deficits, and number of domains affected varies among different subgroups of children (Belman, 1994). Neuropsychological changes observed in pediatric HIV infection range from subtle declines in psychomotor speed and attention (Brouwers, Moss, Wolters, Eddy, & Pizzo, 1989; Loveland & Stehbens, 1990) to differential impairments in selective domains, such as expressive language (Wolters, Brouwers, Moss, & Pizzo, 1995) or motor skills (Belman, 1994; Hittelman, 1990) to global and severe neurodevelopmental deficits in children with encephalopathy (Belman, 1994; Brouwers, Belman, & Epstein, 1994). Brain imaging of children with HIV disease also shows evidence of various abnormalities, including cortical atrophy, white matter lesions, basal ganglia calcifications, and cerebellar atrophy (DeCarli, Civitello, Brouwers, & Pizzo, 1993), which are correlated with neuropsychological deficits (Brouwers, DeCarli, et al., 1995; Wolters, Brouwers, et al., 1995).

During the first decade of pediatric acquired immune deficiency syndrome (AIDS), estimates projected that as many as 50–90% of infected children developed progressive encephalopathy, the most severe form of HIV-related CNS disease (Barnes, 1986; Belman et al., 1988; Epstein et al., 1987). More recent studies suggest that approximately 20–50% of children with HIV infection exhibit some evidence of CNS disease (Cooper et al., 1998; Englund et al., 1996), ranging from mild to severe neurological or neuropsychological abnormalities, with the highest rates in infants (66–75%) (Chase, Vibbert, Pelton, Coulter, & Cabral, 1995; Englund et al., 1996) and the lowest rates in adolescents (30%) (Englund et al., 1996). However, only about 10% of children with HIV disease may display progressive encephalopathy (Lobato, Caldwell, Ng, Oxtoby, & Consortium, 1995). Thus, the prevalence of severe neuropsychological deficits in children appears to be declining over time. The more widespread use and earlier initiation of treatment, particularly with combination antiretroviral therapy, may be preventing, delaying, or reducing the detrimental effects of HIV on the developing brain (McKinney et al., 1997; Pizzo & Wilfert, 1994).

This chapter summarizes the current knowledge regarding the effects of HIV on the neurocognitive functioning of infants, children, and adolescents with HIV infection. The first section presents some background information regarding epidemiology, routes of transmission, and the clinical course of pediatric HIV disease. The main part of the chapter describes the effects of HIV on the developing CNS including neuropathological and neuroradiological findings, various subtypes of HIV-related CNS disease, and associated cognitive and developmental deficits. The effect of current antiretroviral therapies on cognitive function is summarized next. Finally, issues that pertain to the cognitive assessment and education of children with HIV infection are reviewed.

PEDIATRIC HIV INFECTION IN THE UNITED STATES

Epidemiology

As of June 30, 1998, the Centers for Disease Control and Prevention (CDC) reported 8,280 children under 13 years of age and 3,302 adolescents from 13 to 19 years of age with Acquired Immunodeficiency Syndrome (AIDS) in the United States (CDC, 1998). Children and adolescents comprise approximately 2% of all persons with AIDS in this country (CDC, 1998). These data from the CDC only include cases of AIDS, the most severe form of the disease, and do not include the numbers of children thought to be infected with HIV who have not yet experienced an AIDS-defining illness. Most cases of pediatric AIDS are concentrated in the eastern third of the United States, with urban cities reporting a higher concentration than rural areas (CDC, 1998; Scott & Layton, 1997). African American and Hispanic minority groups account for approximately 80% of the total number of children and adolescents with AIDS (CDC, 1998).

Transmission

Ninety-one percent of children with AIDS under 13 years of age acquired HIV disease through vertical transmission from a mother infected with the virus (CDC, 1998). The majority of these children were born to mothers who became infected through intravenous drug use or from sexual contact with an HIV-positive person (injecting drug user, bisexual male, transfusion recipient, etc.) (CDC, 1998). Vertical transmission may occur *in utero* by transplacental passage, during the intrapartum period by exposure to maternal secretions, or through breast feeding (Friedland & Klein, 1987). Approximately 25% of children born to HIV-positive mothers are infected with the virus (Connor et al., 1994). However, treatment with the anti-retroviral agent zidovudine (AZT) during pregnancy and labor and to the newborn has been found to reduce the vertical transmission rate to 8–10% (Aleixo, Goodenow, & Sleasman, 1997; Connor et al., 1994). Factors associated with the probability that a mother infected with HIV will transmit the virus to her infant include the mother's immunological status (Mayaux et al., 1995), levels of maternal viral load (Aleixo et al., 1997; Blanche et al., 1997), biological characteristics of the virus (Douglas, 1994), and obstetrical factors related to the delivery (Landesman et al., 1996; Mayaux et al., 1995).

Blood transfusion (5%) or exposure to blood products for treatment of hemophilia (3%) account for the remaining pediatric AIDS cases reported to the CDC, but these are no longer risk factors due to the increased safety of the blood supply. In adolescents, HIV infection also may be acquired through sexual contact and intravenous drug use (CDC, 1998). In fact, adolescents are considered to be at particular risk for HIV infection due to the high rates of risk-taking behavior, sexual activity, and sexually transmitted diseases found in this age group (Biglan et al., 1990). It is hypothesized that young adults, ages 20–29 years, who account for approximately 20% of the total number of AIDS cases (CDC, 1998), may be infected during adolescence, given the long latency period from HIV infection to AIDS (Gayle & D'Angelo, 1991).

Clinical Course

The clinical course of HIV disease in children is variable among different subgroups. For example, the latency period between initial infection and the onset of clinical symptoms is shorter in children with vertically acquired infection compared to children with transfusion-acquired disease and adults (Frederick et al., 1994; Mintz, 1994). In addition, several studies of children with vertical HIV infection have indicated a bimodal distribution in the onset of symptoms and a distinction between rapid and slow disease progression (Auger et al., 1988; Blanche et al., 1990; Galli et al., 1995;

Scott et al., 1989). One subgroup of children exhibits an early onset of symptoms, usually within the first year of life, and has a rapid disease progression with a higher incidence of opportunistic infections, encephalopathy, and a shorter survival time. In contrast, another subgroup has a later onset of symptoms and slow disease progression, without either opportunistic infections or encephalopathy in the early years of life (Auger et al., 1988; Blanche et al., 1990). Therefore, age of first symptom onset is an important prognostic marker of clinical progression and HIV-related CNS disease in children with vertically acquired HIV infection (Scott et al., 1989). Other symptoms associated with early onset and faster disease progression include low birth weight (Galli et al., 1995), growth failure, hepatitis, fever, diarrhea, anemia (Italian Register for HIV Infection in Children, 1994; Tovo et al., 1992), and severe immunosuppression (Galli et al., 1995). The factors that cause rapid versus slow disease progression in children with vertical HIV infection are not clear; however, potential mediators include host immune response, timing of infection (Galli et al., 1995), genetic factors, different strains of the virus, and effects of antiretroviral therapy (Italian Register for HIV Infection in Children, 1994; Pizzo & Wilfert, 1990).

CENTRAL NERVOUS SYSTEM DISEASE IN PEDIATRIC HIV INFECTION

The manifestations of HIV-related CNS disease in pediatric AIDS have changed somewhat over time and are variable among different subgroups of children. Most of the early studies in the mid- to late 1980s included a large proportion of children with progressive encephalopathy, who exhibited severe and pervasive neuropsychological deficits and were naive to antiretroviral therapy (Belman et al., 1985; Epstein et al., 1986). More recently, however, studies from both the United States and Europe suggest that fewer children are developing severe HIV-related CNS disease (Blanche et al., 1997; Lobato et al., 1995). This reduction in the encephalopathy may be associated with medical advances and more widespread treatment (Pizzo & Wilfert, 1990).

The prevalence and severity of HIV-related CNS disease appear to vary according to the age, disease stage, and treatment history of the child. Encephalopathy tends to be more prevalent in infants and young children with vertically acquired HIV infection (Blanche et al., 1990; Lobato et al., 1995; Tardieu et al., 1995), particularly in those who are naive to antiretroviral therapy (Englund et al., 1996). In fact, CNS disease may be one of the first signs of HIV infection in pediatric patients (Scott et al., 1989). Recent studies have shown that significantly more children under 3 years of age have evidence of CNS disease, compared to children over 6 years of age (Blanche et al., 1997; Englund et al., 1996; McKinney et al., 1997; Tardieu et al., 1995). Neurological abnormalities also are more likely in advanced stages of the disease (Brouwers, Tudor-Williams et al., 1995; Tovo et al., 1992). Vertically infected children with early onset of CNS symptoms and severe immunodeficiency often exhibit the most severe neurodevelopmental impairments (Blanche et al., 1990). HIV-related encephalopathy also is associated with a high viral load (Cooper et al., 1998), rapid and severe clinical course, and shortened survival (Blanche et al., 1990; Cooper et al., 1998; Lobato et al., 1995). On the other hand, most children who have slower progression of their systemic HIV disease, without severe immunodeficiency, tend to have fewer neurological and cognitive abnormalities (Blanche et al., 1990; Tardieu et al., 1995).

Finally, children with HIV infection often have other medical or environmental risk factors that may affect cognitive development in addition to the effects of the virus, including premorbid medical complications, maternal drug abuse, other infections, or exposure to various environmental influences. Thus, the determination of the HIV-related CNS manifestations in children is complex, due to the number of factors that may contribute to cognitive deficits in HIV-infected children and the varying presentations of CNS disease. The cause of the variability observed in the onset, severity, and range of affected developmental domains in children with HIV infection has not been determined. Hypotheses and supporting evidence regarding the neuropathogenesis of the disease are reviewed next.

Neuropathogenesis

The neurodevelopmental deficits in children with HIV infection appear to be caused primarily by the indirect effects of the virus on the CNS (Epstein & Gendelman, 1993; Lipton, 1992). Adult studies suggest that HIV may enter the CNS, probably through HIV-infected blood-derived macrophages, shortly after systemic HIV infection (Davis et al., 1992). Productive HIV infection in the brain has been identified in blood-derived macrophages, resident microglia, and multinucleated giant cells formed by the fusion of these cell types (Sharer, 1992). Limited infection of brain capillary endothelial cells (Moses et al., 1996) and astrocytes (Tornatore, Chandra, Berger, & Major, 1994) also has been observed; however, evidence for the infection of neurons remains sparse (Dickson et al., 1994). The number of HIV-infected cells and viral load within the CNS probably are positively related with the degree of interference with CNS processes (Tornatore, Meyers, Atwood, Conant, & Major, 1994). HIV strains that have increased virulence also may result in more rapid disease progression (Tersmette et al., 1989), and, thus, more severe CNS disease. Host-mediated factors that are produced in response to HIV infection, such as cytokines or other cellular products of the immune system, may cause inflammation and neurotoxic effects in the CNS (Merrill & Chen, 1991) and contribute to neurodevelopmental abnormalities. In addition, the dysfunction of neurotransmitters such as dopamine may be involved in producing some neurological and motor abnormalities (Berger, Kumar, Kumar, Fernandez, & Levin, 1994; Mintz et al., 1996; Vreugdenhil, Brouwers, Wolters, Bakker, & Moss, 1997).

The timing of productive HIV CNS infection and periods of maximum interference during the development of the immature brain may significantly influence the neuropathogenesis (Civitello, Brouwers, DeCarli, & Pizzo, 1994; DeCarli et al., 1993) and impact on the pattern and degree of neurodevelopmental abnormalities (Brouwers, van der Vlugt, Moss, Wolters, & Pizzo, 1995). For example, assuming that structures within the CNS are most vulnerable when they are still being formed, perinatal interference with myelination could affect projection fibers as well as association and commissural connections, resulting in global patterns of deficits with motor abnormalities. Interference later in development would largely affect the commissural connections and the connections with the poles of the cerebral lobes (particularly frontal and temporal) affecting higher cognitive function. Pathological evidence of primary HIV-related effects on the CNS is as follows.

Neuropathology

At autopsy, children often have acquired microcephaly and low brain weight (Burns, 1992) as well as enlarged ventricles and widened sulci that tend to be of equal severity in the left and right hemispheres (Belman et al., 1988). Neuropathological abnormalities are most frequent in the central white matter and the deep gray matter (Epstein, Sharer, & Goudsmit, 1988), but also can be found in the neocortex, accompanied by neocortical cell loss (Masliah, Achim, Ge, De Teresa, & Wiley, 1994). Mineralizations of the walls of the small blood vessels in the basal ganglia and frontal white matter are the most common pathological abnormality in infants and children (Kure et al., 1991). White matter changes with reactive astrocytosis and myelin pallor are the second most notable abnormality, seen in more than 80% of the pediatric cases at autopsy (Budka, 1991). Corticospinal tract degeneration also is found at autopsy in the majority of children (Dickson, Belman, Kim, Horoupian, & Rubinstein, 1989). In general, the pathological manifestations of HIV parallel the clinical and neuropsychological severity of the disease in children (Wiley, Belman, Dickson, Rubinstein, & Nelson, 1990).

Structural Brain Imaging Findings

Computed tomography (CT) and magnetic resonance imaging (MRI) studies of children with HIV infection have shown that global cerebral atrophy, including both symmetric enlargement of cerebral ventricles as well as sulcal prominence, is the most common abnormality (Chamberlain, Nichols, & Chase, 1991; DeCarli et al., 1993). Cerebellar atrophy also has been noted but occurs less frequently (DeCarli et al., 1993). Global attenuation of cerebral white matter is the second most common finding, and the severity tends to correlate with the degree of cerebral atrophy (Belman et al., 1988; DeCarli et al., 1993). Multiple small white matter lesions also may be found on MRI, but the clinical significance of these abnormalities remains uncertain (Mitchell et al., 1993; Tardieu, Blanche, & Brunelle, 1991). Cerebral calcifications occur less frequently and are generally seen in the basal ganglia, and, in more severe cases, in the periventricular white matter of the frontal lobes (Belman et al., 1986; DeCarli et al., 1993). Calcifications are more likely in infants and young children with vertically acquired infection, compared to patients with transfusion-acquired disease, and may indicate intrauterine rather than intra- or postpartum HIV infection (Civitello et al., 1994).

Secondary HIV-Related Central Nervous System Manifestations

HIV significantly reduces the ability of the immune system to fight infection or cancer, and as a result, infections, neoplastic disease, or stroke are secondary manifestations of HIV that also may affect the CNS. Such secondary CNS manifestations are not frequent in pediatric AIDS and tend to be found more often in older children and adolescents. However, when they do occur, infections, tumors, or cerebral vascular disease in the CNS can cause significant neuropsychological impairments. The more common secondary causes of CNS dysfunction in children with HIV are discussed briefly in this section.

In contrast to adults with AIDS, opportunistic and bacterial infections of the CNS, such as toxoplasmosis, cytomegalovirus (CMV), and JC virus (Berger et al., 1992), are uncommon and occur in less than 10% of children with HIV infection (Civitello, Brouwers, & Pizzo, 1993; Krasinski, 1994). However, CNS opportunistic infections that occur in adults with HIV disease are primarily reactivations of latent childhood infections and are likely to become more frequent in children with HIV as they live longer, possibly as primary infections.

Primary CNS lymphoma and systemic lymphoma metastatic to the CNS are rare secondary complications of HIV infection in children (Dickson et al., 1990). Mental status and behavioral changes, seizures, and the onset of focal neurological signs tend to be the presenting symptoms. Neurological deterioration is usually rapid, but sometimes early symptoms of CNS lymphoma can be hard to distinguish from the more insidious course of HIV-associated encephalopathy (Shah, Zimmerman, Rorke, & Vezina, 1996).

Children with HIV infection also may experience cerebrovascular complications. Strokes, due to ischemia or hemorrhage, are the most common cause of focal neurological deficits, such as hemiparesis, in pediatric AIDS patients (Dickson et al., 1990). HIV antigen has been found in endothelial cells from vessel walls of autopsied patients with strokes, suggesting that the virus itself may cause a cerebral vasculopathy. Headaches occur in approximately 33% of pediatric AIDS patients (Civitello, 1996), with vascular headaches being the most frequent type, especially in adolescents. Headaches, however, may be an early symptom of any of the preceding secondary HIV-related CNS manifestations and should be investigated.

Clinical Presentation of Central Nervous System Disease

In children with HIV infection, three main neuropsychological profiles have emerged: (1) encephalopathy, (2) CNS compromise, and (3) apparently unaffected functioning (Wolters & Brouwers, 1998, 1999). *HIV-related encephalopathy* tends to cause pervasive and severe CNS dysfunction in which most brain structures appear to be equally compromised by HIV. Children with HIV-related encephalopathy usually exhibit global deficits in cognitive, language, motor, and social skills, although they may show variability within some affected functions; for example, expressive language is often more impaired than receptive language. HIV-related encephalopathy may be either progressive (subacute and plateau subtypes) or static (Belman, 1994; Brouwers, Belman, & Epstein, 1994). Children with subacute progressive encephalopathy characteristically show a loss of previously acquired developmental milestones. In children with the plateau subtype, the development of new skills slows significantly compared to their previous rate or stops but they do not lose already attained abilities. Both subacute and plateau progressive encephalopathy result in a significant drop in standard scores on developmental or general intelligence tests, but only children with the subacute subtype will lose raw score points due to a regression in skills. Children with static encephalopathy continue to gain new skills but at a consistently slower rate than expected for their age; thus, their scores on standardized tests are usually below average but show no evidence of decline. In addition to global cognitive deficits, children with encephalopathy also may display other CNS signs, such as moderate to severe brain scan abnormalities and significant neurological problems. Finally, behavioral abnormalities, such as flattened affect, apathy, dysprosody, reduced goal-directed behavior, and impaired social and daily living skills may develop in children with severe HIV-related CNS disease (Moss et al., 1994; Roelofs et al., 1996; Wolters, Brouwers, Moss, & Pizzo, 1994).

Children with *HIV-related CNS compromise* exhibit neurocognitive impairments associated with HIV disease, which are milder in severity and less global than the deficits observed in encephalopathic children (Wolters

& Brouwers, 1998, 1999). CNS compromise is characterized by overall cognitive functioning that is typically within normal limits but with impairments in selective neurodevelopmental functions or a decline in one or more areas of functioning that do not fall into the delayed range. These children continue to have adequate functioning in school, social activities, and daily living skills. Children with HIV-related CNS compromise rarely exhibit significant brain scan or neurological abnormalities. However, they may exhibit mild abnormalities observed on brain scans or neurological exams that do not appear to significantly affect their day-to-day functioning.

Other children exhibit *apparently unaffected functioning* in which their cognitive abilities are at least within normal limits without evidence of significant deficits, decline in functioning, or other brain scan or neurological abnormalities that can be attributed to HIV disease. These children also demonstrate age-appropriate academic, social, and daily living skills.

Finally, some children may have a *non-HIV-related CNS impairment*. In this category of CNS disease, children may exhibit overall cognitive functioning below normal limits, selective areas of significant developmental delays, or brain scan or neurological abnormalities. However, careful review of their medical, developmental, and family history suggests that their deficits are most likely explained by factors other than HIV disease. In some cases, children may exhibit both HIV and non-HIV-related impairments.

Domains of Neuropsychological Impairments

The majority of research evaluating the neuropsychological functioning of infants, children, and adolescents with HIV infection utilizes composite measures of general cognitive function. These measures have been effective in assessing the global impact of HIV disease on the CNS as reflected in brain imaging lesions, cerebrospinal fluid abnormalities, and various disease parameters. However, children with HIV infection also may exhibit selective and subtle impairments, and global measures of cognitive function may mask the effects of HIV on separate domains (Wolters, Brouwers, Civitello, & Moss, 1997). Only a few studies have used specific function tests to more comprehensively assess selective domains of cognitive ability. Results of both types of research are presented next to describe the cognitive manifestations of pediatric HIV disease.

General Cognitive Functions

Neurodevelopmental Deficits in Infants

Infants are at risk for early neurodevelopmental manifestations associated with HIV that are distinctive from the effects of prematurity and prenatal drug exposure. Studies consistently have found impaired cognitive as well as motor development, as measured by the Bayley Scales of Infant Development, in infants with HIV infection, compared to infants born to HIV-positive mothers who are not infected (seroreverters) or to unexposed (seronegative) controls (Aylward, Butz, Hutton, Joyner, & Vogelhut, 1992; Chase et al., 1995; Drotar et al., 1997; Gay et al., 1995; Hittelman, Nelson, Shah, Gong, & Peluso, 1993; Nozyce et al., 1994; Pollack et al., 1996). Different patterns of neurodevelopmental impairment are observed in infants with HIV infection. For example, the age of onset of developmental delays tend to range from as early as 3 months (Gay et al., 1995) to as late as 24 months (Chase et al., 1995) and cognitive impairments tend to develop later and be somewhat less prevalent than motor deficits (Chase et al., 1995; Drotar et al., 1997; Englund et al., 1996). By 2 years of age, approximately one-quarter to one-third of infants with HIV infection exhibit moderate to severe cognitive and motor disabilities, as measured by standardized test scores at least 2 standard deviations below the mean (Chase et al., 1995; Drotar et al., 1997; Englund et al., 1996; Gay et al., 1995). On the other hand, approximately one-quarter to one-third of infants with HIV infection exhibit normal development at 24 months of age (Chase et al., 1995; Englund et al., 1996; Gay et al., 1995), while the remaining proportion exhibit mild developmental delays. In some cases, both cognitive and motor functioning may be impaired, or, in other instances, marked motor deficits may be present with relatively spared cognitive abilities (Belman, 1994). In addition, a loss of previously acquired developmental skills or a significant and consistent decline in standard scores on the Mental Bayley Scales is associated with rapid disease progression and a shorter survival time (Brouwers, Wolters, Moss, & Pizzo, 1993). Since the Bayley Scales measure sensorimotor function, the motor deficits of these infants may confound the assessment of their cognitive abilities. Other studies, therefore, have evaluated infants with HIV infection with the Fagan Test of Infant Intelligence, which assesses visual recognition memory using an infant habituation task not requiring a motor response (Drotar et al., 1997; Swales, Scott, & Cohen, 1990). Drotar et al. (1997) found no difference between HIV-infected seroreverters and seronegative controls from Uganda, while Swales (1990) found that 33% of the HIV-positive infants exhibited decreased cognitive function on the Fagan Test, compared to 8% of the HIV-negative controls.

School-Age Children and Adolescents

Cognitive deficits are less prevalent in school-age children and adolescents compared to younger children and infants. In a multicenter clinical trial of pediatric patients naive to antiretroviral therapy, only about 9% of older vertically infected children from 6 to 18 years of age exhibited standard scores of less than 70 on general intelligence tests, compared to 25% of children less than 6 years of age (Englund et al., 1996). A number of studies investigating the neuropsychological functioning of HIV-positive and HIV-negative school-age children and adolescents with hemophilia have not found overall cognitive deficits attributable to HIV disease at baseline evaluations (Loveland et al., 1994; Sirois & Hill, 1993; Whitt et al., 1993). Longitudinal assessments of these patients have produced mixed results. One study identified subtle declines in the cognitive scores of HIV-positive hemophiliacs over time, compared to the HIV-negative hemophiliacs who showed the expected practice effects (Sirois & Hill, 1993), while another study found no systematic differences in the neuropsychological functioning between these groups (Smith et al., 1997). In addition, those children infected with HIV at a younger age exhibited more difficulty on perceptual tasks than those infected at an older age (Sirois & Hill, 1993). Thus, in a small sample of children with hemophilia and HIV infection, subtle problems in learning were becoming apparent over time. Results from studies of HIV-infected children with hemophilia, however, cannot be generalized to children who were vertically infected because hemophiliacs typically acquired HIV later in life, when the brain was more developed. In another study of children transfused at birth (Cohen et al., 1991), children with HIV infection did not differ in overall cognitive function from children who were seronegative, yet slight but significant differences were found in a few selective functions. Finally, Tardieu and colleagues (1995) found that most vertically infected school-age children exhibited overall cognitive abilities in the average range with impairments in selected areas of cognitive function in some patients. The findings from research examining specific cognitive domains in children with HIV disease are described later in the chapter.

Correlation with Brain Imaging Lesions

Greater overall severity of CT brain scan abnormalities has been significantly related to lower levels of general cognitive ability in children with symptomatic HIV disease (see Figure 6.1) (Brouwers, DeCarli et al., 1995). Particularly for vertically infected children, CT brain scan abnormalities accounted for more than 65% of the variance in general cognitive function (Brouwers, DeCarli et al., 1995). Moreover, no differential associations were found between specific CT brain scan abnormalities, such as cortical atrophy and white matter abnormalities, and verbal or perceptual–spatial deficits derived from the IQ test of children older than 3 years of age (Brouwers, DeCarli, et al., 1995). Very few of these children showed any evidence on CT scan of differential laterality or an anterior–posterior gradient of the abnormalities, which further confirmed the global character of the disease in children with symptomatic HIV infection. In older children without encephalopathy, however, CNS compromise may be manifested by a pattern of selective or more subtle neurocognitive deficits. Similarly, brain

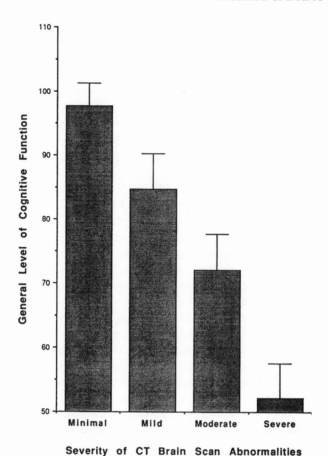

FIGURE 6.1. Relation between overall severity of computed tomographic brain scan abnormalities and general level of cognitive function in 58 children with vertically acquired HIV infection ($r = .81$; $p < .001$).

imaging studies have shown that when cortical atrophy was minimal it tended to be more prominent anteriorly (DeCarli et al., 1993).

Correlations with Cerebrospinal Fluid Abnormalities

As stated earlier, HIV-associated CNS manifestations most likely are caused by the indirect effects of HIV infection of the brain (Epstein & Gendelman, 1993; Lipton, 1992). A potential pathogenic host factor is quinolinic acid (QUIN), an excitatory neurotoxin produced by stimulated macrophages. QUIN levels in the cerebrospinal fluid (CSF) of children with symptomatic HIV disease were significantly elevated, compared to a control group comprised of age-matched pediatric cancer patients (Brouwers, Heyes, et al., 1993). In the group of children with HIV, elevated CSF QUIN levels were correlated with lower levels of general cognitive functioning at baseline. After 6 months of antiretroviral treatment, children had a significant decrease in CSF QUIN, which was associated with a concurrent increase in general cognitive function (Brouwers, Heyes, et al., 1993). Higher brain QUIN levels also were noted in children with encephalopathy at autopsy (Sei et al., 1995).

Correlations with HIV Disease Parameters

In infants and children with symptomatic HIV infection, various disease parameters have been associated with neurodevelopmental function. In infants, the presence of an AIDS-defining illness (excluding lymphoid interstitial pneumonitis) (Nozyce et al., 1994) in the first 2 years of life and high plasma HIV RNA concentration (Pollack et al., 1996) appear to be prognostic markers that are associated with more severe cognitive and motor delays. Moreover, lower levels of general cognitive functioning have been associated with more progressed disease, as defined by low plasma CD4 leukocyte count and elevated p24 antigen levels, in children with symptomatic HIV infection (Brouwers, DeCarli, et al., 1995; Brouwers, Tudor-Williams, et al., 1995).

Recent studies also have investigated the relationship of the level of cognitive dysfunction with the amount of viral replication in the CNS, since the degree of viral activity in the peripheral blood may not reflect what is occurring in the brain. HIV DNA has been identified in brain tissue of children and adults with HIV disease (Sei et al., 1994). The amount of viral DNA in the brain was much higher in encephalopathic compared to nonencephalopathic pediatric AIDS patients, while levels of viral DNA in lymph nodes and spleen were very similar in these subgroups (Sei et al., 1995). In a follow-up study, HIV RNA was evaluated in the CSF and plasma from HIV-infected children (Sei et al., 1996). HIV RNA was more frequently detected in the CSF of children who had abnormal cognitive function compared to those who did not. Furthermore, the level of HIV RNA in CSF was higher in children with a greater severity of CNS dsyfunction (Pratt et al., 1996; Sei et al., 1996). There was no correlation, however, between HIV RNA levels from the CSF and from plasma. Thus, no differences were found in the level of plasma HIV RNA or in the amount of HIV DNA in lymph nodes and spleen between encephalopathic and nonencephalopathic children, but significant differences were found in these levels from the CSF and brain. These findings suggest that the activity of the virus within the CNS may be independent of that in rest of the body, at least in the later stages of the disease.

Attention

Deficits in the ability to pay attention may cause significant problems in learning and school performance. Attention has many dimensions, such as divided, focused, and sustained attention, which can be associated with different brain areas (Mirsky, Anthony, Duncan, Ahearn, & Kellam, 1991). Certain subcomponents of attention therefore may be more at risk than others, due to the differential neuropathology of HIV infection. Attention deficits have been reported in pediatric patients with HIV disease (Brouwers et al., 1989; Hittelman et al., 1993; Lifschitz, Hanson, Wilson, & Shearer, 1989). It is unclear, however, whether an increased prevalence of attentional difficulties exists in these children compared to an uninfected population and whether these problems are directly attributable to HIV infection.

Studies that compare children with HIV infection to other chronically ill children have not found differential attentional problems between the two groups. For example, HIV-positive and HIV-negative males with hemophilia both exhibited subtle deficits on tasks requiring sustained attention, but the performance of the two groups on these measures did not differ (Whitt et al., 1993). In another study of males with hemophilia, neither the HIV-positive nor the HIV-negative patients demonstrated any impairments on the attentional tasks (Loveland et al., 1994). Similarly, in a comparison between school-aged children with symptomatic HIV infection and long-term survivors of acute lymphoblastic leukemia, approximately equal proportions of the two patient samples were classified as having attention deficits based on their subtest profile on the Wechsler Intelligence Scale for Children—Revised (Brouwers et al., 1992). These data suggest that attentional problems in HIV-infected patients may not be related to HIV per se, but rather to having a chronic illness affecting the CNS.

On the other hand, evidence of attentional deficits was found in HIV-infected children with CNS compromise compared to children without CNS compromise using a simple alerted visual reaction time (RT) and a go–no-go choice reaction time task (Appels, 1996). CNS-compromised patients reacted slower and with larger variability on the simple RT test, compared to the noncompromised patients. Both subgroups reacted progressively faster as the preparatory interval increased from 500 milliseconds to a maximum of 2,000 milliseconds. In the choice reaction time task, CNS-compromised patients also reacted significantly slower. Moreover, their decision time (difference between the choice RT and the simple RT for the same preparatory interval) was significantly longer than for the noncompromised patients, suggesting a mental slowing that was independent from a possible motor slowing. In another study using reaction time (Hittelman et al., 1993) severe attentional deficits were reported in 53% of HIV-infected children.

In summary, attentional deficits, particularly in sustained attention, may be associated with HIV disease in children, but most likely are only evident in the later stages of the disease or in cases with clear CNS compromise. More research is needed to further investigate the effects of HIV on attentional processes, using appropriate control groups and direct assessment procedures that measure different types of attention.

Language

Receptive and Expressive Verbal Language

Early studies investigating the neurodevelopmental function of children with HIV infection suggested that deficits in expressive language were more common and of greater severity than delays in receptive language (Condini et al., 1991; Epstein et al., 1986; Wolters et al., 1994). More recent studies have further explored the effect of HIV on expressive language by evaluating children with standardized comprehensive language measures assessing both receptive and expressive domains (Wolters, Brouwers, et al., 1995, Wolters et al., 1997). Results indicated that receptive language abilities were significantly higher than expressive skills in both encephalopathic and nonencephalopathic children with symptomatic HIV disease at the baseline evaluation (Wolters, Brouwers, et al., 1995) and also after 6 and 24 months of antiretroviral therapy (Wolters et al., 1997). Furthermore, overall language function declined over 24 months despite treatment. In contrast, uninfected siblings of the HIV-infected patients did not show a discrepancy between expressive and receptive language function (see Figure 6.2) (Wolters, Brouwers, et al., 1995). Both lower receptive and expressive language scores were correlated with overall severity of abnormalities on CT brain scans in the patient group at baseline. In the encephalopathic children, the magnitude of the discrepancy between receptive and expressive language was related to the degree of CT brain scan abnormality (Wolters, Brouwers, et al., 1995). In addition, poorer immune status was associated with more impaired language function. The data from these studies suggest that the observed language impairments are associated with the direct effects HIV on the CNS rather than with the influence of environmental factors.

Analyses comparing the subtests scores also were performed to examine specific areas of language impairment. School-age children demonstrated significantly more difficulty with the generation of spontaneous sentences than with repeating sentences (Wolters, Brouwers, et al., 1995), suggesting that underlying deficits may be related to problems with the retrieval of information, semantic knowledge base, or syntax, rather than with motor or working memory systems.

Expressive Emotional Language

In addition to deficits in expressive symbolic language, studies have found that children with HIV infection also may display impairments in other areas

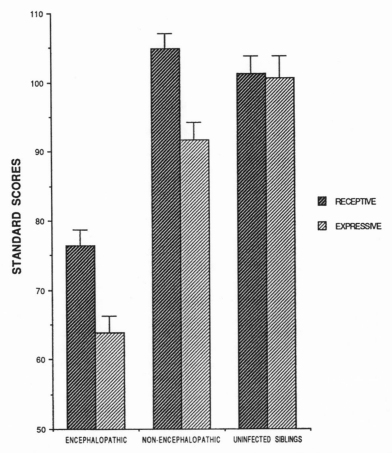

FIGURE 6.2. Comparison of the mean receptive and expressive language standard scores (mean = 100, *SD* = 15) between encephalopathic (*n* = 21) and non-encephalopathic (*n* = 15) pediatric patients with symptomatic HIV infection and an uninfected sibling control group (*n* = 20).

of expressive behavior (Moss, Wolters, Brouwers, Hendricks, & Pizzo, 1996) including emotional language (Roelofs et al., 1996). Previously obtained videotaped samples of behavior (Moss et al., 1996) were rated using a new procedure to evaluate various aspects of expressive emotional nonverbal language (facial expression, emotional gesturing, and prosody), expressive symbolic language (verbal language and pantomime), expressive motor function (facial, limb, and body movement), and irrelevant movement (Wolters, Roelofs, & Fernandez-Hall, 1995). Results indicated that children with HIV-related encephalopathy exhibited less expressive behavior in all domains except for pantomime and irrelevant movement

(Wolters, Roelofs, Fernandez-Hall, Moss, & Brouwers, 1999). Moreover, ratings of various CT brain scan abnormalities negatively correlated with all the expressive behavior variables except for pantomime and irrelevant movement. Thus, expressive emotional language, verbal language, and functional behaviors appear to be affected by HIV-related CNS disease in children. However, pantomime, which consists of communication through simple one-word gestures, and irrelevant movements, such as hyperactive behaviors, did not appear to distinguish between encephalopathic and nonencephalopathic patients.

Other Specific Cognitive Functions

Verbal memory (Skoraszewski, Ball, & Mikulka, 1991) and visual–spatial memory deficits (Van Gorp, Miller, Satz, & Visscher, 1989) have been documented in adults with HIV infection. Some evidence suggests that memory impairments may be a specific neuropsychological manifestation of pediatric HIV disease as well. Visual–spatial memory and immediate rote recall deficits have been documented in school-age children with HIV infection (Boivin et al., 1995; Diamond et al., 1987). However, such memory deficits are not consistently observed (Drotar et al., 1997; Loveland et al., 1994; Sirois & Hill, 1993) and may be more frequent in children who also have accompanying neurological impairment indicative of HIV-related CNS disease (Levenson, Mellins, Zawadzki, Kairam, & Stein, 1992; Perez, Wolters, Moss, & Brouwers, 1998). Visual scanning, cognitive flexibility (Cohen et al., 1991), and visual perception (Boivin et al., 1995; Diamond et al., 1987) are other areas of cognitive functioning that may be impaired in children with HIV infection.

Academic Achievement

Children with HIV infection may be at risk for academic difficulties associated with the effects of HIV on the CNS and with frequent school absences due to acute illnesses. Most studies of academic achievement in school-age children with HIV disease have included children with transfusion-acquired HIV infection (Cohen et al., 1991; Loveland et al., 1994; Sirois & Hill, 1993; Smith et al., 1997). Although results indicated lower achievement scores than expected based on intelligence test scores (Loveland et al., 1994; Sirois & Hill, 1993; Smith et al., 1997), mean academic achievement scores were within the average range (Cohen et al., 1991; Loveland et al., 1994; Sirois & Hill, 1993; Smith et al., 1997). Similarly, in a study of academic achievement in school-age children with vertically acquired HIV infection, two thirds of the children assessed demonstrated normal school achievement as well as normal function on tests of general cognitive abilities, language, and motor functions (Tardieu et al., 1995). Those children with normal academic achievement had a higher percentage of CD4 lymphocytes, indicating better immune function, than the other children. Thus, current studies indicate that the majority of school-age children with HIV infection exhibit generally age-appropriate learning and academic performance; however, they may not be learning at a level commensurate with their IQ.

Associated Developmental Domains

In addition to cognitive deficits, children with HIV-related CNS disease also may exhibit impairments in other domains, particularly motor and behavioral functioning. Deficits in these areas can interfere with the development and assessment of cognitive function, and therefore, are discussed briefly here.

Motor Functioning

Another frequent manifestation of pediatric HIV infection, which frequently co-exists with cognitive deficits, is motor dysfunction (Aylward et al., 1992; Englund et al., 1996; Gay et al., 1995; Nozyce et al., 1994). In a large multicenter study of symptomatic pediatric patients naive to antiretroviral therapy, approximately 23% exhibited some type of motor dysfunction (Englund et al., 1996). Infants less than 1 year of age, however, were at particularly high risk for developing motor impairments (45%) compared to older school-age children and adolescents (9%) (Englund et al., 1996).

Specific motor impairments that are common in infants and young children include abnormalities in gait, strength, coordination, and, particularly, muscle tone (Belman, 1994; Englund et al., 1996; Ultmann et al., 1987). Common changes in muscle tone include hypertonia in the upper and/or lower extremities or mixed tone consisting of axial hypotonia and hyperreflexia in the lower extremities (Lord, Danoff, & Smith, 1995; Ultmann et al., 1987). In progressive encephalopathy, children frequently exhibit severe motor involvement, including spastic diparesis or quadriparesis; movement disorders, such as rigidity and tremors (Belman, 1994); and loss of previously acquired skills (Belman et al., 1988; Epstein et al., 1986; Hittelman, 1990; Ultmann et al., 1987). School-age children tend to develop less severe motor problems due to the lower prevalence of encephalopathy, but they may manifest more subtle disturbances in higher gross motor functions of the lower extremities, such as running agility and speed (Parks, 1994). Older children and adolescents also may exhibit subtle perceptual–motor difficulties (Epstein et al., 1986; Parks, 1994) and psychomotor slowing (Belman, 1994; Cohen et al., 1991). In addition to fine and gross motor abnormalities, oral–motor functioning may be impaired, which may result in articulation problems, expressive language deficits, and feeding and swallowing difficulties (Pressman, 1992).

Such motor involvement may limit children's verbal communication and functional motor output, interfering with their learning and development over time and thereby making a valid assessment of their cognitive abilities difficult. The extent of the child's physical limitations should be evaluated prior to planning the cognitive assessment. Specific tests and subtests can be selected when needed to minimize the impact of motor impairments on the evaluation of cognitive function. (More details on assessment issues are provided later in this chapter). Referral to physical, occupational, and speech therapy for assessment and rehabilitation services is recommended for infants and children with motor and expressive language impairments (Lord et al., 1995; Parks, 1994; Pressman, 1992).

Behavioral Functioning

Direct behavioral effects that are associated with the impact of HIV on the CNS may develop in children with advanced HIV-related CNS disease in addition to cognitive, language, and motor impairments. Such behavioral abnormalities may include impaired adaptive behavior (Wolters et al., 1994), apathy, reduced goal-directed behavior, vacant staring, and flat affect that resembles various psychiatric syndromes (Moss et al., 1994). The number of children exhibiting such severe HIV-related behavioral effects, however, is now relatively low, since severe encephalopathy appears to be less common now than in the first few years of the epidemic. In addition, indirect behavioral effects, which refer to maladaptive psychological reactions, such as anxiety and depression, may result when children and their families face a number of psychosocial and medical stressors as they live with the disease (Brouwers, Moss, Wolters, & Schmitt, 1994; Moss et al., 1994; Wiener, Moss, Davidson, & Fair, 1992).

The daily functioning of children with HIV infection may be influenced by the interaction of both the direct and indirect behavioral effects of the disease. Studies investigating the daily functioning of children with HIV infection suggest that some behavioral impairments appear to be associated with the effects of HIV on the CNS because they are more severe in children with encephalopathy, improve with antiretroviral therapy (Moss et al., 1994; Wolters et al., 1994), and are associated with CT brain scan abnormalities (Brouwers, DeCarli, et al., 1995; Brouwers, van der Vlugt, et al., 1995; Wolters et al., 1994). Other studies have reported increased anxiety (Battles, Sherman, & Wiener, 1997; Havens, Whitaker, Feldman, & Ehrnhardt, 1994), hyperactive behaviors (Moss et al., 1999), poor social competence (Bose, Moss, Brouwers, Pizzo, & Lorion, 1994), and impaired adaptive behavior in children with HIV disease (Loveland et al., 1994; Wolters et al., 1994). However, the proportion of children with HIV infection that exhibited such problem behaviors was not significantly different from comparison groups (Havens et al., 1994; Loveland et al., 1994; Moss et al., 1999). Furthermore, a greater number of behavior problems in children with HIV infection was associated with more adverse life events (Bose et al., 1994), suggesting that other, non-disease-related factors may impact upon their psychological and behavioral functioning.

In children with HIV infection, more impaired adaptive behavior is predicted by lower levels of cognitive ability, more severe deficits in motor skills, and poorer social–emotional adjustment (Bose, 1996). In turn, behavioral abnormalities, either from the direct or indirect effects of HIV disease, may affect a child's cognitive functioning through diminished or impaired interaction with the environment. Behavioral abnormalities such as apathy, lack of expressiveness, depression, or increased anxiety also can negatively affect test performance and interfere with obtaining a valid assessment of the child's cognitive functioning. Thus, professionals working with HIV-infected children should be aware of the possibility of both the direct and indirect behavioral effects of the disease and their possible impact on cognitive function. Differentiating between direct versus indirect behavioral abnormalities is complex but critical for selecting the appropriate psychosocial, behavioral, and medical interventions.

Overview of Treatment and Effects on Cognitive Functioning

A number of antiretroviral drugs currently are available and approved for use in both children and adults with HIV infection. Recommendations indicate that all persons with symptomatic disease should be treated with these agents. Antiretroviral therapy has been found to improve neurobehavioral dysfunction in adults (Brouwers et al., 1997; Yarchoan et al., 1987) and particularly in children with HIV infection (Brouwers et al., 1990; Pizzo et al., 1988). A number of studies, including randomized controlled clinical trials, have shown that zidovudine (azidothymidine, AZT) (McKinney et al., 1991; Schmitt et al., 1988; Sidtis et al., 1993) and didanosine (dideoxy-inosine, ddI) (Butler et al., 1991; Yarchoan et al., 1990) as single agents may benefit neurobehavioral function. The effects of treatment have been most clearly reflected in increases in the general levels of mental abilities of infants and children (McKinney et al., 1991; Pizzo et al., 1988), although improvements in other behavioral domains have also been noted (Moss et al., 1994; Wolters et al., 1994).

Current treatments emphasize combination therapy with various drugs. The effects of combination antiretroviral therapies on neurocognitive function have been studied primarily in children. For example, ddC (dideoxy-cytidine, zalcitabine) was administered as a single agent for 8 weeks, followed at 12 weeks by an alternating schedule with AZT (Pizzo et al.,

1990). Although a response in immunological and virological parameters was observed during the first 8 weeks on ddC alone, neurocognitive functioning declined. However, after 12 weeks on the alternating schedule that included both AZT and ddC, neurocognitive functioning recovered to baseline levels. In addition, recent double-blind randomized clinical trials (AIDS Clinical Trials Group, ACTG 152 and ACTG 300) have shown an advantage of combination therapy (AZT/ddI and AZT/3TC [lamivudine]) over monotherapy with respect to neurobehavioral outcome in children with HIV disease (Englund et al., 1996; McKinney et al., 1998). Preliminary pediatric Phase I–II studies of the new protease inhibitor drugs, which were used in combination with two reverse transcriptase inhibitors, have shown mixed results regarding their effect on cognitive function: one study found a possible CNS benefit while the other did not (Mueller, Sleasman, et al., 1998; Mueller, Nelson, et al., 1998).

The optimal systemic antiretroviral therapy for HIV disease, based on virological or immunological markers, might not necessarily be optimal therapy for CNS disease (Brouwers et al., 1997; Pizzo et al., 1990). The effectiveness of antiretroviral drugs against CNS disease is in part related to their ability to inhibit HIV replication in relevant HIV-infected target cells in the brain, such as macrophages and microglia. Thus, pharmacological parameters, such as dose, route, and schedule of administration, and degree of CNS penetration play an important role. For example, adult patients with AIDS-related dementia receiving a higher dose of AZT were found to have greater neuropsychological improvements (Sidtis et al., 1993) than those patients receiving a lower dose. Similarly, in children, greater improvement in neurocognitive function was associated with higher absorption of ddI over time (Butler et al., 1991). In another study, the importance of the route and schedule of administration was demonstrated. Children with symptomatic HIV disease treated with continuous intravenous infusion of AZT showed much greater improvements in neurobehavioral function than children treated on an intermittent oral schedule (Brouwers et al., 1990). The penetration of antiviral agents into the CNS is quite variable. A number of studies have shown that AZT, which penetrates the CNS relatively well, is particularly effective in the treatment of HIV-associated CNS disease (Pizzo et al., 1988). On the other hand, ddI and ddC, which have only limited CNS penetration, show less beneficial effect on cognitive function (Brouwers, DeCarli, et al., 1994).

The issue of CNS therapy may become even more important as protease inhibitors and other classes of drugs are introduced that may have only limited penetration into the CNS, but which may significantly prolong the lives of people living with AIDS. It will be critically important to study the long-term effects of such therapies, which may leave the CNS relatively unprotected, on the developing brain.

Issues in the Cognitive Assessment
of Children with HIV Disease

Due to the high risk of developing neuropsychological impairments, the progressive nature of the disease, and the possibility of improvement in functioning with the administration of antiretroviral treatment, serial assessments are necessary to appropriately monitor the cognitive status of children with HIV infection over time. Such repeated evaluations are important for identifying the child's current strengths and weaknesses and monitoring longitudinal changes in the child's cognitive functioning. The results of the serial neuropsychological assessments should be used in conjunction with other data from the multidisciplinary team evaluation to assist in planning rehabilitative, educational, psychological, and medical interventions. When conducting longitudinal assessments of children with HIV disease, several areas to consider include the specific domains to assess; procedures of test administration; methodological issues regarding repeated assessments, such as developmental change over time, frequency of serial testing, and practice effects; and interpretation of test results for planning interventions.

Domains to Assess

An optimal neurocognitive assessment of infants, children, and adolescents with HIV disease should assess a wide range of abilities known to be vulnerable to the effects of HIV as described earlier in this chapter, including general cognitive function, language, perceptual–motor and motor skills, attention, and memory. The test battery should include an age-appropriate intelligence test that yields a composite measure of general cognitive function because it is relatively stable and has good validity and reliability (Appelbaum & Tuma, 1977; Neisser et al., 1996). Various studies of these tests report intertest correlations and the expected mean change in standard scores that help interpret interval change when transferring from one general cognitive test to another (Wechsler, 1991). Furthermore, global measures of cognitive function have been associated with measures of disease progression and neurological status in children with HIV infection (Brouwers, Tudor-Williams, et al., 1995), indicating the validity of this approach. On the other hand, a composite score of cognitive function may mask the separate effects of HIV on individual domains of functioning (Wolters et al., 1997). Therefore, it is also useful to include tests in the battery that comprehensively assess other specific functions to evaluate subtle changes that may develop over time. This approach is particularly important in school-age children and adolescents with HIV infection, who tend to exhibit less severe CNS manifestations, most likely due to advances in treatment. Thus, administering tests that more comprehensively evaluate various aspects of specific abilities such as language (receptive, expressive), attention (sustain, shift), or memory (visual, verbal) are useful for identifying the more subtle effects of HIV on the CNS that may not be found when using an overall general cognitive index. The subdomains or subtest scores from such comprehensive tests may be reviewed to further investigate the underlying mechanism of impairment; strengths and weaknesses in various domains; the CNS disease stage of the patient; and whether the deficits may be due to HIV or other etiologies.

In addition to cognitive domains, adaptive behavior should be assessed to obtain a measure of the child's daily behavioral functioning and quality of life in the home environment. If the child is exhibiting behavioral problems, a screening of social–emotional functioning is warranted to aid in the differential diagnosis of whether the difficulties may be attributed to the direct or indirect behavioral effects of HIV. Furthermore, infants and young children should have regular follow-up evaluations by physical, occupational, and speech therapy, due to the high risk of HIV-related language and fine and gross motor deficits in this population.

Developmental Change over Time

Children are constantly learning new skills, and various cognitive functions develop at different rates over time. Therefore, the longitudinal assessment of children with HIV disease is contingent upon using standardized tests with reliable age norms, preferably with small age increments, so that appropriate comparisons can be made from one assessment to another. Interpretation of the interval change in test scores between repeated evaluations should be done by considering the child's abilities in relation to normal developmental growth, the possible effects of HIV disease or antiretroviral treatment on the developing brain, and the impact of environmental and educational factors on the child's functioning.

Most commonly used and standardized psychometric tests for children have restricted age ranges, for which age-scaled deviation norms are available. Therefore, changing test instruments will be necessary when conducting longitudinal assessments to utilize age-appropriate tests and norms as the child grows older. Some area of overlap exists between the majority of tests that are most often used to assess cognitive functioning during childhood, which allows for some flexibility in changing to the next age-appropriate test. When changing tests, however, it will be difficult to interpret any interval change occurring at that assessment. If possible, the change to a new instrument should be done shortly after the child was previously assessed (i.e., within 6 months) and when the child is considered healthy, with no new developmental concerns. However, if the child is assessed as part of a longitudinal study, it is best to continue using the same test (as administered at baseline) for as long as possible so congruent comparisons can be made over time. If a decline in functioning is suspected due to HIV-related CNS disease, the test that was previously administered should be given again if enough overlap exists between the two tests. This approach should also be used for children with significant developmental deficits if the test for the younger population may assess the delayed skills more appropriately. Changing over from one test to another may be associated with some difference in scores, even in children without CNS involvement. However, when the scores are significantly lower than those obtained previously, the examiner needs to reassess the observed decline in scores. The examiner can either readminister the former test if the two measures have enough overlap or give the new test for the older age range again as soon as repeat testing would be considered valid for a chronically ill population (i.e., in 6 months).

Frequency of Repeated Assessments and Practice Effects

Several factors need to be considered when planning the frequency of serial assessments, including the risk and rate of progression of the disease in different ages of children, the estimated timing of therapeutic effect of the treatment, and the amount of practice effects on the tests to be administered. In infants and young children with HIV infection, the possibility of CNS disease is high and the rate of progression is often rapid, which may result in a loss of developmental milestones. Furthermore, the effects of antiretroviral treatment on developmental function may begin within a brief period of time. Therefore, in younger children and those with encephalopathy, shorter intervals between testing are often needed to assess possible changes in functioning. In school-age children and adolescents with HIV infection, the probability of developing CNS disease is somewhat lower and the neurocognitive symptoms tend to be manifest more gradually with subtle changes in function. Thus, test–retest intervals may be longer in older children and adolescents, particularly in those without evidence of HIV-related CNS disease. Unfortunately, few psychological tests have multiple or alternate forms; thus, the possibility of practice effects with repeated administration of similar tests is a problem. The degree of possible practice effects is associated with the child's rate of development, comparative level of functioning, health status, and potential for latent learning. In younger children and infants, practice effects are less of a concern. For example, 1-month test–retest data on the McCarthy Scales of Children's Abilities indicate that practice effects for healthy preschool children with normal IQs average 4.5 points (McCarthy, 1972), while on the Wechsler Intelligence Scale for Children—3rd edition (WISC-III) these effects for approximately the same time period average at least 7 points (Wechsler, 1991). Practice effects also are smaller with longer test–retest intervals, and in children with lower IQs (Tuma & Appelbaum, 1980) or with medical conditions (Farwell et al., 1990; Moss, Nannis, & Poplack, 1981).

In consideration of these various assessment issues, the following general guidelines for determining repeated testing for various age groups are suggested: (1) infants under 1 year should be evaluated every 3 months because they are at high risk for developing CNS disease; (2) children from 1 to 3 years of age should be evaluated every 6 months unless they exhibit neurodevelopmental deficits, in which case they should be assessed every 3 months; and (3) children who exhibit stable functioning in the average range should be evaluated annually from 3 to 10 years of age and every 2 years when older than 10 years of age; if they have deficits, however, they should be evaluated every 6 and 12 months, respectively (Wolters & Brouwers, 1999). To further decrease the testing burden on children while still monitoring the effects of the disease, shorter batteries of individual subtests and specific function tests can be administered between major evaluations in which a measure of general cognitive functioning is obtained.

Special Test Administration Procedures

In addition to cognitive deficits, children with HIV infection may have special needs that require novel approaches or modification of standard psychological testing procedures. For example, physical impairments in gross and fine motor skills, sensory defects in hearing or vision, or diminished expressive language due to HIV may limit a child's ability to respond to cognitive test items. Children with HIV infection also may exhibit unmodulated activity levels, short attention spans, and uncooperative behaviors, or become easily fatigued, which will make the evaluation process difficult. Finally, some children may be bilingual or not experienced in the English language.

For children who cannot be assessed with the standard instruments, alternative tests (i.e., designed specifically for children with visual, hearing, or physical impairments) or assessment procedures (i.e., use of interpreters or eye gaze instead of a pointing response) should be used to assess cognitive functioning. The administration of such tests and procedures will help to ensure that the child's physical problems or language differences do not significantly interfere with the evaluation of his or her cognitive abilities. For a child who is easily fatigued or exhibits behavioral difficulties, the examiner may need to use various behavior management techniques or multiple test sessions in order complete a valid assessment. Thus, the examiner must have the knowledge and skill to select and administer the most appropriate tests and administration procedures depending on the child's special needs to obtain an optimal assessment of cognitive functioning.

Interpretation of Neuropsychological Test Results
for Planning Appropriate Interventions

The results of the neuropsychological evaluation should be integrated and interpreted together with other information obtained from parents and other multidisciplinary team members to determine whether any developmental impairments are likely to be related to HIV disease or to other factors. Such a determination is important for planning appropriate medical, educational, rehabilitative, and psychological interventions. Areas of information to be considered when interpreting test results include the child's birth, medical, developmental, and educational history; environmental and family factors; neurological and neuroimaging findings; results from the medical exam and other evaluations (i.e., audiology, speech, physical, and occupational therapy); behavioral observations; and psychometric test scores. Comparison of longitudinal psychometric test results helps identify possible changes in developmental functioning and the need for modifications in educational services over the course of the disease. For example, a child may be functioning in the normal range and performing well in a regular classroom but later may develop HIV-related CNS compromise and require special education services. In any case, HIV-infected children require appropriate educational services based on their individual needs to facilitate optimal functioning.

SUMMARY AND FUTURE DIRECTIONS

Cognitive dysfunction in pediatric HIV infection is associated primarily with the effects of HIV on the CNS. Younger children and pediatric patients in later stages of the disease tend to be at the highest risk for developing CNS complications. Manifestations of HIV-related CNS disease are variable and may range from subtle weaknesses in one or two domains such as attention, memory, or expressive language, to global cognitive deterioration in children with progressive encephalopathy. Motor and behavioral impairments also are observed in pediatric HIV infection and may interfere with the development and assessment of cognitive function. Due to the dynamic and pervasive nature of HIV-related CNS disease in children, a comprehensive, longitudinal, and multidisciplinary approach to assessment and management is warranted. More widespread treatment with combination antiretroviral therapies appear to be reducing the prevalence and severity of HIV-related developmental deficits in the pediatric population.

Future directions for research investigating the neurocognitive functioning of pediatric HIV disease include examining the effects of HIV in asymptomatic children to identify subtle changes that will help identify initial signs of CNS disease (Wolters et al., 1997), distinguishing the effects of HIV from other confounding factors such as maternal drug abuse (Chase et al., 1995), identifying various patterns of neurodevelopmental function and systemic disease parameters that are prognostic of the rate of disease progression (Chase et al., 1995), and exploring the academic and vocational needs of older children and adolescents, all of which are important for early identification and remedial, therapeutic, and preventative efforts. Since most antiretroviral therapies have minimal penetration into the CNS, other medical treatments specific to HIV-related CNS symptoms and combinations of drugs that do have some potential CNS effects also need to be explored. Finally, advances in research and medicine are gradually changing HIV infection from a terminal disease to a chronic illness as children infected at birth are functional and living well into adolescence. Thus, the investigation of long-term survivors of pediatric HIV infection is necessary to understand the longitudinal effects of the disease and treatment on the CNS in order to provide infants, children, and adolescents the medical, educational, rehabilitative, and psychosocial services that most appropriately meet their needs.

ACKNOWLEDGMENTS

Support for this chapter was provided in part by Reseach Contract Nos. NCI CM 87263-19, NCI-CM-17529-41, N01-SC-47002, and N01-SC-71102 awarded to the Medical Illness Counseling Center, Chevy Chase, Maryland. We wish to thank the children and families treated at the 13th-floor outpatient clinic, NCI; the staff of the Rainbow Team, and all members of the NCI-MICC neuropsychology group for their assistance with the pediatric HIV research conducted over the past several years that served as a basis for this chapter.

REFERENCES

Aleixo, L. F., Goodenow, M. M., & Sleasman, J. W. (1997). Zidovudine administered to women infected with human immunodeficiency virus type 1 and to their neonates reduces pediatric infection independent of an effect on levels of maternal virus. *Journal of Pediatrics, 130*(6), 906–914.

Appelbaum, A. S., & Tuma, J. M. (1977). Social class and test performance: Comparative validity of the Peabody with the WISC and WISC-R for two socioeconomic groups. *Psychological Reports, 40,* 139–145.

Appels, M. (1996). *Assessment of attentional functioning in children with HIV-1 infection.* Unpublished master's thesis, University of Utrecht, The Netherlands.

Auger, I., Thomas, P., De Gruttola, V., Morse, D., Moore, D., Williams, R., Truman, B., & Lawrence, C. E. (1988). Incubation periods for paediatric AIDS patients. *Nature, 336,* 575–577.

Aylward, E. H., Butz, A. M., Hutton, N., Joyner, M. L., & Vogelhut, J. W. (1992). Cognitive and motor development in infants at risk for human immunodeficiency virus. *American Journal of Diseases of Children, 146,* 218–222.

Barnes, D. M. (1986). Brain function decline in children with AIDS. *Science, 232,* 1196.

Battles, H. B., Sherman, B. F., & Wiener, L. S. (1997, February 10). *Changes in psychological functioning over a period of one year in long-term survivors of pediatric HIV.* Paper presented at the NIH Clinical Research Day, National Institutes of Health, Bethesda, MD.

Belman, A. L. (1994). HIV-1-associated CNS disease in infants and children. In R. W. Price & S. W. Perry (Eds.), *HIV, AIDS and the brain* (pp. 289–310). New York: Raven Press.

Belman, A. L., Diamond, G., Dickson, D., Horoupian, D., Liena, J., Lantos, G., & Rubinstein, A. (1988). Pediatric acquired immunodeficiency syndrome: Neurologic syndromes. *American Journal of Diseases of Children, 142,* 29–35.

Belman, A. L., Lantos, G., Horoupian, D., Novick, B. E., Ultmann, M. H., Dickson, D. W., & Rubinstein, A. (1986). AIDS: Calcification of the basal ganglia in infants and children. *Neurology, 36,* 1192–1199.

Belman, A. L., Ultmann, M. H., Horoupian, D., Novick, B., Spiro, A. J., Rubinstein, A., Kurtzberg, D., & Cone-Wesson, B. (1985). Neurological complications in infants and children with acquired immune deficiency syndrome. *Annals of Neurology, 18,* 560–566.

Berger, J. R., Kumar, M., Kumar, A., Fernandez, J. B., & Levin, B. (1994). Cerebrospinal fluid dopamine in HIV-1 infection. *AIDS, 8,* 67–71.

Berger, J. R., Scott, G., Albrecht, J., Belman, A. L., Tornatore, C., & Major, E. O. (1992). Progressive multifocal leukoencephalopathy in HIV-1-infected children. *AIDS, 6,* 837–841.

Biglan, A., Metzler, C. W., Wirt, R., Ary, D., Nowell, J., Ochs, L., French, C., & Hood, D. (1990). Social and behavioral factors associated with high-risk sexual behavior among adolescents. *Journal of Behavioral Medicine, 13,* 245–261.

Blanche, S., Newell, M., Mayaux, M., Dunn, D., Teglas, J., Rouzioux, C., & Peckham, C. (1997). Morbidity and mortality in European children vertically infected by HIV-1. *Journal of Acquired Immune Deficiency Syndromes and Human Retrovirology, 14,* 442–450.

Blanche, S., Tardieu, M., Duliege, A., Rouzioux, C., Le Deist, F., Fukunaga, K., Caniglia, M., Jacomet, C., Messiah, A., & Griscelli, C. (1990). Longitudinal study of 94 symptomatic infants with perinatally acquired human immunodeficiency virus infection: Evidence for a bimodal expression of clinical and biological symptoms. *American Journal of Diseases of Children, 144*(11), 1210–1215.

Boivin, M., Green, S., Davies, A., Giordani, B., Mokili, J., & Cutting, W. (1995). A preliminary evaluation of the cognitive and motor effects of pediatric HIV infection in Zairian children. *Health Psychology, 14,* 13–21.

Bose, S. (1996). *An examination of adaptive functioning in HIV infected children: Exploring the relationships with HIV disease, neurocognitive functioning and psychosocial characteristics.* Unpublished doctoral dissertation, University of Maryland, College Park.

Bose, S., Moss, H., Brouwers, P., Pizzo, P., & Lorion, R. (1994). Psychologic adjustment of human immunodeficiency virus-infected school-age children. *Journal of Developmental and Behavioral Pediatrics, 15*(3), S26–S33.

Brouwers, P., Belman, A. L., & Epstein, L. (1994). Central nervous system involvement: Manifestations, evaluation, and pathogenesis. In P. A. Pizzo & C. M. Wilfert (Eds.), *Pediatric AIDS: The challenge of HIV infection in infants, children, and adolescents*, (2nd ed., pp. 433–455). Baltimore: Williams & Wilkins.

Brouwers, P., DeCarli, C., Civitello, L., Moss, H., Wolters, P., & Pizzo, P. (1995). Correlation between computed tomographic brain scan abnormalities and neuropsychological function in children with symptomatic human immunodeficiency virus disease. *Archives of Neurology, 52*, 39–44.

Brouwers, P., DeCarli, C., Tudor-Williams, G., Civitello, L., Moss, H., & Pizzo, P. (1994). Interrelations among patterns of change in neurocognitive, CT brain imaging, and CD4 measures associated with antiretroviral therapy in children with symptomatic HIV infection. *Advances in Neuroimmunology, 4*, 223–231.

Brouwers, P., Hendricks, M., Lietzau, J. A., Pluda, J. M., Mitsuya, H., Broder, S., & Yarchoan, R. (1997). Effect of combination therapy with zidovudine and didanosine on neuropsychological functioning in patients with symptomatic HIV disease: A comparison of simultaneous and alternating regimens. *AIDS, 11*, 59–66.

Brouwers, P., Heyes, M. P., Moss, H. A., Wolters, P. L., Poplack, D. G., Markey, S. P., & Pizzo, P. A. (1993). Quinolinic acid in the cerebrospinal fluid of children with symptomatic human immunodeficiency virus type 1 disease: Relationship to clincal status and therapeutic response. *Journal of Infectious Diseases, 168*, 1380–1386.

Brouwers, P., Moss, H., Wolters, P., Eddy, J., Balis, F., Poplack, D. G., & Pizzo, P. A. (1990). Effect of continuous infusion zidovudine therapy on neuropsychologic functioning in children with symptomatic human immunodeficiency virus infection. *Journal of Pediatrics, 117*, 980–985.

Brouwers, P., Moss, H., Wolters, P., Eddy, J., & Pizzo, P. (1989). Neuropsychological profile of children with symptomatic HIV infection prior to antiretroviral therapy [Abstract No. TBP 179]. *Proceedings of the V International Conference on AIDS* (Vol. 1, p. 316), Montreal, Canada.

Brouwers, P., Moss, H., Wolters, P., El-Amin, D., Tassone, E., & Pizzo, P. (1992). Neurobehavioral typology of school-age children with symptomatic HIV disease[Abstract]. *Journal of Clinical and Experimental Neuropsychology, 14*, 113.

Brouwers, P., Moss, H., Wolters, P., & Schmitt, F. (1994). Developmental deficits and behavioral change in pediatric AIDS. In I. Grant & A. Martin (Eds.), *Neuropsychology of HIV infection* (pp. 310–338). New York: Oxford University Press.

Brouwers, P., Tudor-Williams, G., DeCarli, C., Moss, H. A., Wolters, P., Civitello, L., & Pizzo, P. (1995). Relation between stage of disease and neurobehavioral measures in children with symptomatic HIV disease. *AIDS, 9*, 713–720.

Brouwers, P., van der Vlugt, H., Moss, H., Wolters, P., & Pizzo, P. (1995). White matter changes on CT brain scan are associated with neurobehavioral dysfunction in children with symptomatic HIV disease. *Child Neuropsychology, 1*(2), 93–105.

Brouwers, P., Wolters, P., Moss, H., & Pizzo, P. (1993). Encephalopathy in vertically acquired pediatric HIV disease. *Journal of Clinical and Experimental Neuropsychology, 15*, 95.

Budka, H. (1991). Neuropathology of human immunodeficiency virus infection. *Brain Pathology, 1*, 143–152.

Burns, D. K. (1992). The neuropathology of pediatric acquired immunodeficiency syndrome. *Journal of Child Neurology, 7*(4), 332–346.

Butler, K. M., Husson, R. N., Balis, F. M., Brouwers, P., Eddy, J., El-Amin, D., Gress, J., Hawkins, M., Jarosinski, P., Moss, H., Poplack, D., Santacroce, S., Venzon, D., Wiener, L., Wolters, P., & Pizzo, P. A. (1991). Dideoxyinosine in children with symptomatic human immunodeficiency virus infection. *New England Journal of Medicine, 324*(3), 137–144.

Centers for Disease Control and Prevention (CDC). (1998). *HIV/AIDS Surveillance Report, 10*(1), 1–40.

Chamberlain, M. C., Nichols, S. L., & Chase, C. H. (1991). Pediatric AIDS: Comparative cranial MRI and CT scans. *Pediatric Neurology, 7,* 357–362.

Chase, C., Vibbert, M., Pelton, S. I., Coulter, D. L., & Cabral, H. (1995). Early neurodevelopmental growth in children with vertically transmitted human immunodeficiency virus infection. *Archives of Pediatric and Adolescent Medicine, 149,* 850–855.

Civitello, L. (1996). Headache in pediatric human immunodeficiency virus disease. *Annals of Neurology, 40,* 310.

Civitello, L., Brouwers, P., DeCarli, C., & Pizzo, P. (1994). Calcification of the basal ganglia in children with HIV infection. *Annals of Neurology, 36,* 506.

Civitello, L. A., Brouwers, P., & Pizzo, P. A. (1993). Neurological and neuropsychological manifestations in 120 children with symptomatic human immunodeficiency virus infection [Abstract]. *Annals of Neurology, 34,* 481.

Cohen, S. E., Mundy, T., Karassik, B., Lieb, L., Ludwig, D. D., & Ward, J. (1991). Neuropsychological functioning in human immunodeficiency virus type 1 seropositive children infected through neonatal blood transfusion. *Pediatrics, 88*(1), 58–68.

Condini, A., Axia, G., Cattelan, C., D'Urso, M., Laverda, A., Viero, F., & Zacchello, F. (1991). Development of language in 18–30-month- old HIV-1-infected but not ill children. *AIDS, 5,* 735–739.

Connor, E. M., Sperling, R. S., Gelber, R., Kiselev, P., Scott, G., O'Sullivan, M. J., VanDyke, R., Bey, M., Shearer, W., Jacobson, R. L., Jiminez, E., O'Neill, E., Bazin, B., Delfraissy, J.F., Culnane, M., Coombs, R., Elkins, M., Moye, J., Stratton, P., & Balsley, J. (1994). Reduction of maternal–infant transmission of human immunodeficiency virus type 1 with zidovudine treatment. *New England Journal of Medicine, 331*(18), 1173–1180.

Cooper, E. R., Hanson, C., Diaz, C., Mendez, H., Abboud, R., Nugent, R., Pitt, J., Rich, K., Rodriguez, E. M., & Smeriglio, V., for the Women and Infants Transmission Study Group. (1998). Encephalopathy and progression of human immunodeficiency virus disease in a cohort of children with perinatally acquired human immunodeficiency virus infection. *Journal of Pediatrics, 132*(5), 808–812.

Davis, L., Hjelle, B. L., Miller, V. E., Palmer, C. L., Llewellyn, A. L., Merlin, T. L., Young, S. A., Mills, R. G., Wachsman, W., & Wiley, C. A. (1992). Early viral brain invasion in iatrogenic human immunodeficiency virus infection. *Neurology, 42,* 1736–2739.

DeCarli, C., Civitello, L. A., Brouwers, P., & Pizzo, P. A. (1993). The prevalence of computed azial tomographic abnormalities of the cerebrum in 100 consecutive children symptomatic with the human immunodeficiency virus. *Annals of Neurology, 34,* 198–205.

Diamond, G. W., Kaufman, J., Belman, A. L., Cohen, L., Cohen, H. J., &

Rubinstein, A. (1987). Characterization of cognitive functioning in a subgroup of children with congenital HIV infection. *Archives of Clinical Neuropsychology, 2,* 1–16.

Dickson, D. W., Belman, A. L., Kim, T. S., Horoupian, D., & Rubinstein, A. (1989). Spinal cord pathology in pediatric acquired immunodeficiency syndrome. *Neurology, 39,* 227–235.

Dickson, D. W., Lee, S. C., Hatch, W., Mattiace, L. A., Brosnan, C. F., & Lyman, W. D. (1994). Macrophages and microglia in HIV-related CNS neuropathology. *Research Publications of the Association for Research on Nervous and Mental Disorders, 72,* 99–118.

Dickson, D. W., Llena, J. F., Weidenheim, K. M., Kure, K., Goldstein, J., Park, Y. D., & Belman, A. L. (1990). Central nervous system pathology in children with AIDS and focal neurologic signs—stroke and lymphoma. In P. Kozlowski, D. A. Snider, P. M. Vietze, & H. M. Wisniewski (Eds.), *Brain in pediatric AIDS* (pp. 147–157). Basel: Karger.

Douglas, S. D. (1994). Immunological and virological clues for mother-to-child transmission of HIV-1 and HIV-2. *Journal of the American Medical Association, 272*(6), 487–488.

Drotar, D., Olness, K., Wiznitzer, M., Guay, L., Marum, L., Svilar, G., Hom, D., Fagan, J. F., Ndugwa, C., & Kiziri-Mayengo, R. (1997). Neurodevelopmental outcomes of Ugandan infants with human immunodeficiency virus Type 1 infection. *Pediatrics, 100*(1), e5.

Englund, J., Baker, C., Raskino, C., McKinney, R., Lifschitz, M., Petrie, B., Fowler, M., Connor, J., Mendez, H., O'Donnell, K., Wara, D., & AIDS Clinical Trials Group Protocol 152 Study Team. (1996). Clinical and laboratory characteristics of a large cohort of symptomatic, human immunodeficiency virus-infected infants and children. *Pediatric Infectious Disease Journal, 15*(11), 1025–1035.

Epstein, L. G., & Gendelman, H. E. (1993). Human immunodeficiency virus type 1 infection of the nervous system: Pathogenetic mechanisms. *Annals of Neurology, 33,* 429–436.

Epstein, L. G., Goudsmit, J., Paul, D. S., Morrison, S. H., Connor, E. M., Oleske, J. M., & Holland, B. (1987). Expression of human immunodeficiency virus in cerebrospinal fluid of children with progressive encephalopathy. *Annals of Neurology, 21,* 397–401.

Epstein, L. G., Sharer, L. R., & Goudsmit, J. (1988). Neurological and neuropathological features of human immunodeficiency virus infection in children. *Annals of Neurology, 23*(Suppl.), S19–S23.

Epstein, L. G., Sharer, L. R., Oleske, J. M., Connor, E. M., Goudsmit, J., Bagdon, L., Robert-Guroff, M., & Koenigsberger, M. R. (1986). Neurologic manifestations of human innumodeficiency virus infection in children. *Pediatrics, 78*(4), 678–687.

Farwell, J. R., Lee, Y. J., Hirtz, D. G., Sulzbacher, S. I., Ellenberg, J. H., & Nelson, K. B. (1990). Phenobarbital for febrile seizures—effects on intelligence and on seizure recurrence. *New England Journal of Medicine, 322,* 364–369.

Frederick, T., Mascola, L., Eller, A., O'Neil, L., Byers, B., & Los Angeles County Pediatric AIDS Consortium. (1994). Progression of human immunodeficiency virus disease among infants and children infected perinatally with human immunodeficiency virus or through neonatal blood transfusion. *Pediatric Infectious Disease Journal, 13,* 1091–1097.

Friedland, G., & Klein, R. (1987). Transmission of the human immunodeficiency virus. *New England Journal of Medicine, 317*(18), 1125–1135.

Galli, L., de Martino, M., Tovo, P., Gabiano, C., Zappa, M., Giaquinto, C., Tulisso, S., Vierucci, A., Guerra, M., Marchisio, P., Plebani, A., Zuccotti, G. V., Martino, A., Dallacasa, P., Stegagno, M., & Italian Register for HIV Infection in Children. (1995). Onset of clinical signs in children with HIV-1 perinatal infection. *AIDS, 9*, 455–461.

Gay, C. L., Armstrong, F. D., Cohen, D., Shenghan, L., Hardy, M. D., Swales, T. P., Morrow, C. J., & Scott, G. B. (1995). The effects of HIV on cognitive and motor development in children born to HIV-seropositive women with no reported drug use: Birth to 24 months. *Pediatrics, 96*(6), 1078–1082.

Gayle, H. D., & D'Angelo, L. J. (1991). Epidemiology of acquired immunodeficiency syndrome and human immunodeficiency virus infection in adolescents. *Journal of Pediatric Infectious Diseases, 10*, 322–328.

Havens, J. H., Whitaker, A. H., Feldman, J. F., & Ehrnhardt, A. A. (1994). Psychiatric morbity in school-age children with congenital human immunodeficiency virus infection. *Journal of Developmental and Behavioral Pediatrics, 15*, 518–525.

Hittelman, J. (1990). Neurodevelopmental aspects of HIV infection. In P. B. Kozlowski, D. A. Snider, P. M. Vietze, & H. M. Wisneiwski (Eds.), *Brain in pediatric AIDS* (pp. 64–71). Basel: Karger.

Hittelman, J., Nelson, N., Shah, V., Gong, J., & Peluso, F. S. (1993). Neurodevelopmental disabilities in infants born to HIV-infected mothers. *The AIDS Reader, July/August*, 126–132.

Italian Register for HIV Infection in Children. (1994). Features of children perinatally infected with HIV-1 surviving longer than 5 years. *Lancet, 343*, 191–195.

Krasinski, K. (1994). Bacterial infections. In P. A. Pizzo & C. M. Wilfert (Eds.), *Pediatric AIDS* (2nd ed., pp. 241–253). Baltimore: Williams & Wilkins.

Kure, K., Llena, J. F., Lyman, W. D., Soeiro, R., Weidenheim, K. M., Hirano, A., & Dickson, D. (1991). Human immunodeficiency virus1 infection of the nervous system. *Human Pathology, 22*, 700–710.

Landesman, S. H., Kalish, L. A., Burns, D. N., Minkoff, H., Fox, H. E., Zorrilla, C., Garcia, P., Fowler, M. G., Mofenson, L., Tuomala, R., & Women and Infants Transmission Study. (1996). Obstetrical factors and the transmission of human immunodeficiency virus type 1 from mother to child. *New England Journal of Medicine, 334*(25), 1617–1623.

Levenson, R., Mellins, C., Zawadzki, R., Kairam, R., & Stein, Z. (1992). Cognitive assessment of human immunodeficiency virus-exposed children. *American Journal of Diseases of Children, 146*, 1479–1483.

Lifschitz, M., Hanson, C., Wilson, G., & Shearer, W. T. (1989). Behavioral changes in children with human immunodeficiency virus (HIV) infection [Abstract No. TBP 175]. *Proceedings of the V International Conference on AIDS* (Vol. 1, pp. 316), Montreal, Canada.

Lipton, S. A. (1992). Models of neuronal injury in AIDS: another role for the NMDA receptor? *Trends in Neuroscience, 15*, 75–79.

Lobato, M. N., Caldwell, M. B., Ng, P., Oxtoby, M. J., & Pediatric Spectrum of Disease Clinical Consortium. (1995). Encephalopathy in children with perinatally acquired human immunodeficiency virus infection. *Journal of Pediatrics, 126*, 710–715.

Lord, D., Danoff, J., & Smith, M. (1995). Motor assessment of infants with human immunodeficiency virus infection: A retrospective review of multiple cases. *Pediatric Physical Therapy, 7*, 9–13.

Loveland, K. A., & Stehbens, J. A. (1990). Early neurodevelopmental signs of HIV infection in children and adolescents. In P. B. Kozlowski, D. A. Snider, P. M. Vietze, & H. M. Wisneiwski (Eds.), *Brain in pediatric AIDS* (pp. 72–79). Basel: Karger.

Loveland, K. A., Stehbens, J., Contant, C., Bordeaux, J. D., Sirois, P., Bell, T. E., & Hill, S. (1994). Hemophilia growth and development study: Baseline neurodevelopmental findings. *Journal of Pediatric Psychology, 19*, 223–239.

Masliah, E., Achim, C. L., Ge, N., De Teresa, R., & Wiley, C. A. (1994). Cellular neuropathology in HIV encephalitis. *Research Publications of the Association for Research in Nervous and Mental Disorders, 72*, 119–31.

Mayaux, M. J., Blanche, S., Rouzioux, C., Le Chenadec, J., Chambrin, V., Firtion, G., Allemon, M., Vilmer, E., Vigneron, N. C., Tricoire, J., Guillot, F., Courpotin, C., & French Pediatric HIV Infection Study Group. (1995). Maternal factors associated with perinatal HIV-1 transmission: The French cohort sutdy. 7 years of follow-up observation. *Journal of Acquired Immune Deficiency Syndromes and Human Retrovirology, 8*, 188–194.

McCarthy, D. (1972). *McCarthy Scales of Children's Abilities.* San Antonio, TX: Psychological Corporation.

McKinney, R. E., Johnson, G. M., Stanley, K., Yong, F., Keller, A., O'Donnell, K. J., Brouwers, P., Mitchell, W., Yogev, R., Wara, D. W., Wiznia, A., & Spector, S. (1998). A randomized study of combined zidovudine-lamivudine versus didanosine monotherapy in children with symptomatic therapy-naive HIV-1 infection. *Journal of Pediatrics, 133*, 500–508.

McKinney, R. E., Maha, M. A., Connor, E. M., Feinberg, J., Scott, G. B., Wulfsohn, M., McIntosh, K., Borkowsky, W., Modlin, J. F., Weintrub, P., O'Donnell, K., Gelber, R. D., Rogers, G. K., Lehrman, S. N., & Wilfert, C. M. (1991). A multicenter trial of oral zidovudine in children with advanced human immunodeficiency virus disease. *New England Journal of Medicine, 324*(15), 1018–1025.

Merrill, J. E., & Chen, I. S. Y. (1991). HIV-1, macrophages, glial cells, and cytokines in AIDS nervous system disease. *Federation of American Societies for Experimental Biology Journal 5*, 2391–2397.

Mintz, M. (1994). Clinical comparison of adult and pediatric neuroAIDS. *Advances in Neuroimmunology, 4*, 207–221.

Mintz, M., Tardieu, M., Hoyt, L., McSherry, G., Mendelson, J., & Oleske, J. (1996). Levodopa therapy improves motor function in HIV-infected children with extrapyramidal syndromes. *Neurology, 47*, 1583–1585.

Mirsky, A. F., Anthony, B. J., Duncan, C. C., Ahearn, M. B., & Kellam, S. G. (1991). Analysis of the elements of attention: A neuropsychological approach. *Neuropsychology Review, 2*, 109–145.

Mitchell, W. G., Nelson, M. D., Contant, C. F., Bale, J. F., Wilson, D. A., Bohan, T. P., & Fernstermacher, M. J. (1993). Effects of human immunodeficiency virus and immune status on magnetic resonance imaging of the brain in hemophilic subjects: Results from hemophilic growth and development study. *Pediatrics, 91*, 742–746.

Moses, A. V., Stenglein, S. G., Strussenberg, J. G., Wehrly, K., Chesebro, B., & Nelson, J. A. (1996). Sequences regulating tropism of human immunodeficiency virus type 1 for brain capillary endothelial cells map to a unique region on the viral genome. *Journal of Virology, 70*, 3401–3406.

Moss, H. A., Brouwers, P., Wolters, P. L., Wiener, L., Hersh, S., & Pizzo, P. A. (1994). The development of a Q-sort behavioral rating procedure for pediatric HIV patients. *Journal of Pediatric Psychology, 19*(1), 27–46.

Moss, H. A., Nannis, E. D., & Poplack, D. G. (1981). The effects of prophylactic treatment of the central nervous system on the intellectual functioning of children with acute lymphocytic leukemia. *American Journal of Medicine, 71*, 47–52.

Moss, H. A., Wolters, P. L., Brouwers, P., Bartels Kuster, C., Hersh, S. P., & Pizzo, P. A. (1999). *Comparison of HIV-infected children and their uninfected siblings on the Conners Parent Rating Scales*. Manuscript submitted for publication.

Moss, H. A., Wolters, P. L., Brouwers, P., Hendricks, M. L., & Pizzo, P. A. (1996). Impairment of expressive behavior in pediatric HIV-infected patients with evidence of CNS disease. *Journal of Pediatric Psychology, 21*(3), 379–400.

Mueller, B. U., Nelson, R. P., Sleasman, J., Zuckerman, J., Heath-Chiozzi, M., Steinberg, S. M., Balis, F. M., Brouwers, P., Hsu, A., Saulis, R., Sei, S., Wood, L. V., Zeichner, S., Katz, T.K., Highham, C., Aker, D., Edgerly, M., Jarosinski, P., Serchuck, L., Whitcup, S. M., Pizzuit, D., & Pizzo, P. A. (1998). A phase I/II study of the protease inhibitor Ritonavir in children with HIV infection. *Pediatrics, 101*(3), 335–343.

Mueller, B. U., Sleasman, J., Nelson, R. P., Smith, S., Deutsch, P. J., Ju, W., Steinberg, S. M., Balis, F. M., Jarosinski, P. F., Brouwers, P., Mistry, G., Winchell, G., Zwerski, S., Sei, S., Wood, L. V., Zeichner, S., & Pizzo, P. A. (1998). A phase I/II study of the protease inhibitor Indinavir in children with HIV infection. *Pediatrics, 102*(1), 101–109.

Neisser, U., Boodoo, G., Bouchard, T. J., Boykin, A. W., Brody, N., Ceci, S. J., Halpern, D. F., Loehlin, J. C., Perloff, R., Sternberg, R. J., & Urbina, S. (1996). Intelligence: Knowns and unknowns. *American Psychologist, 51*(2), 77–101.

Nozyce, M., Hittelman, J., Muenz, L., Durako, S. J., Fischer, M. L., & Willoughby, A. (1994). Effect of perinatally acquired human immunodeficiency virus infection on neurodevelopmment in children during the first two years of life. *Pediatrics, 94*(6), 883–891.

Parks, R. A. (1994). Occupational therapy with children who are HIV positive. *Developmental Disabilities, 4*, 5–6.

Perez, L. A., Wolters, P. L., Moss, H. A., & Brouwers, P. (1998). Verbal learning and memory in children with HIV infection [Abstract]. *Journal of NeuroVirology, 4*(3), 362.

Pizzo, P., Butler, K., Balis, F., Brouwers, P., Hawkins, M., Eddy, J., Einloth, M., Falloon, J., Husson, R., Jarosinski, P., Meer, J., Moss, H., Poplack, D., Santacroce, S., Wiener, L., & Wolters, P. (1990). Dideoxycytidine alone and in an alternating schedule with zidovudine in children with symptomatic human immunodeficiency virus infection. *Journal of Pediatrics, 117*, 799–808.

Pizzo, P., Eddy, J., Falloon, J., Balis, F., Murphy, R., Moss, H., Wolters, P., Brouwers, P., Jarosinski, P., Rubin, M., Broder, S., Yarchoan, R., Brunetti, A., Maha, M., Nusinoff-Lehrman, S., & Poplack, D. (1988). Effect of continuous intravenous infusion of zidovudine (AZT) in children with symptomatic HIV infection. *New England Journal of Medicine, 319*(14), 889–896.

Pizzo, P., & Wilfert, C. (1990). Treatment considerations for children with HIV infection. In P. Pizzo & C. Wilfert (Eds.), *Pediatric AIDS: The challenge of HIV infection in infants, children, and adolescents* (pp. 478–494). Baltimore: Williams & Wilkins.

Pizzo, P., & Wilfert, C. (1994). Antiretroviral therapy for infection due to human immunodeficiency virus in children. *Clinical Infectious Diseases, 19*, 177–196.

Pollack, H., Kuchuk, A., Cowan, L., Hacimamutoglu, S., Glasberg, H., David, R., Krasinski, K., Borkowsky, W., & Oberfield, S. (1996). Neurodevelopment, growth, and viral load in HIV-infected infants. *Brain, Behavior, and Immunity, 10,* 298–312.

Pratt, R. D., Nichols, S., McKinney, N., Kwok, S., Dankner, W. M., & Spector, S. A. (1996). Virologic markers of human immunodeficiency virus type 1 in cerebrospinal fluid of infected children. *Journal of Infectious Diseases, 174,* 288–293.

Pressman, H. (1992). Communication disorders and dysphagia in pediatric AIDS. *ASHA, 34*(1), 45–47.

Roelofs, K., Wolters, P., Fernandez-Carol, C., van der Vlugt, H., Moss, H., & Brouwers, P. (1996). Impairments in expressive emotional language in children with symptomatic HIV infection: Relation to brain abnormalities and immune function. *Journal of the International Neuropsychological Society, 2*(3), 193.

Schmitt, F., Bigley, J., McKinnis, R., Logue, P., Evans, R., Drucker, J., & AZT Collaboration Group. (1988). Neuropsychological outcome of zidovudine (AZT) treatment of patients with AIDS and AIDS-related complex. *New England Journal of Medicine, 319*(24), 1573–1578.

Scott, G. B., Hutto, C., Makuch, R. W., Mastrucci, M. T., O'Connor, T., Mitchell, C. D., Trapido, E. J., & Parks, W. P. (1989). Survival in children with perinatally acquired human immunodeficiency virus type 1 infection. *New England Journal of Medicine, 321*(26), 1791–1796.

Scott, G. S., & Layton, T. L. (1997). Epidemiological principles in studies of infectious disease outcomes: Pediatric HIV as a model. *Journal of Communication Disorders, 30,* 303–324.

Sei, S., Kleiner, D. E., Kopp, J. B., Chandra, R., Klotman, P. E., Yarchoan, R., Pizzo, P. A., & Mitsuya, H. (1994). Quantitative analysis of viral burden in tissues from adults and children with symptomatic human immunodeficiency virus type 1 infection assessed by polymerase chain reaction. *Journal of Infectious Diseases, 170,* 325–333.

Sei, S., Saito, K., Stewart, S. K., Crowley, J. S., Brouwers, P., Kleiner, D. E., Katz, D. A., Pizzo, P. A., & Heyes, M. P. (1995). Increased HIV-1 DNA content and quinolinic acid concentration in brain tissues obtained from AIDS patients with HIV-encephalopathy. *Journal of Infectious Diseases, 172,* 638–647.

Sei, S., Stewart, S. K., Farley, M., Mueller, B. U., Lane, J. R., Robb, M. L., Brouwers, P., & Pizzo, P. A. (1996). Evaluation of HIV-1 RNA levels in cerebrospinal fluid and viral resistance to Zidovudine in children with HIV-encephalopathy. *Journal of Infectious Diseases, 174,* 1200–1206.

Shah, S. S., Zimmerman, R. A., Rorke, L. B., & Vezina, L. G. (1996). Cerebrovascular complications of HIV in children. *American Journal of Neuroradiology, 17,* 1913–1917.

Sharer, L. R. (1992). Pathology of HIV-1 infection of the central nervous system: A review. *Journal of Neuropathology and Experimental Neurology, 51,* 3–11.

Sidtis, J. J., Gatsonis, C., Price, R. W., Singer, E. J., Collier, A. C., Richman, D. D., Hirsch, M. S., Schaerf, F. W., Fischl, M. A., Kieburtz, K., Simpson, D., Koch, M. A., Feinberg, J., & Dafni, U. (1993). Zidovudine treatment of the AIDS dementia complex: Results of a placebo-controlled trial. *Annals of Neurology, 33,* 343–349.

Sirois, P. A., & Hill, S. D. (1993). Developmental change associated with human immunodeficiency virus infection in school-age children with hemophilia. *Developmental Neuropsychology, 9*(3 & 4), 177–197.

Skoraszewski, M., Ball, J., & Mikulka, P. (1991). Neuropsychological functioning of HIV-infected males. *Journal of Clinical and Experimental Neuropsychology, 13,* 278–290.

Smith, M. L., Minden, D., Nteley, C., Read, S. E., King, S. M., & Blanchette, V. (1997). Longitudinal investigation of neuropsychological functioning in children and adolescents with hemophilia and HIV infection. *Developmental Neurospychology, 13*(1), 69–85.

Swales, T. P., Scott, G. B., & Cohen, D. (1990, June). *Neurocognitive functioning among infants exposed to prenatally to HIV.* Paper presented at the International Conference on AIDS, San Francisco.

Tardieu, M., Blanche, W., & Brunelle, F. (1991). Cerebral magnetic resonance imaging studies in HIV-1 infected children born to seropositive mothers [Abstract]. *Neuroscience of HIV-1 infection* (p. 60). Padova, Italy: Satellite Conference of Seventh International Conference on AIDS.

Tardieu, M., Mayaux, M., Seibel, N., Funck-Brentano, I., Straub, E., Teglas, J., & Blanche, S. (1995). Cognitive assessment of school-age children infected with maternally transmitted human immunodeficiency virus type 1. *Pediatrics, 126*(3), 375–379.

Tersmette, M., Gruters, R. A., de Wolf, F., deGoede, R. E., Lange, J. M., Schellekens, P. T., Goudsmit, J., Huisman, H. G., & Miedema, F. (1989). Evidence for a role of virulent human immunodeficiency virus (HIV) variants in the pathogenesis of acquired immunodeficiency syndrome: Studies on sequential HIV isolates. *Journal of Virology, 63*(5), 2118–2125.

Tornatore, C., Chandra, R., Berger, J. R., & Major, E. O. (1994). HIV-1 infection of subcortical astrocytes in the pediatric central nervous system. *Neurology, 44,* 481–487.

Tornatore, C., Meyers, K., Atwood, W., Conant, K., & Major, E. O. (1994). Temporal patterns of human immunodeficiency virus type 1 transcripts in human fetal astrocytes. *Journal of Virology, 68,* 93–102.

Tovo, P. A., de Martino, M., Gabiano, C., Cappello, N., D'Elia, R., Loy, A., Plebani, A., Zuccotti, G. V., Dallacasa, P., Ferraris, G., Caselli, D., Fundaró, C., D'Argenio, P., Galli, L., Principi, N., Stegagno, M., Ruga, E., Palomba, E., & Children, Italian Register for HIV Infection in Children. (1992). Prognostic factors and survival in children with perinatal HIV-1 infection. *Lancet, 339,* 1249–1253.

Tuma, J. M., & Appelbaum, A. S. (1980). Reliability and practice effects of WISC-R IQ estimates in a normal population. *Educational and Psychological Measurement, 40,* 671–678.

Ultmann, M. H., Diamond, G. W., Ruff, H. A., Belman, A. L., Novick, B. E., Rubinstein, A., & Cohen, H. J. (1987). Developmental abnormalities in children with acquired immunodeficiency syndrome (AIDS): A follow up study. *International Journal of Neuroscience, 32,* 661–667.

Van Gorp, W., Miller, E., Satz, P., & Visscher, B. (1989). Neuropsychological performance in HIV-1 immunocompromised patients: A preliminary report. *Journal of Clinical and Experimental Neuropsychology, 11,* 763–773.

Vreugdenhil, H., Brouwers, P., Wolters, P., Bakker, D., & Moss, H. (1997). Spontaneous eye blinking, a measure of dopaminergic function, in children with acquired immunodeficiency syndrome. *Archives of Pediatric and Adolescent Medicine, 151,* 1025–1032.

Wechsler, D. (1991). *Wechsler Intelligence Scale for Children—3rd edition.* San Antonio, TX: Psychological Corporation.

Whitt, J. K., Hooper, S. R., Tennison, M. B., Robertson, W. T., Gold, S. H., Burchinal, M., Wells, R., McMillan, C., Whaley, R. A., Combest, J., & Hall, C. (1993). Neuropsychologic functioning of human immunodeficiency virus-infected children with hemophilia. *Journal of Pediatrics, 122,* 52–59.

Wiener, L., Moss, H., Davidson, R., & Fair, C. (1992). Pediatrics: The emerging psychosocial challenges of the AIDS epidemic. *Child and Adolescent Social Work Journal, 9*(5), 381–407.

Wiley, C. A., Belman, A. L., Dickson, D. W., Rubinstein, A., & Nelson, J. A. (1990). Human immunodeficiency virus within the brains of children with AIDS. *Clinical Neuropathology, 9,* 1–6.

Wolters, P. L., & Brouwers, P. (1998). Evaluation of neurodevelopmental deficits in children with HIV infection. In H. E. Gendelman, S. Lipton, L. Epstein, & S. Swindells (Eds.), *Neurological and neuropsychiatric manifestations of HIV-1 infection* (pp. 425–442). Philadelphia: Chapman & Hall.

Wolters, P. L., & Brouwers, P. (1999). Neurodevelopmental function and assessment of children with HIV-1 infection. In S. Zeichner & J. Read (Eds.), *Handbook of pediatric HIV care* (pp. 210–227). Philadelphia, PA: Lippincott Williams & Wilkins.

Wolters, P. L., Brouwers, P., Civitello, L., & Moss, H. (1997). Receptive and expressive language function of children with symptomatic HIV infection and relationship with disease parameters: A longitudinal 24-month follow-up study. *AIDS, 11,* 1135–1144.

Wolters, P. L., Brouwers, P., Moss, H. A., & Pizzo, P. A. (1994). Adaptive behavior of children with symptomatic HIV infection before and after zidovudine therapy. *Journal of Pediatric Psychology, 19*(1), 47–61.

Wolters, P. L., Brouwers, P., Moss, H. A., & Pizzo, P. A. (1995). Differential receptive and expressive language functioning of children with symptomatic HIV disease and relation to CT scan brain abnormalities. *Pediatrics, 95*(1), 112–119.

Wolters, P. L., Roelofs, K., & Fernandez-Hall, C. (1995). *Rating Scale of Expressive Emotional Language and Behavior.* Unpublished manuscript, National Cancer Institute, Bethesda, MD.

Wolters, P. L., Roelofs, K., Fernandez-Hall, C., Moss, H. A., & Brouwers, P. (1999). *Expressive emotional language impairments in children with symptomatic HIV infection: Relation with brain abnormalities and immune function.* Manuscript submitted for publication.

Yarchoan, R., Berg, G., Brouwers, P., Fischl, M., Spitzer, A., Wichman, A., Grafman, J., Thomas, R., Safai, B., Brunetti, A., Perno, C., Schnidt, P., Larson, S., Myers, C., & Broder, S. (1987). Response of human immunodeficiency virus-associated neurological disease to 3′azido-3′deoxythymidine. *Lancet, 1,* 132–135.

Yarchoan, R., Pluda, J. M., Thomas, R. V., Mitsuya, H., Brouwers, P., Wyvill, K., Hartman, N., Johns, D. G., & Broder, S. (1990). Long-term toxicity/activity profile of 2′,3′-dideoxyinosine in AIDS or AIDS-related complex. *Lancet, 336,* 526–529.

CHAPTER SEVEN

Insulin-Dependent Diabetes Mellitus

JOANNE ROVET

CHERYL FERNANDES

Insulin-dependent diabetes mellitus (IDDM) is one of the commonest chronic illnesses of childhood. In North America, IDDM affects about 1 in 600 children below the age of 12 (Traisman, 1980), while in some countries such as Finland, the incidence can be as high as 1 in 250 (LaPorte et al., 1985; Reunanen, Akerblom, & Kaar, 1982). Recently, there has been the added concern that the incidence of diabetes in children may in fact be increasing worldwide (Gardner, Bingley, Sawtell, Weeks, & Gale [the Bart's–Oxford Study Group] 1997). Thus, a major recent thrust in diabetes research is toward its prevention; there are presently several international clinical prevention trials underway. These are aimed at using therapeutic agents to prevent diabetes in high-risk individuals, who typically are the siblings of children already affected by diabetes.

IDDM is caused by the autoimmune destruction of pancreatic beta cells in genetically predisposed individuals (Atkinson & Maclaren, 1994). It is triggered by an environmental event such as an infection or exposure to an antigen. One such antigen that has received considerable attention recently is cows' milk protein, which is directly associated with increased risk of diabetes (Karjalainen et al., 1992). The onset of diabetes is a relatively slow and insidious process that extends over a number of years, while the beta cells are being destroyed. The symptoms of diabetes, which include polydypsia (thirst), polyuria (frequent urination), and fatigue, and in some children more severe illness, only become manifested once the number of beta cells becomes inadequate.

Beta cells are critical for life because they are responsible for the production of insulin, a hormone that is essential for glucose metabolism. Without insulin, glucose accumulates in the urine and bloodstream as the body draws on other sources of energy until it eventually starves to death. Since the discovery of insulin in 1922 (Banting, 1929), individuals with IDDM have been able to lead long and productive lives with exogenous insulin therapy, which requires several daily insulin injections. As the dose of insulin has to be closely regulated with food intake and activity levels, diabetes is a relatively complex disease that requires assiduous and continuous monitoring for its close control. However, once diabetes is stabilized, children with IDDM are generally healthy and develop normally, with the exception of the need to follow a tedious and relentless treatment regimen for the rest of their lives.

Unfortunately, levels of insulin administered exogenously never perfectly mimic normal physiological insulin production. As a result, children with IDDM are constantly exposed to perturbations of blood glucose and insulin outside the normal range. When blood glucose levels are above normal limits, this is known as hyperglycemia, and below normal limits, hypoglycemia. During hyperglycemia, insulin levels are correspondingly low and, conversely, during hypoglycemia they are correspondingly high. A number of complications are associated with both high and low glucose levels and with high and low insulin levels, all of which can affect a number of different organ systems including the central nervous system (CNS). Diabetes has been shown to have both transient and permanent effects on the brain, and these are associated with a variety of neuropsychological sequelae (Holmes, 1990). As considerable brain development occurs throughout childhood and into adolescence, pediatric patients with diabetes are at elevated risk of neurocognitive impairment from this disease.

Some diabetes-related events that are quite severe affect the brain permanently. For example, the seizures associated with severe hypoglycemia, which are especially prevalent in very young children with diabetes (Bergada, Suissa, Dufresne, & Shiffrin, 1989; Casparie & Elving, 1985; Davis & Jones, 1998), lead to impaired psychomotor efficiency and poorer attention and memory (Rovet, Ehrlich, & Hoppe, 1987; Ryan, Vega, & Drash, 1985). While the effects of other diabetes-related events may be less severe, they are nonetheless cumulative and so associated with poorer outcome, most notably in the language domain. Still other events are transient, but may affect the amount of material retained during class time, or lead to greater school absence due to frequent clinic visits, hospitalizations, and increased rates of illness (Ryan, Longstreet, & Morrow, 1985). However, the latter does not fully explain why diabetes affects cognition to a greater degree than diseases with similar numbers of clinic appointments and missed school (Fowler, Johnson, & Atkinson, 1985). Finally, there is also the effect of having a chronic disease itself, which impacts on the child's psychological well-being and psychosocial development and so constricts neurocognitive development.

Not only can diabetes impede neurocognitive functioning, poorer cognitive abilities can adversely affect diabetes management. As adequate management of diabetes requires the satisfactory performance of a number of mental activities (e.g., perceptual abilities, memory, fine motor skills, and organizational abilities), it is necessary that adequate levels of these skills be maintained. However, one of the ironies of diabetes is that assiduous control to prevent later physical complications (e.g., nephropathy, retinopathy) also increases the risk of hypoglycemia, which in turn affects cognitive functioning in children (Bjorgaas, Gimse, Vik, & Sand, 1997; Golden et al., 1989; Rovet et al., 1987) and adults (Langan, Deary, Hepburn, & Frier, 1991; MacLeod, Hepburn, & Frier, 1993). Thus, diabetes involves a vicious cycle whereby it impairs cognition, and poorer cognitive skills affect diabetes. This issue is especially critical later in life because diabetes accelerates the aging process and normal cognitive decline (Ryan & Williams, 1993). As cognitive impairments can impede diabetes management, diabetes complications are further exacerbated and outcome is further deteriorated in the elderly (Meneilly, Cheung, & Tuokko, 1994). While parents are the primary caregivers of children with diabetes, the issue of cognitive dysfunction may be less relevant for diabetes management; however, it does still affect children's school performance and quality of life.

Over the past several decades, a number of studies have been conducted on children with diabetes. This chapter will serve to review the literature on how diabetes affects children's cognitive abilities. It will also highlight relevant studies from our own research program. Three issues will be addressed in particular: (1) how diabetes affects children's cognitive abilities and school performance; (2) how different diabetes-related factors affect specific abilities, which has important implications for treating diabetes in childhood; and (3) how cognitive abilities and other behavioral characteristics including temperament affect diabetes control.

OVERVIEW OF DIABETES MANIFESTATIONS

In diabetes, morbidity and mortality are increased, and adverse effects can arise from either hyperglycemic or hypoglycemic states. Typically, these effects were thought to reflect abnormal glucose levels; however, some complications have more recently been linked directly to abnormal insulin levels, particularly the role of insulin in the CNS, where it is involved in neurotransmitter pathway regulation (McCall, 1992).

Hyperglycemia

Hyperglycemia occurs when glucose availability exceeds glucose needs. Hyperglycemia affects a number of metabolic systems including glucagon and growth hormone secretion, the breakdown of fats, and catecholamine release. In normal individuals, hyperglycemia stimulates increased insulin production in order to bring about a return to homeostasis. However, among patients with diabetes who receive insulin exogenously, homeostasis cannot be achieved as easily. As a result, diabetes increases the risk of macrovascular disturbances such as heart disease, stroke, and peripheral vascular occlusion leading to limb amputations, and it also leads to microvascular changes in the kidney (nephropathy), eye (retinopathy), and autonomic and peripheral nervous systems (neuropathy). In fact, diabetes is one of the leading causes of heart and kidney disease, as well as blindness. As diabetes complications are associated with chronic blood glucose elevations over time, such complications do not normally become evident until much later in life, although recent studies suggest they may begin during puberty (Lindgren, Dahlquist, Efendic, Persson, & Skottner, 1990; Rogers et al., 1986). As a result of elevated blood glucose levels associated with increased gonadotropin and sex-steroid levels and increased insulin resistance at this time (Amiel et al., 1991; Bloch, Clemons, & Sperling, 1987; Caprio et al., 1989), puberty is thought to trigger the onset of complications (Kostraba et al., 1989). Indeed, evidence is now accumulating showing mild manifestations of diabetes-related complications in adolescent patients (Donaghue et al., 1993; Krolewski, Laffel, Krolewski, Quinn, & Warram, 1995; Lawson, Sochett, Chait, Balfe, & Daneman, 1996).

A number of studies have shown that brain function is impaired in both children (Davis, Soong, Byrne, & Jones, 1996) and adults (Skenazy & Bigler, 1984). Animal models and human evidence from neuropathological and neuroimaging studies also demonstrate that brain changes arise from glucose toxicity associated with hyperglycemia. These changes include degeneration of ganglion cells, demyelination, neuronal damage, and biochemical changes (McCall & Figlewicz, 1997; Merali & Ahmad, 1985). Also, hyperglycemia affects cell signaling and rates of neurotransmission.

Prolonged severe hyperglycemia is associated with poor compliance, and nonadherence can lead to a serious and debilitating condition known as diabetic ketoacidosis (DKA). DKA is a chemical imbalance that leads to acute illness, unconsciousness, and coma and causes permanent CNS dysfunction (Tsalikian, Daneman, Becker, Crumrine, & Drash, 1980) and death ultimately.

Hypoglycemia

Hypoglycemia occurs when blood glucose concentrations fall below the normal range. This is caused by a high insulin dosage, inadequate food intake, or prolonged exercise. Hypoglycemia is more common in patients with better than with poorly controlled diabetes (Davis, Keating, Byrne, Russell, & Jones, 1998). When blood glucose levels fall, patients experience physiological reactions such as tremor, weakness, confusion, and lack of concentration, to name a few, which are due to excess secretion of counterregulatory hormones (e.g., epinephrine, cortisol) in response to lowered blood glucose. When hypoglycemia becomes very severe, the patient with diabetes can become unconscious or experience seizures or coma. Severe hypoglycemia, in fact, accounts for about 3–4% of IDDM-related deaths. Treatment of hypoglycemia requires an immediate glucose supplement (e.g., juice, candy).

Severe hypoglycemia affects between 6 and 16% of children yearly (Bergada et al., 1989) and as many as 2% over a 3-month period (Dammacco et al., 1998). About 31% of children experience severe hypoglycemia at some time during childhood (Daneman et al., 1989). A greater number of severe hypoglycemic incidents are reported during spring and summer months, and this is attributed to increased exercise during the warmer weather (Daneman, Frank, Perlman, Tamm, & Ehrlich, 1989). Severe hypoglycemia is also common during sleep (Porter, Keating, Byrne, & Jones, 1997). Children who experience severe hypoglycemia at a younger age (below 5 years of age) are thought to be at greater risk for brain damage (Eeg-Olofsson & Petersen, 1966) and permanent neurocognitive impairment (Goldstein, England, Hess, Rawlings, & Walker, 1981). Very young children who experience moderate hypoglycemia frequently also show permanent selective neurocognitive deficits (Golden et al., 1989).

In some individuals with diabetes, the physiological responses to hypoglycemia are obtunded, which is known as hypoglycemia unawareness. As a result of frequent hypoglycemia, these individuals fail to experience the physiological warning signs of a forthcoming episode and so do not take corrective measures to counteract it. This in turn increases the risk of very severe hypoglycemia and the associated brain damage (Amiel, 1996; Tribl et al., 1996) or cognitive impairment and brain dysfunction (Amiel & Gale, 1993).

As a result of two very large-scale clinical trials conducted on adults and older adolescents in North America and Sweden (Diabetes Control and Complications Trial Research Group, 1993; Reichard, Berglund, Britz, Levander, & Rosenqvist, 1991), the benefits of intensive diabetes management (i.e., three or more daily insulin injections) for reducing complications associated with hyperglycemia have been firmly established. As a consequence, this mode of therapy is now prescribed regularly for most individuals with diabetes. However, for the pediatric population the virtues of intensive therapy are still undecided and of great concern, given the potential for brain damage from hypoglycemia. Although studies of neuropsychological outcome in adult patients receiving intensive diabetes therapy have not shown any associated neurocognitive deterioration, it is not clear whether children are similarly affected, as their brains are continuing to develop during this period. (Further, there are a number of expressed methodological concerns about the validity of the adult findings; e.g., see Deary & Frier, 1996.) Children with seizures from hypoglycemia demonstrate abnormalities in brain function (Auer & Siesjo, 1988; Haumont, Dorchy, &

Pelc, 1979; Soltesz & Acsadi, 1989), but the long-term impact of these seizures has not been adequately addressed in empirical research, although work currently in our laboratory is attempting to deal with this issue (Rovet & Ehrlich, 1999).

NEUROCOGNITIVE SEQUELAE OF DIABETES IN CHILDHOOD

Originally diabetologists believed that children with diabetes had at least average intelligence, if not above average (Grishaw, West, & Smith, 1939), and that they performed adequately in school (Weil & Ack, 1964). With the exception of an early study by Shirley and Greer (1940), most earlier papers reported IQ levels well within the normal range (Brown, 1938; Kubany, Danowski, & Moses, 1956; McGavin, Schultz, Peden, & Bowen, 1940). However, the majority were limited methodologically due to lack of premorbid measurements, use of poor measures or global indices only, sampling difficulties, small sample sizes, and no control groups. It is interesting to note that Shirley and Greer, the only early research group to report poorer outcome, in fact tested a very large group of 155 patients.

With the exception of a controlled study by Ack, Miller, and Weil in 1961 showing that children who developed diabetes at an early age did poorly on intelligence tests, the bulk of research showing diabetes-related neurocognitive sequelae dates back only to the mid-1980s. In 1984, Ryan and his associates reported that adolescents with diabetes evidenced more difficulty on selective neurocognitive tests than did their siblings and showed an increasing number of impairments with age (Ryan, Vega, Longstreet, & Drash, 1984). These investigators subsequently found the patients who developed their diabetes prior to age 5 were at greater risk of impairment than were those whose diabetes developed later, who did not differ from controls (Ryan, Vega, & Drash, 1985). Contemporaneously, Holmes and Richman (1985) reported that children with both early age of onset and longer disease durations were more affected. In a review of nine studies up to 1993, Rovet, Ehrlich, Czuchta, and Akler (1993) reported that children with diabetes achieved a mean IQ level of 106.1, in contrast to controls who achieved 111.3. As studies indicate no evidence of any intellectual impairment predating illness (Kovacs, Goldston, Iyengar, 1992; Northam, 1996; Northam, Anderson, Werther, Adler, & Andrewes, 1995; Rovet, Ehrlich, & Czuchta, 1990), the intellectual functioning of children with diabetes appears to have been reduced by their disease.

In recent years, a number of studies have been conducted on children and adolescent samples of patients with diabetes. The findings show that various diabetes-related factors or events compromise cognitive functioning in multiple domains. We review the findings by ability domain.

Verbal Skills

Deficits in the verbal domain of cognitive functioning have been noted in pediatric diabetes patients (Northam, Bawden, Anderson, & Court, 1992; Hagen et al., 1990; Rovet et al., 1988b; Ryan et al., 1984). Word knowledge and general store of information are the most severely affected, while language difficulties per se are not usually seen. Ryan (1990) has attributed the verbal deficits in older diabetic children to external factors that compromise the child's capacity to learn at school, including erratic school attendance, attentional inconsistencies in class related to continuous alterations in blood glucose levels, and the emotional impact of the disease itself as an inhibiting factor on cognitive development. Unfortunately, there are no detailed studies of specific language abilities in diabetes subjects, including no assessments on preschool children who developed diabetes before their language skills were fully consolidated, or on older children whose abilities were compromised by poor school attendance or decreased attentiveness in the classroom.

Several studies have now indicated that, in diabetes, children's verbal skills deteriorate with duration of illness. Kovacs, Ryan, and Obrosky (1994) followed a group of pediatric patients with diabetes for 6 years and found their verbal abilities declined significantly, whereas their visuospatial abilities improved somewhat from baseline. Similarly, as part of two independent studies, we recently had the opportunity to follow 16 patients with newly diagnosed diabetes over an extended 7-year period. Longitudinal evaluations revealed a decline in their verbal skills, particularly word knowledge. In contrast, their verbal reasoning skills and global knowledge abilities were relatively unaffected, while their visuospatial abilities remained constant (see Figure 7.1). A recent study by Northam (1996) following children from time of diagnosis over a 2-year period showed verbal fluency skills declined in these children. However, it is not clear whether this was due to poorer language or poorer executive processing skills and to what degree baseline testing was lowered by the psychological impact of diagnosis and concurrent illness.

Visuospatial Abilities

Ryan, Vega, and Drash (1985) were the first to observe lower visuospatial ability in adolescent patients whose diabetes had developed at a very early age. Their performance was poorer on tasks of Block Design, Embedded Figures, and Road Map. Rovet et al. (1987) subsequently observed similar deficits in younger patients, particularly girls who developed diabetes at a young age. They were significantly outperformed by their sibling controls on tasks of block construction, copying, and spatial relations. In contrast, Holmes, Dunlap, Chen, and Cornwell, (1992) also found visuospatial diffi-

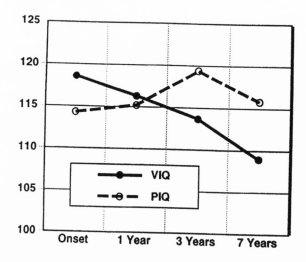

FIGURE 7.1. IQ levels as a function of diabetes duration in children followed prospectively. VIQ, Verbal IQ; PIQ, Performance IQ.

culties, but only among boys with early-onset diabetes. To this date, the gender issue has not been resolved and may be a result of sampling differences, the specific tasks used to assess visuospatial abilities, or a differential psychosocial impact of diabetes on boys and girls at different stages of development (Rovet, Ehrlich, & Hoppe, 1988b).

Holmes, Cornwall, Dunlap, Chen, and Lee (1992) have described an anomalous Wechsler Intelligence Scale for Children—Revised (WISC-R) factor structure in children with IDDM. Typically, three factors characterize children's WISC-R performance (i.e., Verbal Comprehension, Perceptual Organization, and Freedom from Distractibility), but in diabetes four factors were observed. This was because the visuospatial factor was divided in two, with one factor representing visual discrimination and the other, spatial abilities. Holmes and her colleagues attributed this to reduced visual discrimination ability from associated retinal nerve damage diabetes. Using a large sample of prepubertal and pubertal children with and without diabetes, Rovet (in press) reported that diabetes in childhood affects both spatial and perceptual domains of cognitive function.

Recent studies examining children with diabetes over time have generally reported no change in visuospatial abilities (e.g., Kovacs, Goldston, Iyengar, 1992; Northam, 1996; Rovet, in press; Rovet & Ehrlich, 1998), which is inconsistent with the earlier findings showing reduced functioning in this domain (Holmes & Richman, 1985; Rovet et al. 1987; Ryan, Vega, & Drash, 1985). The current lack of effect in visuospatial processing may be attributed to a secular change in treating diabetes with the advent of self-monitoring blood glucose technologies, which allow for better diabetes control. However, the different findings may also reflect the shorter illness durations in the later studies.

Attention

Problems with attention are often recognized by teachers and parents of children with diabetes (Holmes, 1990; Northam et al., 1992; Ryan, 1990). Attention problems are also frequently observed in adults with diabetes (Langan et al., 1991; Ryan, Williams, Finegold, & Orchard, 1993; Wredling, Levander, Adamson, & Lins, 1990). Studies using both clinical tests (Rovet et al., 1987) and laboratory-based instruments (Hagen et al., 1990) have reported that the attentional capacities of diabetes patients are definitely compromised.

Comparing multiple aspects of attentional processing in children with diabetes to controls, Rovet and Alvarez (1997) found that attention was mildly and selectively disrupted by diabetes. Selective attention was weaker in all children with diabetes, whereas focused attention was weaker only in children with early disease onset or seizures from hypoglycemia. The ability to inhibit attention was lower only in children with seizures. The results from a computerized test of attention in addition showed children with a seizure history were more likely to err because they had greater difficulty holding in memory information from a previous item in order to compare it with an upcoming stimulus (Rovet & Alvarez, 1997). Although Northam (1996) reported that attention was not affected by diabetes, her subjects were tested after just 2 years of illness, in contrast to our study, which tested subjects after 3 to 10 years of having diabetes.

Memory and Learning

The effects of diabetes on memory are generally mixed, in part due to the multicomponential nature of this ability and the types of tasks given. In adults with diabetes, few effects if any are seen (Dejgaard et al., 1991; Langan et al., 1991; Ryan et al, 1984; Skenazy & Bigler, 1984), whereas in children subtle impairments are observed, although there are inconsistencies across the studies. For example, Ryan, Vega, and Drash (1985) reported that adolescents with diabetes showed memory deficits in the visual but not the verbal domain, whereas Kovacs et al. (1994) noted that diabetes affected children's verbal memory on tasks of associative and working memory but not recall of prose material. Deficits in short-term or immediate memory have been reported by Ryan et al. (1990) in older but not younger adolescent patients, whereas Northam (1996) observed such deficits in children who had had diabetes for 2 years. Rovet and Ehrlich (1998) reported deficits in short-term memory, but only in children who experienced hypoglycemic seizures. Deficits in long-term or delayed memory tasks have not been observed (Northam, 1996; Rovet & Ehrlich, 1998).

Hagen and his colleagues (1990) explored memory processes systematically in children with diabetes using experimental paradigms. The children used less efficient organization and recall strategies and had a greater "primacy" deficit. The latter indicates that they had more difficulty recalling material from the beginning than the end of an array (Hagen et al., 1990), which suggests more difficulty retaining information on-line, as also observed by Rovet and Ehrlich (1998). However, in a subsequent recent paper aimed at extending these findings, Hagen and his colleagues failed to replicate these effects, although some correlations were noted between certain diabetes variables and selective aspects of performance (Wolters, Yu, Hagen, & Kail, 1996). Therefore, findings from memory studies of children with diabetes suggest some difficulty in initially encoding novel verbal or visual information, whereas recall of semantically meaningful information is unaffected.

Several studies specifically examining verbal learning skills have reported that children with diabetes take longer than normal to learn and are less efficient on learning tasks (Hagen et al., 1990; Northam, 1996; Rovet & Ehrlich, 1998). This suggests diabetes has a mild effect on learning capacity.

Psychomotor Efficiency

On speeded tasks, children with diabetes have been shown to respond slower than normal (Holmes, 1980), although their accuracy is usually preserved (Ryan et al., 1984). Those tasks that are particularly sensitive to diabetes require rapid analysis of visual detail, decision making, and motor responding, as well as verbal fluency.

Executive Functioning

Executive functions refer to the higher-order cognitive skills necessary for purposeful, goal-directed activity. Executive function skills include flexibility, fluency, and planning and are thought to involve the prefrontal cortex (Dennis, 1991). Decreased mental flexibility (Dejgaard et al., 1991; Ryan, Williams, Finegold, & Orchard, 1993; Ryan, Williams, Orchard, & Finegold, 1992; Skenazy & Bigler, 1984) and poorer conceptual reasoning (Franceschi et al., 1984; Skenazy & Bigler, 1984) have been observed among adults with diabetes, while children have been reported to show reduced fluency in addition (Northam, 1996). However, in our analysis of a variety of executive function skills in preadolescent and adolescent subjects with IDDM, no effects were observed in any aspect (Rovet, 1998).

School Achievement

Diabetes is associated with generally poorer scholastic performance (Fowler et al., 1985; Sansbury, Brown, & Meacham, 1997), as well as with underachievement in reading or spelling (Gath, Smith, & Baum, 1980; Holmes & Richman, 1985; Ryan, Longstreet, & Morrow, 1985) and arithmetic (Northam, 1996), and a greater need for special education and remedial help (Anderson et al., 1984; Rovet et al., 1988b). As Rovet et al. (1993) observed some improvement in achievement in children with diabetes over the first 3 years from diagnosis, this suggests that their subsequent underachievement may take a number of years to manifest, if it actually does exist. As well, their performance at baseline, when they were ill and adjusting to the diagnosis, may have been less than optimum.

DIABETES-RELATED FACTORS AND NEUROCOGNITIVE OUTCOME

A large number of studies indicate that poorer outcome in children with diabetes is directly associated with several diabetes-related factors. Early age at onset and seizures from hypoglycemia appear to be greater culprits than hyperglycemic-associated events. The effects appear to be both transient and permanent.

Age at Onset

Children who developed diabetes prior to age 5 are at increased risk of neurocognitive impairment in many domains of function. Primarily affected by early diabetes onset are abilities in perceptual (Ryan, Vega, & Drash, 1985), spatial (Rovet et al., 1987), fine motor (Rovet & Ehrlich, 1998), visual memory (Rovet, in press), verbal learning (Ryan, Vega, & Drash, 1985), verbal fluency (Northam, 1996), and attention (Rovet & Alvarez, 1997) domains. Regarding attention, children with early onset of diabetes also have greater difficulty on tasks of focused and selective attention than children with later onset. As well, verbal abilities are associated with early onset in some (Hagen et al., 1990; Rovet & Ehrlich, 1998) but not in all studies (e.g., Rovet et al., 1988b). The early onset effect has been attributed to manifestations of diabetes on the young developing brain and the increased risk of severe hypoglycemia in younger patients, given the greater difficulty associated with controlling blood glucose levels in very small children (Ryan, 1990).

Duration of Illness

A longer duration of illness in childhood is also associated with poorer outcome in diabetic children (Holmes & Richman, 1985; Sansbury et al., 1997). Verbal skills appear to be more sensitive to duration effects than visuospatial (Kovacs et al., 1994). As shown in Figure 7.1, verbal abilities declined to a greater degree over the first 7 years of diabetes than did visuospatial ones. Duration effects are usually attributed to the cumulative impact of mild hyperglycemia over time.

Hypoglycemia

A number of studies have employed a technique using the insulin-glucose infusion clamp system to examine the direct effects of hypoglycemia on cognitive functioning. While this technique has mostly been used on adult patients with diabetes (e.g., Herold, Polonsky, Cohen, Levy, & Douglas, 1985; Holmes, Hayford, Gonzalez, & Weydert, 1983; Widom & Simonson, 1990), as well as adults without diabetes (Ipp & Forster, 1987; McCrimmon, Deary, Huntly, MacLeod, & Frier, 1996; Mitrakou et al., 1991; Stevens et al., 1989), several investigators have in fact studied children in this way (Davis et al., 1996; Gschwend, Ryan, Atchison, Arslanian, & Becker, 1995; Ryan et al., 1990). The findings indicate that several attentional parameters, namely those reflecting vigilance and the ability to sustain attention over time, are especially sensitive to hypoglycemia. In addition, an inverse relationship exists between the number of attentional demands of a task and the degree to which blood glucose must be experimentally lowered to cause dysfunction (Holmes, Koepke, & Thompson, 1986). As a rule, only a slight degree of hypoglycemia can impair performance on tasks involving several attentional demands, whereas more extreme blood glucose lowering is necessary to affect performance on simple attention tasks that involve only single attentional demands (Holmes, 1990). While these effects are usually transient, Reich et al. (1990) have shown the recovery of attention following hypoglycemia lags behind return to euglycemia (i.e., normal blood glucose levels).

Normally, mild hypoglycemia is seldom associated with permanent deficits unless children are very young when they experience this condition (Golden et al., 1989). In fact, in our prospective study of newly diagnosed patients whose 3-year histories were closely and continuously studied by us, children with more frequent low blood-glucose recordings actually obtained higher scores in the verbal and memory domains (see also Northam et al., 1995). Although this is seemingly counterintuitive, it may be a marker for children having stronger linguistic abilities also better communicating their symptoms to their parents (who were also more adept at reporting these in their child's diabetes diaries). Alternatively, the positive effect of lower blood sugar readings may be a by-product of overall better diabetic control (i.e., less high blood-sugar readings). It is interesting to note that Northam (1996) also found that fewer errors on an executive processing task were associated with lower blood-glucose readings, suggesting that more episodes of mild hypoglycemia may lead to a more cautious decision-making response style.

In contrast to mild hypoglycemia, severe hypoglycemia contributes to a variety of cognitive deficits and poorer arithmetic skills (Rovet, in press), particularly if there were seizures. Seizures from hypoglycemia have been associated with poorer performance on tasks of focused and selective attention, inhibitory control, short-term memory, and visual recognition, as well as poorer verbal, perceptual, and spatial skills (Rovet, in press). In a group of children followed for 7 years prospectively, those most affected by diabetes had a positive seizure history (Rovet & Ehrlich, 1998). The pattern of memory deficit in these children reflected their greater difficulty on tasks of episodic memory, which is known to involve the hippocampus, than on semantic or working memory tasks that involve other surrounding structures (Squire & Zola, 1996) or the frontal lobes. The pattern of memory deficit seen in diabetic children who had hypoglycemic seizures is comparable to that of children with hippocampal damage from other kinds of seizures (Vargha-Khadem et al., 1997). However, the severity may be less in children with diabetes. The possibility of hippocampal dysfunction in diabetes following severe hypoglycemia is not surprising given the abundance of insulin receptors in the hippocampus (Baskin, Figlewicz, Woods, Porte, & Dorsa, 1987; Havrankova, Roth, & Brownstone, 1983) and that the pyramidal layer of the hippocampus (which is important for memory and human learning) is particularly sensitive to hypoglycemia (Brierley, Brown, & Meldrum, 1971).

Hyperglycemia

There is relatively little research on the effects of acute hyperglycemia on cognitive functioning. In fact, studies involving both animal and human evidence show moderate hyperglycemia may actually enhance performance (Gold, Vogt, & Hall, 1986). Two studies have used the glucose-clamp procedure to investigate how transient hyperglycemia affects pediatric patients with diabetes. Davis, Soong, Byrne, and Jones (1996) reported a deterioration in function when blood-glucose levels were between 20 to 30 mmol/liter, whereas Gschwend et al. (1995) found no negative effects of milder elevations in blood glucose (20 mmol/liter), suggesting there may be a glycemic threshold for deteriorating function on certain cognitive tasks. Rovet (in press) reported that performance on tasks of verbal, visuomotor, attention, and executive processing was better when ambient blood-glucose levels during testing were in the higher ranges.

In adults with a history of poor control, neurophysiological and neuroimaging changes (Dejgaard et al., 1991) and cognitive deficits (Lichty & McGill, 1989) are associated with chronic hyperglycemia from a history of poor control. Chronically elevated blood-glucose levels are associated with poorer learning and memory, reduced psychomotor speed, and spatial deficits (Franceschi et al., 1984; Holmes, 1986; Lichty & McGill, 1989; Ryan et al., 1992). These effects may reflect decreased myelin in the cerebral structures that underlie these abilities since *in vitro* studies show that myelin production is impeded in the presence of excess glucose (Vlassara, Brownlee, & Cerami, 1983). In pediatric patients, in whom myelin formation is still occurring well into the second decade of life (Yakovlev & Lecours, 1967), elevations in blood glucose may impede such development.

Rovet and Ehrlich (1997) conducted a study to examine this effect. As it was known that the frontal lobes and reticular formation (which are involved in executive processing and attention) have protracted periods of myelination that extend into adolescence and also that blood-glucose levels are normally elevated during puberty (Bloch et al., 1987; Caprio et al., 1989), it was hypothesized that those brain structures undergoing myelination in pubertal patients would be most affected by diabetes during adolescence. It was also hypothesized that with advancing pubertal development, the difference between nondiabetic and diabetic subjects would increase in attention and executive-processing domains but not in other domains of cognitive function. These predictions were mostly borne out, as there was an increasing differential on most of the attention and executive processing tasks examined and almost none on the others. Figure 7.2, which presents the results for the Matching Familiar Figures Test and the Wisconsin Card Sorting Tasks, shows that the difference between children with diabetes and controls increased with advancing pubertal stage. The only exception on other tasks was a pubertal-status effect on a mental rotation spatial task, which is known to depend heavily on working memory and to involve frontal lobe structures (Cohen et al., 1996; Corballis, 1997).

Severe hyperglycemia leading to DKA definitely affects brain function and causes permanent EEG changes (Tsalikian et al., 1980). However, to our knowledge no studies have as yet reported an association between DKA and specific neurocognitive impairment.

Summary

Diabetes affects cognitive abilities through several different mechanisms that can affect the CNS both transiently and permanently. Among the factors examined, seizures from hypoglycemia appear to have the greatest impact on the later functioning of the child with diabetes. In light of the recent recommendations following the Diabetes Control and Complications Trial (Diabetes Control and Complications Trial Research Group, 1993) DCCT

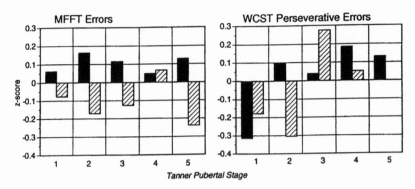

FIGURE 7.2. Test results as a function of pubertal status in adolescents with diabetes. Subjects with diabetes shown with black bars, controls with striped bars. MFFT, Matching Familiar Figures Test; WCST, Wisconsin Card Sorting Test.

study, which supports treating diabetes patients intensively with insulin to minimize or delay later severe physical complications, the risk of seizures from hypoglycemia is increased. While the benefits of intensified therapy for morbidity may outweigh the harms associated with hypoglycemic seizures in adults, this may not be the case in children whose brains are developing (Geffner, 1994; Sperling, 1997). Further study is warranted to determine the specific and long-term consequences of lowered blood-glucose levels in children, particularly if convulsions occur. Given that certain brain structures (e.g., the hippocampus) are especially vulnerable to hypoglycemia (Auer, 1986) and given the importance of such structures for essential cognitive activities (e.g., memory), it is important to discern how hypoglycemic seizures affect neurodevelopment using neuroimaging techniques and clinically sensitive test procedures. As preliminary research comparing directly intensive and conventional insulin therapies shows that selective verbal memory skills are compromised with an intensive approach (Hershey, Bhargava, White, & Craft, 1998), it is important to continue this line of investigation.

THE ROLE OF COGNITIVE ABILITIES AND BEHAVIOR IN DIABETES MANAGEMENT

Diabetes is a complex disease with a complicated treatment regimen that is potentially iatrogenic for neurocognitive functioning, yet these are the neurocognitive skills that are essential for good diabetes control. Optimal compliance and adherence each demand good skills in perceptual, fine motor, mathematical, organizational, attention, and memory areas. Studies with pediatric patients show that those children with better knowledge and ability (La Greca, Follansbee, & Skyler, 1990) achieve better control. Also, those who were better able to cope with problematic issues related to having diabetes and who reported less stress related to the disease showed more acceptable metabolic control (Fernandes, 1997). There is additionally an effect of the child's behavior, including temperament, on glycemic control.

Knowledge and Diabetes

One issue that is highly relevant for adequate diabetes management is one's understanding of the disease. Furthermore, there are changes in cognitive development and one's conceptualization of illness that can directly impact on diabetes control (Glasgow & Anderson, 1995; Johnson, 1984). Older children are both more knowledgeable about their diabetes and have better problem-solving skills (Auslander, Haire-Joshu, Rogge, & Santiago, 1991; Johnson et al., 1982), which are correlated with better diabetes management (Ingersoll, Orr, Herrold, & Golden, 1986). Interestingly, the duration of illness is not typically associated with diabetes knowledge (Wysocki et al., 1992)

Several authors have shown changes in diabetes knowledge and skill throughout childhood and into adolescence. Johnson et al. (1982) reported that 6- to 8-year-old children were knowledgeable about the dietary restrictions and how to deal with an insulin reaction but lacked knowledge and understanding of important diabetes-related practices such as urine testing and insulin injections, which was attributed to the role parents play in their diabetes management. Between 9 and 13 years of age, Johnson and colleagues found that diabetes knowledge became constant across all facets of diabetes care. More recently, Auslander et al. (1991) studied changes in diabetes-related abilities in preadolescent and adolescent patients. These investigators found that diabetes-related problem-solving skills showed a definite improvement between 11 and 12 years of age, whereas knowledge about exercise, diet, anxiety, illness, and insulin reactions improved steadily to age 15.

In an unpublished PhD dissertation, Bauer (1990) examined children's understanding of diabetes in relation to their general conceptual development. She questioned 119 children between 4 and 14 years of age as to their understanding of diabetes and its causes and analyzed their responses qualitatively. Bauer found significant age differences in children's causal explanations of diabetes. These reflected both their current stage of cognitive development and, to a lesser degree, age at which their diabetes developed. Four- to five-year-olds, who were predominantly at the preoperational stage of cognitive development, gave primarily finalistic explanations eliciting a single cause that was artificialistic in nature or implied an external causative agent (e.g., "Diabetes comes from God"). Six-year-olds were quite variable in their levels of causal reasoning, with the majority attributing their illness to an external but now natural agent (e.g., "Diabetes comes from a germ"). With increasing age to 9 years, there was a decrease in the number of finalistic responses and an increase in the number of physicalistic. At age 10, Bauer noted a qualitative shift in thinking about diabetes, as children gained a deeper understanding of disease etiology of diabetes and provided responses similar to knowledgeable adults involving a physiological basis (e.g., "The pancreas usually keeps your sugars low, but since it doesn't really work, the insulin from the needle has to do that" and "You might get it in your family because a gene passes it on to your family"). After this age, children were able to integrate their understanding of diabetes into a greater whole.

Bauer also found that the age when children develop diabetes affects their causal reasoning about this disease. Those who developed diabetes at a later age (and higher stage of cognitive development) were more advanced in their understanding of diabetes than were children whose schemata of diabetes were less developed when they were first introduced to the disease. Regardless of age of onset, all children seemed to pass through the same orderly sequence of stages of conceptualizing diabetes.

In the studies by Johnson et al. (1982) and Auslander et al. (1991) described earlier, some of the age differences in diabetes knowledge and skill were attributed to the greater role that parents of younger children played in children's diabetes care, particularly with regard to injections and blood-glucose testing. Auslander et al. (1991) observed an interesting phenomenon whereby parents of children who were younger at time of diagnosis had greater knowledge of diabetes than parents of older children at diagnosis. This was attributed to the greater role that parents of younger children play in their child's diabetes care and their greater attempts to maintain this knowledge as their child grows. As children who were older at diagnosis are themselves more responsible for their own care, there is less necessity for their parents to gain further diabetes knowledge. Unfortunately, it has also been shown that in families where parents assume greater responsibility regardless of the child's age, better control is achieved (Anderson, Auslander, Jung, Miller, & Santiago, 1990).

More recently, Wysocki et al. (1996) studied the role of children's self-care autonomy in understanding their diabetes and showed that this was a complex phenomenon intimately connected with the role parents play in their child's disease. Children whose parents were more involved in their diabetes care were themselves more constrained in their self-care management, and although more adherent and better controlled metabolically, they were less knowledgeable about their disease. Diabetes knowledge was also associated with child's age but not disease duration. Because children with greater health care autonomy who developed diabetes at a very young age did not get knowledge from their parent and so were not able to refine their initial knowledge with age, their understanding of diabetes was immature, consistent with Bauer's (1990) findings. Wysocki et al. (1992, 1996) emphasized the need for a clear definition of self-care responsibilities, which must take into account the child's social and emotional maturity as well as stage of cognitive development. In addition, the appropriate level of autonomy in self-care must be redefined so that older children and adolescents are not ascribed excessive levels of self-care autonomy before they are psychologically mature enough to assume or understand it.

Brandt and Magyary (1993) have demonstrated the importance of diabetes education and reeducation programs. In their study evaluating the long-term benefits of a diabetes education program for school-age children and their mothers, there were immediate improvements on many facets of diabetes knowledge (e.g., diabetes information, problem solving, insulin injection) by diabetes education At 3-month follow-up, children's specific diabetes knowledge and perception of their abilities in managing their disease increased, whereas their problem-solving and injection skills remained stable, failing to make comparable developmental gains.

Fernandes (1997) also found that during adolescence, patients who were more confident in their abilities to manage the disease showed better metabolic control and claimed to be better at controlling their disease. Adolescents who were more knowledgeable about their diabetes obtained higher self-efficacy ratings for dealing with diabetes. Interestingly, adherence and specific diabetes knowledge were not directly associated with metabolic control but rather were mediated by stress and coping factors. Thus, it appears that knowing how to cope with this disease, as well as how to control the effects of stress, are important for managing diabetes in adolescence.

Cognition and Diabetes Control

The importance of cognitive variables in diabetes management cannot be underestimated. However, this issue has received very little attention. Holmes, Overstreet, and Greer (1997) recently showed that level of cognitive functioning actually affects diabetes control. These investigators observed that the performance of children with diabetes on a memory task predicted better self-care behaviors in diabetes than intelligence or achievement levels. Different memory processes were correlated with different aspects of health care.

In a study of diabetes symptomatology, Eastman, Johnson, Silverstein, Spillar, and McCallum (1983) found that young children with diabetes were unable to attend to internal events and so were less able to predict their current blood-glucose levels. Some of the symptoms traditionally reported by physicians as signifying hyperglycemia were reported by patients as symptoms of hypoglycemia, while patients often used the same symptoms to describe opposite states. These authors suggested that "classic" symptomatology of diabetes events may not actually be "classic" for all patients. Thus, it is important for health care providers to work closely with patients to identify their individual symptoms and then train them how to attribute these symptoms to specific diabetes states and also to realize when certain symptoms result from factors other than altered glycemia.

Temperament and Diabetes

Temperament refers to a constellation of behavioral traits that include activity and arousal levels, adaptive style, organization of routines, mood, persistence, and distractibility. In the light of the role of some of these traits for diabetes management and for differences in metabolic function, it is not surprising that temperament and glycemic control are related. Indeed, there are several studies which have examined these issues directly.

Rovet and Ehrlich (1988) examined the relationships between temperament and metabolic control in children. While there was no distinctive temperament profile characteristic of children with diabetes, better metabolic control was related to certain temperament traits. Typically, better control was exhibited by children who were more active and better at following routines, whose responses to external stimuli were milder, and who were less attentive and more often showed negative moods. Highest hemoglobin A_{1C} levels (signifying poorest control) were obtained by the least active children, whereas best control was reflective of normal activity levels rather than overactivity. The association between being better able to follow routines and better glycemic control is obvious, given the great demands for following a prescribed health care regimen in diabetes. However, this means that greater attention should be paid to children who are naturally less organized in their routines and schedules. The fact that children who typically displayed more intense reactions to stimulation displayed poorer control most likely reflects physiological differences in regulating stress, which in turn impacts directly on glucose metabolism. The association between metabolic control and mood was interpreted to reflect a trade-off between general happiness and better diabetes control.

More recently, Garrison, Biggs, and Williams (1990) examined the temperaments of both children with diabetes and their mothers in relation to compliance and metabolic control. Better compliance was predicted by children's lower activity levels, rhythmicity of routines, and good attention span. Poor metabolic control was also associated with characteristics of both child and mother. In both the child and mother, poor control was associated with social withdrawal, lack of flexibility, and a negative mood, while in the child poor control was additionally associated with a shorter attention span and less adherence.

Summary

This section has shown that optimal diabetes management is a complex multidimensional phenomenon that reflects developmental, family, and inherent temperamental factors. Although diabetes control and cognitive level are intimately linked, these are mediated by family factors, particularly parental style in managing diabetes.

CONCLUSIONS AND FUTURE DIRECTIONS

In North America, a significant number of children suffer from diabetes, a highly complex disorder with a complicated treatment regimen that places a significant burden on the mental and emotional resources of the child and family. Optimal diabetes management involves a number of cognitive skills that require an adequate level of brain functioning. While diabetes can have profound effects on a number of organ systems that become evident mainly later in life, in children its effects are mainly on the brain. One of the most distressing aspects of diabetes is that the regions of the brain targeted mostly by diabetes are those that that underlie the very skills essential for good diabetes management (Rovet, 1998).

In children, therefore, low as well as high blood-glucose levels must be prevented, which means increasing the restrictions on blood-glucose elevations. However, it is not certain how this will impact on later health and prevention of medical complications. Preventing hypoglycemia is a particularly difficult task for young children who may not be able to communicate these effects or who are unaware of changes in internal states and who are also more active, which is associated with poorer control. Furthermore, it is not known what level of hypoglycemia must be prevented. Several of the studies described have suggested that asymptomatic hypoglycemia was not harmful for cognitive development, unlike moderate to severe hypoglycemia, which were associated with impairment, particularly if seizures occurred. Future studies are therefore needed to differentiate the effects of mild from severe hypoglycemia and severe hypoglycemia per se from severe hypoglycemia with seizures, particularly in light of recent findings showing *less* cortical dysfunction in intensively than conventionally treated patients (Borg, Borg, & Tamborlane, 1997), but greater memory impairments (Hershey et al., 1998).

Parents play a significant role in diabetes control and, indeed, parent factors such as level of intellectual functioning and personality and temperament may be important. However, parents may be responsible for overcontrolling their child's diabetes, which in turn predisposes the child to more hypoglycemic events and poorer neurocognitive outcome. The degree to which this needs to monitored will also depend on future studies and related intervention programs.

What is the bottom line? Should control be looser in children, whose brains are still developing? It is clear from our review that the issue of hypoglycemia in children with diabetes needs to be revisited with better designed studies that directly examine the effects (both permanent and transient) of varying degrees of hypoglycemia, and that more sensitive measures as well as newer technologies, including neuroimaging, be used. It is also important to evaluate more thoroughly those areas of cognitive function that are most likely to be affected (e.g., memory), rather than to sample broadly global abilities.

Surprisingly, despite the prevalence of diabetes and the relatively large number of studies that have been conducted on the behavioral aspects of managing diabetes, this disease has largely been understudied from a neuropsychological perspective. Yet, this is a disease that profoundly affects the CNS, as well as the associated cognitive functions. We have shown here that diabetes has both direct and indirect effects on the brain, including neuropathology from glucose toxicity and insulin insufficiency as well as the secondary effects of altered vascularity (mainly in older patients) and peripheral hyperinsulinism. Moreover, diabetes can affect neurotransmission because insulin plays an intricate role in neurotransmitter regulation (McCall & Figlewicz, 1997; Wan et al., 1997), which in turn has a bearing on cognitive function. Studies showing a direct link between hypoglycemic seizures and hippocampal functioning (Auer, 1986) and the importance of the hippocampus in memory (Squire & Zola, 1996; Vargha-Khadem et al., 1997) suggest that children with IDDM are in fact an ideal population to address these important neuroscientific issues. Diabetes also provides a theoretically interesting and promising model for the study of neurocognitive processing, especially in children, because of the relative precision with which the timing of particular diabetes-specific events can be recorded. Therefore, not only will future studies of pediatric diabetes patients provide greater clarity about the disease itself and its impact on the brain, future studies of children with diabetes may also increase our understanding of the developing brain.

From the fetus exposed to excess glucose *in utero* due to maternal diabetes (Jovanovic-Petersen, 1997), to the child with diabetes and, ultimately, the elderly patient, it is essential to prevent at all costs the adverse neuropathological consequences from hypoglycemia and hyperglycemia. While a major thrust of future diabetes research should be devoted to diabetes prevention, it is also important to consider how to improve the quality of life in children, in whom diabetes is shockingly on the rise. As quality-of-life issues also include cognitive abilities, every effort should be maintained to ensure adequate brain development during these formative years. This will require establishing optimal treatment protocols that ensure normal glucose and insulin levels at all times so as to allow for normal brain development. While new and improved insulins (e.g., Lyspro) seem to offer this potential, it is important to assess their effectiveness in children from a cognitive as well as metabolic perspective (Holcombe, Zalani, Arora, Headlee, & Gill, 1997)

In short, diabetes involves a highly complex relationship between brain and body, and all efforts should be maintained so that children with diabetes are normalized to prevent any associated brain damage and cognitive dysfunction. This information is both medically and scientifically relevant.

REFERENCES

Ack, M., Miller, I., & Weil, W. (1961). Intelligence of children with diabetes mellitus. *Pediatrics, 28,* 764–770.

Amiel, S. A. (1996). Studies in hypoglycaemia in children with insulin-dependent diabetes mellitus. *Hormone Research, 45*(6), 285–290.

Amiel, S. A., Caprio, S., Sherwin, R. S., Plewe, G., Haymond, M. W., & Tamborlane, W. V. (1991). Insulin resistance of puberty: A defect restricted to peripheral glucose metabolism. *Journal of Clinical Endocrinology and Metabolism, 72*(2), 277–282.

Amiel, S. A., & Gale, E. (1993) Physiological responses to hypoglycemia. Counter-regulation and cognitive function. *Diabetes Care, 16*(Suppl. 3), 48–55.

Anderson, B. J., Auslander, W. F., Jung, K. C., Miller, J. P., & Santiago, J. V. (1990). Assessing family sharing of diabetes responsibilities. *Journal of Pediatric Psychology, 15,* 477–492.

Anderson, B. J., Hagen, J., Barclay, C., Goldstein, G., Kandt, R., & Bacon, G. (1984) Cognitive and school performance in diabetic children. *Diabetes, 33*(Suppl.), 81.

Atkinson, M. A., & Maclaren, N. K. (1994). The pathogenesis of insulin-dependent diabetes mellitus. *New England Journal of Medicine, 331*(21), 1428–1436.

Auer, R. (1986). Progress Review: Hypoglycemic brain damage. *Stroke, 17*(4), 699–708.

Auer, R. N., & Siesjo, B. K. (1988). Biological differences between ischemia, hypoglycemia, and epilepsy. *Annals of Neurology, 24,* 699–707.

Auslander, W. F., Haire-Joshu, D., Rogge, M., & Santiago, J. V. (1991). Predictors of diabetes knowledge in newly diagnosed children and parents. *Journal of Pediatric Psychology, 16*(2), 213–228.

Banting, F. G. (1929). The history of insulin. *Edinburgh Medical Journal, 36,* 1–18.

Baskin, D. G., Figlewicz, D. P., Woods, S. C., Porte, D., & Dorsa, D. M. (1987). Insulin in the brain. *Annual Reviews of Physiology, 49,* 335–347.

Bauer, L. G. (1990). *The development of the understanding of diabetes in children with diabetes.* Unpublished doctoral thesis, University of Toronto.

Bergada, I., Suissa, S., Dufresne, J., & Schiffrin A. (1989) Severe hypoglycemia in IDDM children. *Diabetes Care, 12*(4), 239–244.

Bjorgaas, M., Gimse, R., Vik, T., & Sand, T. (1997). Cognitive function in type 1 diabetes children with and without episodes of severe hypoglycemia. *Acta Pediatrica, 8*(2), 148–153.

Bloch, C. A., Clemons, P., & Sperling, M. A. (1987). Puberty decreases insulin sensitivity. *Journal of Pediatrics, 110,* 481–487.

Borg, W. P., Borg, M. A., & Tamborlane, W. V. (1997). The brain and hypoglycemic counterregulation: Insights from hypoglycemic clamp studies. *Diabetes Spectrum, 10,* 33–38.

Brandt, P. A., & Magyary, D. L. (1993). The impact of a diabetes education program on children and mothers. *Journal of Pediatric Nursing, 8*(1), 31–40.

Brierley, J. B., Brown, A. W., & Meldrum, B. S. (1971). The nature and time course of the neuronal alterations resulting from oligaemia and hypoglycaemia in the brain of *Macaca mulatta. Brain Research, 25,* 483–499.

Brown, G. (1938). The development of diabetic children, with special reference to mental and personality comparisons. *Child Development, 9,* 175–183.

Caprio, S., Plewe, G., Diamond, M. P., Simonson, D. C., Boulwar, S. D., Sherwin, R. S., & Tamborlane, W. V. (1989). Increased insulin secretion in puberty: A compensatory response to reductions in insulin sensitivity. *Journal of Pediatrics, 114,* 963–967.

Casparie, A. F., & Elving, L. D. (1985) Severe hypoglycemia in diabetic patients: Frequency, causes, prevention. *Diabetes Care, 8,* 217–222.

Cohen, M. S., Kosslyn, S. M., Breiter, H. C., DiGirolamo, G. J., Thompson, W. L., Anderson, A. K., Bookheimer, S. Y., Rosen, B. R., & Belliveau, J. W. (1996). Changes in cortical activity during mental rotation. A mapping study using functional MRI. *Brain, 119,* 89–100.

Corballis, M. (1997). Mental rotation and the right hemisphere. *Brain and Language, 57,* 100–121.

Dammacco, F., Torelli, C., Frezza, E., Piccinno, E., Tansella, F., & the Diabetes Study Group of the Italian Society of Pediatric Endocrinology & Diabetes. (1998). Problems of hypoglycemia arising in children and adolescents with insulin-dependent diabetes mellitus. *Journal of Pediatric Endocrinology and Metabolism, 11,* 167–176.

Daneman, D., Frank, M., Perlman, K., Tamm, J., & Ehrlich, R. (1989). Severe hypoglycemia in children with insulin-dependent diabetes mellitus: Frequency and predisposing factors. *Journal of Pediatrics, 115*(5, Pt. 1), 740–742. (Comment in *Journal of Pediatrics, 117*(2, Pt. 1), 340–341.)

Davis, E. A., & Jones, T. W. (1998). Hypoglycemia in children with diabetes: Incidence, counterregulation and cognitive dysfunction. *Journal of Pediatric Endocrinology and Metabolism, 11,* 177–182.

Davis, E. A., Keating, B., Byrne, G. C., Russell, M., & Jones, T. W. (1998). Impact of improved glycaemic control on rates of hypoglycaemia in insulin dependent diabetes mellitus. *Archives of Diseases in Childhood, 78,* 111–115.

Davis, E. A., Soong, S. A., Byrne, G. C., & Jones, T. W. (1996). Acute hyperglycaemia impairs cognitive function in children with IDDM. *Journal of Pediatric Endocrinology and Metabolism, 9*(4), 455–461.

Deary, I. J., & Frier, B. M. (1996). Severe hypoglycaemia and cognitive impairment in diabetes not proven. *British Medical Journal, 313,* 67–68.

Dejgaard, A., Gade, A., Larsson, H., Balle, V., Parving, A., & Parving, H. (1991). Evidence for diabetic encephalopathy. *Diabetic Medicine, 8,* 162–167.

Dennis, M. (1991) Frontal lobe function in childhood and adolescence: A heuristic for assessing attention regulation, executive control, and the intentional states important for social discourse. *Developmental Neuropsychology, 73,* 327–358.

Diabetes Control and Complications Trial Research Group. (1993). The effects of intensive treatment of diabetes on the development and progression of long-term complicationsin insulin-dependent diabetes mellitus. *New England Journal of Medicine, 329,* 977–986.

Donaghue, K. C., Bonney, M., Simpson, J. M., Schwingshandl, J., Fung, A. T., Howard, N. J., & Silink, M. (1993). Autonomic and peripheral nerve function in adolescents with and without diabetes. *Diabetes Medicine, 10,* 664–671.

Eastman, B. G., Johnson, S. B., Silverstein, J., Spillar, R. P., & McCallum, M. (1983). Understanding of hypo- and hyperglycemia by youngsters with diabetes and their parents. *Journal of Pediatric Psychology, 8*(3), 229–243.

Eeg-Olofsson, O., & Petersen, I. (1966). Childhood diabetic neuropathy: A clinical and neuropsychological study. *Acta Pediatrica Scandinavica, 55,* 163–176.

Fernandes, C. B. (1997). *An investigation into the factors predicting blood-glucose control in adolescents with insulin-dependent diabetes mellitus.* Unpublished bachelor's honor thesis, University of Western Ontario.

Fowler, M., Johnson, M., & Atkinson, S. (1985). School achievement and absence in children with chronic health conditions. *Journal of Pediatrics, 106,* 683–687.

Franceschi, M., Cecchetto, R., Minicucci, F., Smizne, S., Baio, G., & Canal, N. (1984). Cognitive processes in insulin-dependent diabetes. *Diabetes Care, 7,* 228–231.

Gardner, S. G., Bingley, P. J., Sawtell, P. A., Weeks, S., & Gale, E. A. (1997). Rising incidence of insulin dependent diabetes in children aged under 5 years in the Oxford region: Time trend analysis. The Bart's–Oxford Study Group. *British Medical Journal, 315,* 713–717.

Garrison, W. T., Biggs, D., & Williams, K. (1990). Temperament characteristics and clinical outcomes in young children with diabetes mellitus. *Journal of Child Psychology and Psychiatry, 31*(7), 1079–1088.

Gath, A., Smith, M. A., & Baum, J. D. (1980). Emotional, behavioural, and educational disorders in diabetic children. *Archives of Diseases in Childhood, 55*(5), 371–375.

Geffner, M. E. (1994). Reviewing the Diabetes Control and Complications Trial: One member of "control panel" speaks out. *Journal of Pediatrics, 125,* 228.

Glasgow, R. E., & Anderson, B. J. (1995). Future directions for research on pediatric chronic disease management: Lessons from diabetes. *Journal of Pediatric Psychology, 20*(4), 389–402.

Gold, P. E., Vogt, J., & Hall, J. L. (1986). Glucose effects on memory: Behavioral and pharmacological characteristics. *Behavioral and Neural Biology, 46*(2), 145–155.

Golden, M. P., Ingersoll, G. M., Brack, C. J., Russell, B. A., Wright, J. C., & Huberty, T. J. (1989). Longitudinal relationship of asymptomatic hypoglycemia to cognitive function in IDDM. *Diabetes Care, 12,* 89–93.

Goldstein, D. E., England, J. D., Hess, R., Rawlings, S. S., & Walker, B. (1981). A prospective study of symptomatic hypoglycemia in young patients. *Diabetes Care, 4*(6), 601–605.

Grishaw, W., West, H., & Smith, B. (1939). Juvenile diabetes mellitus. *Archives of Internal Medicine, 64,* 787–799.

Gschwend, S., Ryan, C., Atchison, J., Arslanian, S., & Becker, D. (1995). Effects of acute hyperglycemia on mental efficiency and counterregulatory hormones in adolescents with insulin-dependent diabetes mellitus. *Journal of Pediatrics, 126,* 178–184.

Hagen, J. W., Barclay, C. R., Anderson, B. J., Freeman, D. J., Segal, S. S., Bacon, G., & Goldstein, G. W. (1990). Intellectual functioning and strategy use in children with insulin-dependent diabetes mellitus. *Child Development, 61,* 1714–1727.

Haumont, D., Dorchy, H., & Pelc, S. (1979). EEG abnormalities in diabetic children. *Clinical Pediatrics, 28,* 750–752.

Havrankova, J., Roth, K., & Brownstone, M. J. (1983). Insulin receptors in brain. *Advances in Metabolic Disorders, 10, 259–268.*

Herold, K. C., Polonsky, K. S., Cohen, R. M. Levy, J., & Douglas, F. (1985). Variable deterioration in cortical function during insulin-induced hypoglycemia. *Diabetes, 34*(7), 677–685.

Hershey, T., Bhargava, N., White, N., & Craft, S. (1998). *Standard vs. intensive insulin treatment in children with insulin-dependent diabetes mellitus (IDDM): Effects on memory and reaction time.* Poster presented at the meeting of the International Neuropsychological Society, Honolulu.

Holcombe, J., Zalani, S., Arora, V., Headlee, S., & Gill, A. (1997). *Diabetes, 46*(Suppl. 1), 329A.

Holmes, C. S. (1980). Prevention: An idea whose time has come? *Western Journal of Medicine, 132*(5), 471–473.

Holmes, C. S. (1986). Neuropsychological profiles in men with insulin dependent diabetes. *Journal of Consulting and Clinical Psychology, 54*(3), 386–389.

Holmes, C. S. (1990). Neuropsychological sequelae of acute and chronic blood glucose disruption in adults with insulin-dependent diabetes. In C. Holmes (Ed.), *Neuropsychological and behavioral aspects of diabetes* (pp. 122–154). New York: Springer-Verlag.

Holmes, C., Cornwell, J., Dunlap, W., Chen, R., & Lee, C. (1992) Anomalous factor structure of the WISC-R for diabetic children. *Neuropsychology, 6,* 341–350.

Holmes, C. S., Dunlap, W. P., Chen, R. S., & Cornwell, J. M. (1992) Gender differences in the learning status of diabetic children. *Journal of Consulting and Clinical Psychology, 60*(5), 698–704.

Holmes, C. S., Hayford, J. T., Gonzalez, J. L., & Weydert, J. A. (1983). A survey of cognitive functioning at different glucose levels in diabetic persons. *Diabetes Care, 6,* 180–185.

Holmes, C. S., Koepke, K. M., & Thompson, R. G. (1986). Simple versus complex performance impairments at three blood glucose levels. *Psychoneuroendocrinology, 11,* 353–357.

Holmes, C. S., Overstreet, S., & Greer, T. (1997). Cognitive predictors of self-care behaviors 3 years later in youth with IDDM. *Diabetes, 46,* 263A.

Holmes, C. S., & Richman, L. C. (1985). Cognitive profiles of children with insulin-dependent diabetes. *Journal of Developmental and Behavioral Pediatrics, 6,* 323–326.

Ingersoll, G. M., Orr, D. P., Herrold, A. J., & Golden, M. P. (1986). Cognitive maturity and self management among adolescents with insulin-dependent diabetes mellitus. *Journal of Pediatrics, 108*(4), 620–623.

Ipp, E., & Forster, B. (1987). Sparing of cognitive function in mild hypoglycemia: Dissociation from the neuroendocrine response. *Journal of Clinical Endocrinology and Metabolism, 65,* 806–810.

Johnson, S. B. (1984). Knowledge, attitudes, and behavior: Correlates of health in childhood diabetes. *Clinical Psychology Review, 4,* 503–524.

Johnson, S. B., Pollak, T., Silverstein, J. H., Rosenbloom, A. L., Spillar, R., Mc-Callum, M., & Harkavay, J. (1982). Cognitive and behavioral knowledge about insulin-dependent diabetes among children and parents. *Pediatrics, 69*(6), 708–713.

Jovanovic-Peterson, L. (1997). The effects of maternal diabetes on the fetal neuro-developmental outcome: A case study and review. *Diabetes Spectrum, 10*(1), 63–68.

Karjalainen, J., Martin, J. M., Knip, M., Ilonen, J., Robinson, B. H., Savilahti, E., Akerblom, H. K., & Dosch, H. M. (1992). A bovine albumin peptide as a possible trigger of insulin-dependent diabetes mellitus. *New England Journal of Medicine, 327*(5), 302–307. (Published erratum appears in *New England Journal of Medicine, 327*(17), 1252.)

Kostraba, J. N., Dorman, J. S., Orchard, T. J., Becker, D. J., Ohki, Y., Ellis, D., Doft, B. H., Lobes, L. A., Laporte, R. E., & Drash, A. L. (1989). Contribution of diabetes duration before puberty to development of microvascular complications in IDDM subjects. *Diabetes Care, 12,* 686–693.

Kovacs, M., Goldston, D., & Iyengar, S. (1992). Intellectual development and academic performance of children with insulin-dependent diabetes mellitus: A longitudinal study. *Developmental Psychology, 28*(4), 676–684.

Kovacs, M., Ryan, C., & Obrosky, D. (1994). Verbal intellectual and verbal memory performance of youths with childhood-onset insulin dependent diabetes mellitus. *Journal of Pediatric Psychology, 19,* 475–483.

Krolewski, A. S., Laffel, L. M., Krolewski, M., Quinn, M., & Warram, J. H. (1995). Glycosylated hemoglobin and the risk of microalbuminuria in patients with insulin-dependent diabetes mellitus. *New England Journal of Medicine, 332*(19), 1251–1255.

Kubany, A. J., Danowski, T. S., & Moses, C. (1956). The personality and intelligence of diabetics. *Diabetes, 5,* 462–467.

La Greca, A. M., Follansbee, D., & Skyler, J. (1990). Developmental and behavioral aspects of diabetes management in youngsters. *Children's Health Care, 19,* 132–139.

Langan, S. J., Deary, I. J., Hepburn, D. A., & Frier, B. M. (1991). Cumulative cognitive impairment following recurrent severe hypoglycaemia in adult patients with insulin-treated diabetes mellitus. *Diabetologia, 34*(5), 337–344.

LaPorte, R. E., Tajima, N., Akerblom, H. K., Berlin, N., Brosseau, J., Christy, M., Drash, A. L., Fishbein, H., Green, A., Hamman, R., Harris. M., King, H., Laron, Z., & Andrew, N. (1985). *Diabetes Care, 8*(Suppl. 1), 101–107.

Lawson, M. L., Sochett, E. B., Chait, P. G., Balfe, J. W., & Daneman, D. (1996). Effect of puberty on markers of glomerular hypertrophy and hypertension in IDDM. *Diabetes, 45*(1), 51–55.

Lichty, W., & McGill, J. (1989). Cognitive deficits of adult diabetics with insulin-dependent diabetes: Relationship of metabolic control and disease duration. *Diabetes, 38,* 125A.

Lindgren, F., Dahlquist, G., Efendic, S., Persson, B., & Skottner, A. (1990). Insulin sensitivity and glucose-induced response changes during adolescence. *Acta Pediatrica Scandinavica, 79*(4), 431–436.

MacLeod, K. M., Hepburn, D. A., & Frier, B. M. (1993). Frequency and morbidity of severe hypoglycemia in insulin treated diabetic patients. *Diabetic Medicine, 10,* 238–245.

McCall, A. L. (1992). The impact of diabetes on the CNS (Review). *Diabetes, 41,* 557–570.

McCall, A. L., & Figlewicz, D. P. (1997). How does diabetes mellitus produce brain dysfunction? *Diabetes Spectrum, 10, 25–32.*

McCrimmon, R. J., Deary, I. J., Huntly, B. J., MacLeod, K. J., & Frier, B. M. (1996) Visual information processing during controlled hypoglycaemia in humans. *Brain, 119*(Pt. 4), 1277–87.

McGavin, A. P., Schultz, K., Peden, G. W., & Bowen, B. D. (1940). The physical growth, the degree of intelligence and the personality adjustment of a group of diabetic children. *New England Journal of Medicine, 223,* 119–127.

Meneilly, G. S., Cheung, E., & Tuokko, H. (1994). Altered responses to hypoglycemia of healthy elderly people. *Journal of Clinical Endocrinology and Metabolism, 78*(6), 1341–1348.

Merali, Z., & Ahmad, Q. (1985). Diabetes-induced alterations in brain monoamine and metabolite levels: Effects of insulin replacement. *Society for Neuroscience Abstracts, 12,* 125.

Mitrakou, A., Ryan, C., Veneman, T., Mokan, M., Jenssen, T., Kiss, I., Durrant, J., Cryer, P., & Gerich, J. (1991). Hierarchy of glycemic threshold for counterregulator hormone secretion, symptoms, and cerebral dysfunction. *American Journal of Physiology, 260,* E67–E74.

Northam, E. (1996). *Neuropsychological changes in children with insulin dependent diabetes mellitus.* Unpublished doctoral thesis, University of Melbourne, Melbourne, Australia.

Northam, E., Anderson, P., Werther, G., Adler, R., & Andrewes, D. (1995). Neuropsychological complications of insulin dependent diabetes in children. *Child Neuropsychology, 1,* 74–87.

Northam, E., Bowden, S., Anderson, V., & Court, J. (1992). Neuropsychological functioning in adolescents with diabetes. *Journal of Clinical and Experimental Neuropsychology, 14,* 884–900.

Porter, P. A., Keating, B., Byrne, G., & Jones, T. (1997). Incidence and predictive criteria of nocturnal hypoglycemia in young children with insulin-dependent diabetes mellitus. *Journal of Pediatrics, 130,* 366–372.

Reich, J. N., Kaspar, J. C., Puczynski, M. S., Puczynski, S., Cleland, J. W., Dell'Angela, K., & Emanuele, M. A. (1990). Effect of a hypoglycemic episode on neuropsychological functioning in diabetic children. *Journal of Clinical and Experimental Neuropsychology, 12,* 613–626.

Reichard, P., Berglund, B., Britz, A., Levander, S., & Rosenqvist, U. (1991). Hypoglycemic episodes during intensified insulin treatment: Increased frequency but not effect cognitive function. *Journal of Internal Medicine, 229,* 9–16.

Reunanen, A., Akerblom, H. K., & Kaar, M. L. (1982). Prevalence and ten-year (1970–1979) incidence of insulin-dependent diabetes mellitus in children and adolescents in Finland. *Acta Paediatrica Scandinavica, 71*(6), 893–899.

Rogers, D. G., White, N. H., Santiago, J. V., Miller, J. P., Weldon, V. V., Kilo, C., &

Williamson, J. R. (1986). Glycemic control and bone age are independently associated with muscle capillary basement membrane width in diabetic children after puberty. *Diabetes Care, 9*(5), 453–459.

Rovet, J. F. (in press). Neurological sequelae of pediatric diabetes. In K. O. Yeates, M. D. Ris, & H. G. Taylor (Eds.), *Pediatric neuropsychology: Research, theory, and practice.* New York: Guilford Press.

Rovet, J. F., & Alvarez, M. (1997). Attentional functioning in children and adolescents with IDDM. *Diabetes Care, 20,* 803–810.

Rovet, J. F., & Ehrlich, R. M. (1988). Effect of temperament on metabolic control in children with diabetes mellitus. *Diabetes Care, 11*(1), 77–82.

Rovet, J. F., & Ehrlich, R. (1997). Predictors of neuropsychological functioning in adolescents with IDDM. *Diabetes, 46*(Suppl. 1), 14A.

Rovet, J. F., & Ehrlich, R. M. (1999). The effect of hypoglycemic seizures on cognitive function in children with diabetes: A 7-year prospective study. *Journal of Pediatrics, 135,* 503–506.

Rovet, J. F., Ehrlich, R. M., & Czuchta, D. (1990). Intellectual characteristics of diabetic children at diagnosis and one year later. *Journal of Pediatric Psychology, 15,* 775–788.

Rovet, J. F., Ehrlich, R. M., Czuchta, D., & Akler, M. (1993) Psychoeducational characteristics of children and adolescents with insulin-dependent diabetes mellitus. *Journal of Learning Disabilities, 26,* 7–22.

Rovet, J. F., Ehrlich, R. M., & Hoppe, M. (1987). Intellectual deficits associated with early onset of insulin-dependent diabetes mellitus in children. *Diabetes Care, 10,* 510–515.

Rovet, J. F., Ehrlich, R. M., & Hoppe, M. (1988). Specific intellectual deficits in children with early onset diabetes mellitus. *Child Development, 59,* 226–234.

Ryan, C. M. (1990). Neuropsychological consequences and correlates of diabetes in childhood. In C. S. Holmes (Ed.), *Neuropsychological and behavioral aspects of diabetes* (pp. 58–84). New York: Springer-Verlag.

Ryan, C. M., Atchison, J., Puczynski, S., Puczynski, M., Arslanian, S., & Becker, D. (1990). Mild hypoglycemia associated with deterioration of mental efficiency in children with insulin-dependent diabetes mellitus. *Journal of Pediatrics, 117,* 32–38.

Ryan, C., Longstreet, C., & Morrow, L. (1985). The effects of diabetes mellitus on the school attendance and school achievement of adolescents. *Child: Care, Health and Development, 11,* 229–240.

Ryan, C., Vega, A., & Drash, A. (1985). Cognitive defects in adolescents who developed diabetes early in life. *Pediatrics, 75,* 921–927.

Ryan, C., Vega, A., Longstreet, C., & Drash, A. (1984). Neuropsychological changes in adolescents with insulin dependent diabetes. *Journal of Consulting and Clinical Psychology, 52,* 335–342.

Ryan, C. M., & Williams, T. M. (1993). Effects of insulin-dependent diabetes on learning and memory efficiency in adults. *Journal of Clinical and Experimental Neuropsychology, 15,* 685–700.

Ryan, C. M., Williams, T. M., Finegold, D. N., & Orchard, T. J. (1993). Cognitive dysfunction in adults with Type 1 (insulin-dependent) diabetes mellitus of long duration: Effects of recurrent hypoglycaemia and other chronic complications. *Diabetologia, 36,* 329–334.

Ryan, C. M., Williams, T. M., Orchard, T. J., & Finegold, D. N. (1992). Psychomotor slowing is associated with distal symmetrical polyneuropathy in adults with diabetes mellitus. *Diabetes, 41,* 107–113.

Sansbury, L., Brown, R. T., & Meacham, L. (1997). Predictors of cognitive functioning in children and adolescents with insulin-dependent diabetes mellitus: A preliminary investigation. *Children's Health Care, 26*(3), 197–210.

Shirley, H., & Greer, I. (1940). Environmental and personality problems in the treatment of diabetic children. *Journal of Pediatrics, 16,* 775–781.

Skenazy, J., & Bigler, E. (1984). Neuropsychological findings in diabetes mellitus. *Journal Clinical Psychology, 40,* 246–258.

Soltesz, G., & Acsadi, G. (1989) Association between diabetes, severe hypoglycaemia and encephalographic abnormalities. *Archives of Diseases in Childhood, 64,* 992–996.

Sperling, M. A. (1997). The Scylla and Charybdis of blood glucose control in children with diabetes mellitus. *Journal of Pediatrics, 130*(3), 339–341.

Squire, L. R., & Zola, S. M. (1996). Structure and function of declarative and nondeclarative memory systems. *Proceedings of the National Academy of Sciences of the United States of America, 93*(24), 13515–13522.

Stevens, A. V., McKane, W. R., Bell, P. M., Bell, P., King, D. J., & Hayes, J. R. (1989). Psychomotor performance and counterregulatory responses during mild hypoglycemia in healthy volunteers. *Diabetes Care, 12,* 12–17.

Traisman, H. S. (1980). *Management of juvenile diabetes* (3rd ed.). St. Louis, MO: Mosby.

Tribl, G., Howorka, K., Heger, G., Anderer, P., Thomas H., & Zeitlhofer. (1996) EEG topography during insulin-induced hypoglycemia in patients with insulin-dependent diabetes mellitus. *European Neurology, 36*(5), 303–309.

Tsalikian, E., Daneman, D., Becker, D. J., Crumrine, P. K., & Drash, A. L. (1980). EEG changes during therapy of diabetic ketoacidosis in children. *Journal of Pediatrics, 96,* 1115–1116.

Vargha Khadem, F., Gadian, D. G, Watkins, K. E, Connelly, A., Van Paesschen, W., & Mishkin, M. (1997). Differential effects of early hippocampal pathology on episodic and semantic memory. *Science, 277,* 376–380.

Vlassara, H., Brownlee, M., & Cerami, A. (1983). Excessive nonenzymatic glycosylation of peripheral and central nervous system myelin components in diabetic rats. *Diabetes, 32,* 670–674.

Wan, Q., Xiong, Z. G., Man, H. Y., Ackerly, C. A., Braunton, J., Lu, W. Y., Becker, L. E., MacDonald, J. F., & Wang Y. T. (1997). Recruitment of functional GABAA receptors to postsynaptic domains by insulin. *Nature, 388,* 686–690.

Weil, W. B., & Ack, M. (1964). School achievement in juvenile diabetes mellitus. *Diabetes, 13,* 303–306.

Widom, B., & Simonson, D. C. (1990). Glycemic control and neuropsychologic function during hypoglycemia in patients with insulin-dependent diabetes mellitus. *Annals of Internal Medicine, 112,* 904–912.

Wolters, C. A, Yu, S. L, Hagen, J. W., & Kail, R. (1996). Short-term memory and strategy use in children with insulin-dependent diabetes mellitus. *Journal of Consulting and Clinical Psychology, 64,* 1397–1405.

Wredling, R., Levander, S., Adamson, U., & Lins, P. E. (1990). Permanent neuropsychological impairment after recurrent episodes of severe hypoglycaemia in man. *Diabetologia, 33,* 152–157.

Wysocki, T., Meinhold, P. A., Abrams, K., Barnard, M. U., Clarke, W. L., Bellando, B. J., & Bourgeois, M. J. (1992). Parental and professional estimates of self-care independence of children and adolescents with IDDM. *Diabetes Care, 15*(1), 43–52.

Wysocki, T., Taylor, A., Hough, B. S., Linscheid, T. R., Yeates, K. O., & Naglieri, J. A. (1996). Deviation from developmental appropriate self-care autonomy: Association with diabetes outcomes. *Diabetes Care, 19*(2), 119–125.

Yakovlev, P. I., & Lecours, A. (1967). The myelogenetic cycles of regional maturation of the brain. In A. Minkowski (Ed.), *Regional Development of the brain in early life* (pp. 3–64). Oxford: Blackwell.

CHAPTER EIGHT

Sickle Cell Disease

NATALIE C. FRANK
SUSANNAH M. ALLISON
M. E. CATHERINE CANT

Sickle cell disease (SCD) is a chronic illness that affects 1 out of every 400–500 African-American babies born in the United States (Tarnowski & Brown, 1995). The disease is caused by an autosomal recessive genetic deficit. Although SCD does occur in other ethnic groups, affecting approximately 1 out of every 9,900 individuals who are not African-Americans (Davis, 1995), the disease occurs most frequently in the African-American population. The high prevalence of the sickle cell trait in this population is due to the adaptive advantage of the heterozygous genotype in conferring a resistance to malarial infections (Lemanek, Buckloh, Woods, & Butler, 1995). It is for this reason that the gene has been maintained in the African-American population despite its deleterious effects in the case of SCD. SCD is caused by a single base pair substitution in the beta-globin chain of hemoglobin (Kunz & Finkel, 1987). Since this is essentially a disease of hemoglobin, which is carried by red blood cells, the disease has multiple effects upon vascular circulation and the oxygen-carrying capacity of blood.

SCD causes normally round red blood cells to assume a rigid crescent or sickle shape (Kunz & Finkel, 1987). The aberration in cell shape and membrane pliability of these sickled cells compromises their ability to flow readily through the vasculature. Blood vessels may become blocked, thereby impeding the delivery of oxygen to the various tissues and organs of the body. When adequate levels of oxygen are not delivered, a person can experience severe pain, swelling, and fatigue. These symptoms are characteristic of the vasoocclusive phenomenon, or sickle cell crisis. The body responds by destroying the abnormal sickled red blood cells. This increase in the destruction of red blood cells is often coupled with the inadequate production of new red blood cells, the result of which can be low hemoglobin or anemia. Other severe manifestations of the disease include vasoocclusive crises, serious infections, cerebral vascular accidents (CVAs) or strokes, anemic episodes, microvascular infarcts or strokes without overt symptoms, and delayed growth and onset of puberty.

With increases in medical technology, more and more children with chronic diseases are surviving into adulthood. Specifically in SCD, the expected life span of an individual with this disease has increased dramatically, with some patients reported to survive into their 50s, 60s, and 70s (Midence, Fuggle, & Davies, 1993). Newborn screening and the implementation of the use of prophylactic penicillin (Sharpe, Brown, Thompson, & Eckman, 1994) and vaccines in the management of SCD have significantly decreased the mortality rate in children. As a result, the long-term psychosocial adjustment of these children is of increasing focus. Research to date has examined such areas as neurocognitive deficits, social functioning, and psychological adaptation; however, the findings from these studies are often equivocal, with some research suggesting difficulties and others finding few differences between children with SCD and typically developing children. More research therefore is needed to further clarify the subsequent long-term effects of living with this chronic condition.

ETIOLOGY OF SICKLE CELL DISEASE

SCD is a hereditary condition caused by a genetic point mutation in an individual's hemoglobin, the oxygen-carrying component of the red blood cells. There are three genotypes of sickle cell syndromes: (1) the homozygous condition (HbSS), known as sickle cell anemia, caused by two abnormal genes for hemoglobin S; (2) a heterozygous condition (HbSC) for hemoglobin S and hemoglobin C; and (3) HbS-beta-thalassemia. The latter two conditions are typically more benign than HbSS sickle cell anemia. There also exists a carrier condition, labeled sickle cell trait, in which there is one normal gene for hemoglobin and one sickle cell gene. Hemoglobin is made up of four protein chains, two alpha chains and two beta chains. The point mutation occurs in one beta chain and leads to an incorrect amino acid being substituted for the correct one. This affects the red blood cell membrane, resulting in a change in the shape and texture of the cells. As a cell changes shape ("sickles"), it becomes a sticky substance that can cling to other cells, creating a mass that can become lodged in the bloodstream. When these lumps become large enough to interrupt or impede blood flow, they are termed vascular occlusions, or vasoocclusions (Embury, Hebbel, Steinberg, & Mohandes, 1994).

Vasoocclusions

Vasoocclusions are one of the core symptoms of SCD and can have serious consequences. They can disrupt and retard blood flow, resulting in the deprivation of oxygen to parts of the body that are "downstream" of the site of the vasoocclusion. These vasoocclusions can occur anywhere in the body and frequently lead to acute pain crises, which are unpredictable and difficult to manage. These crises can be sudden and disruptive to daily functioning and are typically managed with analgesics and warmth, with emphasis on hydration. Vasoocclusions may cause tissue or organ damage due to the lack of oxygen or eventual ischemia. Further, vasoocclusions can lead to increased sickling, as cells tend to sickle when deoxygenated. Vasoocclusions are often caused by sickling, although it appears that there can be other antecedent events, to which the sickling is a secondary event. The mechanism seems to vary over time and depends on a number of factors, including which vascular bed is affected or the presence of concurrent illness, and it can differ greatly among patients. The location of a vasoocclusion can vary over time and also seems to depend on a number of factors. When vasoocclusions occur in the brain, they are referred to as cerebral vascular accidents (CVAs) and may result in many serious consequences, including ischemia (deprivation of oxygen to tissue, which can lead to deadening of tissues or stroke) or infarcts (death of tissue). When a stroke occurs, the symptoms that emerge depend on the part of the brain affected by the deprivation of oxygen (Embury et al., 1994).

Neurophysiological Complications

The potential neurological complications of SCD are vast and can be quite severe. Cerebrovascular disease, including cerebral infarction and intracranial hemorrhage, is a common possibility. Cerebrovascular complications may actually occur at many sites in the central nervous system (CNS) and, thus, various symptoms will result. Oxygen deprivation in the brain due to occlusion of blood cells can lead to an ischemic stroke, which may result in either transient symptoms (e.g., transient ischemic attack [TIA]) or permanent neurological damage. Approximately 6% of children with SCD suffer from strokes, which can lead to a number of permanent neurological impairments (Powars, Wilson, Imbus, Pegelow, & Allen, 1978). For many years, pathology in the CNS has been clearly documented in association with sickle cell disease (Powars et al., 1978; Stockman, Nigro, & Mishkin, 1972; Sydenstricker, Mulhern, & Houseal, 1923). Additional possible neurological manifestations affecting individuals with SCD include hearing loss, neuropathy, and nutritional deficiencies, all of which may result in subtle neurological deficits and infections that can subsequently have an even greater impact on cognitive impairments (Adams, 1994).

Nutrition

Children with SCD may be at increased risk for nutritional deficiencies, which are linked to anemia and neurocognitive impairments. Although iron deficiencies may be seen in some cases, children with SCD seem to be most at risk for protein calorie deficiencies (Brown, Armstrong, & Eckman, 1993). Prolonged or severe protein deficiencies can interfere with the developing nervous system and have a detrimental impact on future cognitive functioning (Evans, Bowie, Hansen, & Moodie, 1980).

Anemia

Patients with SCD are often afflicted with chronic hemolytic anemia, where the body is attempting to compensate for the sickling and its consequences but cannot manage the effect on the red blood cells. The spleen is responsible for filtering blood, but the sickled red blood cells cause the system to have to put forth extra effort for the purpose of breaking them down. Although the body tries to compensate for this overload, as evidenced by an increased reticulocyte count (newly formed, young red blood cells being produced to compensate for the deficits), this is typically difficult. The result is decreased hemoglobin, decreased hematocrit (the portion of the blood that is red blood cells), a diminished red blood cell lifespan, and increased reticulocyte count. Sickling appears to induce cell abnormalities that lead to red blood cell destruction, although there appear to be many mechanisms involved. The symptoms and the degree of anemia can vary widely across individuals and between different genotypes, and, occasionally, it can vary from time to time in the same individual (Mohandes & Hebbel, 1994).

Although it has been suggested that cognitive impairments often associated with iron deficiency anemia may be a factor in the cognitive functioning of patients with SCD with chronic anemia (Swift et al., 1989), this has not been empirically corroborated (Brown et al., 1993). Research that specifically examines the relationship between hemoglobin levels in patients with SCD and cognitive functioning is necessary to determine the extent of the impact anemia has on SCD (Brown et al., 1993).

Ophthalmological Complications

Individuals with SCD often exhibit ophthalmological complications, typically due to vasoocclusions in the blood vessels of the eye. The symptoms depend on the location of the vasoocclusion. For example, if they occur in the retina, which is very sensitive to the loss of oxygen, serious damage can result if the affected vessel is located in the central part of the retina, rather than in the peripheral portion. The central part is responsible for sharp vision, and vasoocclusions within this area that last for as little as 90 minutes can lead to infarction, which can result in unalterable loss of vision. When the vasoocclusion occurs in the peripheral portion, some abnormalities that have an impact on vision can result, but vision is rarely lost. Most frequently, vasoocclusions tend to occur in the peripheral retina, which triggers the onset of sickle cell retinopathy, the mechanisms of which are poorly understood. Vasoocclusions can also occur in the conjunctiva, the mucous membrane covering the surface of the eye, but this does not influence vision, as the conjunctiva is not affected by the loss of oxygen. Other ophthalmological complications may include color vision impairments and delayed adaptation to darkness (Lutty & Goldberg, 1994).

NEUROCOGNITIVE EFFECTS

Few studies exist that address the cognitive functioning of children with SCD. To date, the studies that have been conducted have provided contradictory results as to whether children with SCD do in fact experience problems with cognitive functioning and academic difficulties (Lemanek et al., 1995). In the earliest study of this issue, Chodorkoff and Whitten (1963) asserted that there were no significant intellectual deficits associated with SCD; however, more recent studies have noted some differences between children with SCD and their healthy peers. Flick and Duncan (1973) examined numerous neurological and psychological factors in children with sickle cell trait over a 4-year period and found that the only significant deficit in the children with sickle cell trait compared to their healthy peers was an apparent perceptual–motor deficit, as indicated by greater numbers of errors on the Bender–Gestalt and lower scores on the Draw-a-Person. These results, however, are not generalizable to all patients with SCD as the study included only individuals with sickle cell trait and not children with actual disease genotypes. In a more recent study, Swift et al. (1989) examined neuropsychological functioning in children with SCD and their healthy siblings and found that the subjects with SCD, despite having no evidence of overt neurological disease, had significantly lower Full Scale IQ scores and consistently lower scores than the controls on nearly all measures of cognitive functioning. School achievement for both groups was consistent with their respective cognitive test scores. Similarly, Whitten and Fischoff (1974), found decreased school achievement in children with SCD when compared to healthy controls.

A number of studies have examined the neuropsychological and psychosocial outcomes in children with SCD who have survived CVAs (Armstrong et al., 1996; Craft, Schatz, Glauser, Lee, & DeBaun, 1993; Hariman, Griffith, Hurtig, & Keehn, 1991). Studies in this area have examined the differences in children with SCD with and without CVA stroke. In one such study, Craft et al. (1993) examined whether the presence and location of a CVA as determined by magnetic resonance imaging (MRI) affected specific neuropsychological functions in children with SCD. Results indicated that the pattern of stroke influences the pattern of neuropsychological impairment. Children who were classified as having had a diffuse cortical stroke were found to exhibit impairment on measures of spatial ability, while children with anterior lesions exhibited attentional problems. No significant differences were found on measures of motor, verbal, or memory measures between children with CVAs and sibling controls. However, results from another study (Hariman et al., 1991) that compared children with SCD who had had at least one stroke with children with SCD who had not suffered a stroke found that although patients with stroke had more severe psychosocial impairments, most patients did exhibit impairments in intellectual functioning, language functions, and social and personal adjustment. Psychosocial deficits were found to significantly outweigh any physical disabilities. Powars et al. (1978), in their follow-up investigation of SCD patients who had suffered a stroke, found that although there was some recovery of function immediately following a stroke, patients never regained full recovery of their previous intellectual functioning. Furthermore, multiple strokes over time resulted in furthering of progressive neurological deficits, including decreased scores in intelligence.

In studies using MRI to detect neurological evidence of stroke, many children have been found to have evidence of stroke on MRI without any history of a damaging neurological event as detected by routine examination (Armstrong et al., 1996; Craft et al., 1993). These strokes have been termed silent infarcts or microvascular infarcts. MRI has detected cerebral infarction in 11–20% of children with SCD with no observable neurological deficit. These subtle cerebrovascular infarcts have been hypothesized to be responsible for learning problems in children with SCD (Armstrong et al., 1996). Armstrong et al. (1996) provided data to suggest that silent infarcts result in areas of diminished function, but the outcome is not as severe as is seen in children with CVAs as detected by neurological exam. Neuropsychological impairment appears to become greater with age. CNS abnormalities were found to occur more frequently in children with HbSS when compared to children with HbSC disease.

One intervention that is currently used to prevent recurrent strokes is chronic transfusion therapy (Armstrong et al., 1996). This approach has been shown to be successful in decreasing the number of subsequent strokes.

Fowler et al. (1988) compared the academic performance and neuropsychological functioning in children with SCD and typically developing children, controlling for such factors as socioeconomic status, disease characteristics, and neurological development. Families completed measures that assessed family functioning, stressful life events, and illness severity. Children were administered a screening battery of neuropsychological tests to assess cognitive functioning, language ability, visual–motor integration, and attention. In addition, achievement testing was conducted to assess school functioning. Results indicated that children with SCD scored significantly lower than typically developing controls on the Coding subtest of the Wechsler Intelligence Scale for Children—Revised (WISC-R; Wechsler, 1974), which assesses visual–motor skill and speed. Children with SCD also scored more poorly on the Reading and Spelling tasks of the Wide Range Achievement Test (WRAT; Jastak & Wilkinson, 1984) than did the children who served as controls. When considering age, older children with SCD scored significantly lower on measures of attention in comparison to other children. Interestingly, children with SCD were rated by their teachers as more productive than the typically developing controls. These results suggest that more subtle difficulties in reading, visual–motor ability, and attention may be problems that are not always evident on a standard neurological exam.

In a study conducted by Wasserman, Wilimas, Fairclough, Mulhern, and Wang (1991), children with SCD or thalassemia were compared with siblings who possessed sickle cell trait or who were not identified as having sickle cell disease. Children were administered the Luria–Nebraska (Golden, 1981), the WISC-R, and the WRAT. Results indicated that children with SCD scored lower than their siblings on the WISC-R Performance and Full Scale IQ. No differences were found on the WRAT. On the Luria Nebraska, while there were no differences between children over 13 and their siblings, younger children demonstrated several decrements in performance relative to their younger siblings. Younger children with SCD were found to score significantly lower on tasks involving writing, arithmetic, visual–motor skills, and memory.

Most of the studies to date have only included children with the major (homozygous) trait form of SCD. Reing (1975) utilized genetic theory to link learning disabilities in children at risk for the minor (heterozygous) trait form of SCD and thalassemia to gene-determined neurochemical abnormalities. This is an important investigation in that the minor form of the disease, while frequently undetected, can produce symptoms that have the ability to impede and reduce energy level. Subjects included 191 children referred for learning problems. Subjects were divided into groups based on Mediterranean descent (thalassemia prone), African-American descent (SCD prone), or other descent (controls). Results indicated that children of Mediterranean and African-American descent displayed greater learning difficulties, more fatigue, poorer attention span, and poorer visual–perceptual abilities than the control subjects who were also referred for psychoeducational testing. Although differences were found between the groups, which included children referred for similar problems, a major limitation of the study is that the presence of SCD or thalassemia in these children was not confirmed by laboratory studies.

In the literature, it is frequently assumed that children with SCD are at risk for the development of neurocognitive and academic problems (Goonan, Goonan, Brown, Buchanan, & Eckman, 1994). It is possible that such potential neurological impairments found in these children may be due to physiological processes related to the disease. A vasoocclusion can result in cerebral hemorrhaging (although rare in children with SCD), major cerebral accidents (which occur more frequently in children than in adults; approximately 6%), or microvascular infarcts (where an occlusion precludes oxygen from reaching an area of the brain; these are typically not detected on routine physical exams) (Goonan et al., 1994). A significant percentage of children with SCD experience these phenomena particularly in the frontal lobe area. Other occurrences that could result in neurocognitive deficits in children with SCD include chronic anemia (oxygen deprivation to the brain), nutritional deficiencies, or ischemia (tissue death) (Lemanek et al., 1995). Studies have found that children with SCD score lower on a reading decoding achievement test and a sustained attention task, the latter of which is associated with frontal lobe functioning (for review, see Tarnowski & Brown, 1995). In another study however, social class was found to be the best predictor of cognitive functioning beyond the physiological effects of the disease (Lemanek et al., 1995). Social class therefore may serve as a specific risk factor for the development of cognitive functioning in children with SCD. For this reason, early intervention programs, such as Head Start programs, should be a high priority, particularly for those children who are designated at risk. When controlling for social class, level of hemoglobin has been found to be predictive of intellectual functioning, fine motor skills, and academic achievement (for review, see Lemanek et al., 1995; Tarnowski & Brown, 1995). Since hemoglobin is the oxygen transport molecule in red blood cells, this could be indicative of a chronic reduced level of oxygen delivered to the brain. Reduction in cognitive functioning may also be the result of subclinical strokes, which are typically undetected by routine physical examination.

In summary, while there are a number of studies indicating various subtle neurocognitive deficits in children with sickle cell disease, it is difficult to determine the etiology of such difficulties. Such problems may in fact be due to specific neurological symptoms related to the disease, such as vasoocclusions, or they may be due to other factors, including social class, the stress of coping with a chronic and incurable disease, physical limitations resulting from the disease, increased fatigue, recurring pain crises, hospitalizations, or school absences.

PSYCHOSOCIAL EFFECTS

Currently, there are a number of studies that have examined the ramifications of SCD on the psychological adjustment of children, adolescents, and their families. Many of these studies suggest that there is a broad range of adaptation in children and adolescents with SCD, with only a small segment of the SCD population being at risk for developing serious psychological problems (for review, see Midence et al., 1993; Tarnowski & Brown, 1995). Risk in general has not been found to be associated with disease severity or frequency of pain but instead with the age and sex of the affected child and with the specific coping strategies utilized in adjusting to the stressors associated with the disease (Midence et al., 1993).

Self-Concept

Studies have been conducted to assess the emotional and behavioral adaptation of children and adolescents with SCD. Self-concept of children with SCD has been examined with varying results yielded across studies. Earlier studies found that children with SCD displayed poorer self-concepts (Midence et al., 1993; Schuman, Armstrong, Pegelow, & Routh, 1993), although more recent studies have not distinguished between younger children with and without SCD on measures of self-concept (Lemanek et al., 1995). However, in these later studies, adolescents with SCD were "more susceptible to the negative influences of their medical condition on specific dimensions of their self-concept" (Lemanek et al., 1995, p. 291). Adolescents with SCD reported less satisfaction with their bodies and had more negative views of sexuality and physical development when compared to healthy peers. It is possible that these differences in self-concept may be due to the effect SCD has on growth and puberty.

Social Competence

Social competence has been another area of interest, as it relates to the functioning of children with SCD. Inadequate social competence in healthy children has been found to be associated with a greater prevalence of psychiatric problems, poor adjustment to academic demands, and disruptions to the family system (Cicchetti, Toth, & Bush, 1988). In essence, good peer relationships and meaningful family relationships provide the skills necessary for adequate social competence. Problems with social adjustment appear to affect both boys and girls with SCD. In fact, Hurtig and White (1986) consider SCD to have a greater impact on social adjustment than psychological adjustment. Children with SCD have been found to spend less time in social activities, have less contact with friends and have fewer friends than do their healthy peers (Lemanek et al., 1995; Midence et al., 1993; Schuman et al., 1993). However, the frequency of potentially contagious symptoms was the factor that was most associated with fewer contacts with friends, as opposed to the frequency of pain crises. The greatest impact of disease appears to be in adolescent males (Lemanek et al., 1995). However, other studies have indicated that there are no differences between children with SCD and controls in self-perceived competence and peer acceptance (Schuman et al., 1993). Young children with SCD also have been found to display adequate levels of social competence as rated by parents and teachers (Lemanek, Horwitz, & Ohene-Frempong, 1994; Schuman et al., 1993).

Externalizing Problems

A range of behavior problems of children and adolescents with SCD has been examined in various settings and with different informants, including parents, teachers, and children. Children and adolescents have been found to exhibit more problematic behavior at home, school, and with peers than controls; however, individual ratings were not found to be clinically significant (Lemanek et al., 1995). Both age and sex effects have been reported, with adolescent males being more likely to display somatic, immature, and overactive behavior than girls and younger children with SCD. It is believed that this difference may be due to the general developmental immaturity of boys. The importance society places on male physical strength could also be a contributing factor. Consistent with this hypothesis, one study provided data to show that a significant number of boys with SCD worried more than their healthy counterparts about their ability to play sports (Lemanek et al., 1995). Another study examining preschool children with SCD found no differences in externalizing behavior between the children with SCD and controls (Schuman et al., 1993). These findings support the apparent age effect in externalizing behaviors among children and adolescents with SCD, with older children evidencing a greater frequency of behavior problems relative to their younger peers.

Internalizing Problems

In contrast to the relatively few behavior problems among children with SCD, high rates of internalizing behavior problems have been found. Consistent with the externalizing disorders, there appears to be an effect for age in internalizing disorders, with adolescents being at a greater risk than elementary school-age children for developing difficulties in adjustment (Midence et al., 1993). Symptoms of anxiety and phobias were the most frequent types of child adjustment disorders observed in children with SCD (Thompson et al., 1994). In addition, symptoms of depression have also been found to occur at a higher frequency than in the general population, with more severe symptoms in children with SCD (Lemanek et al., 1995; Midence et al., 1993; Schuman et al., 1993). Internalizing problems have been posited to be associated with the frequency of pain episodes (Tarnowski & Brown, 1995) or specifically to the "unpredictability and uncontrollability" of such pain episodes (Lemanek et al., 1995).

CHILD COPING STYLE

As previously mentioned, coping strategies have been demonstrated to be a good predictor of children's psychological adjustment. A relationship between coping strategies and health-seeking behavior was found among children with SCD (for review, see Tarnowski & Brown, 1995). Children who scored high on negative thinking and passive adherence were found to be less active in school and in social situations, required more health care services, and reported greater psychologically distress during painful episodes (Gil, Williams, Thompson, & Kinney, 1991; Tarnowski & Brown, 1995). Negative thinking also was found to be associated with higher levels of adjustment problems (Lemanek et al., 1995). Gil et al. (1993) found that the frequency of active coping attempts was associated with higher levels of school, household, and social activity during painful episodes, while passive adherence and negative thinking were associated with more frequent health care contacts. An association between parental coping strategies and child behavior also has been demonstrated. For example, parents who score high on passive adherence and negative thinking have children who display a higher incidence of activity reduction and more internalizing and externalizing behavior problems (Gil et al., 1991; Tarnowski & Brown, 1995). Thompson et al. (1994) found that at a 10-month follow-up, children's coping strategies for pain accounted for a significant amount of the variance in child-reported symptoms and internalizing behavior problems as reported by mothers above the contribution of illness and demographic parameters. Unfortunately, there has been a dearth of studies that have examined coping strategies. Thus, there is much to be learned about the stability of coping strategies over time and the direction of the association between parent and child coping strategies.

FAMILY FACTORS

As researchers have been increasingly sensitive to the significant role of the family in mediating the potential effects of a chronic illness, studies have begun to investigate family relationships for children with SCD. In general, it is the parent–parent relationships, not the parent–child relationships, that impact adjustment for children with SCD (Midence et al., 1993). Children's illness significantly impacts psychological adjustment, employment opportunities, and marital functioning and satisfaction. These findings are consistent with the general chronic illness literature (Tarnowski & Brown, 1995). Specific factors, including social support and knowledge, have been identified as contributing to positive family relationships, whereas social class, family structure, and illness severity were not found to be predictive of parental adjustment (Hurtig, 1994). A relationship also has been demonstrated between parent's knowledge about the disease, stability and availability of their social network, parental coping methods, and children's self-esteem (Tarnowski & Brown, 1995). Increased family cohesion and organization also are associated with resilience and coping competency of SCD children (Midence et al., 1993; Tarnowski & Brown, 1995). Families of girls with SCD have been found to have more positive familial relationships, thus suggesting a possible differential influence by gender (Hurtig, 1994).

ASSESSMENT

The number of problems experienced by children with SCD dictate that ongoing and careful assessment must be the standard of care for children with SCD. Basic screening should include questions about the child's academic functioning, along with particular skill strengths and deficits (e.g., math, spelling, reading), and emotional functioning, including self-concept, symptoms of depression, anxiety, behavior problems, and problems with attention and concentration. Such information should be obtained across situations during the clinical interview, as well as from the parent, child, and teacher. It may be useful to send questionnaires to the parents prior to meeting with them so the information is available at the initial meeting. Because children with SCD are at risk, ongoing screening for cognitive and academic problems should be routine.

INTERVENTION

Treatment of SCD involves primarily medical management of the disorder, as to date, no specific cures are available. Information about the patient's medical, neurological, psychological, academic, and social functioning should be integrated to produce a comprehensive intervention plan. The general medical treatments include newborn screening, directed analgesics, blood transfusions, and bone marrow transplants. Psychological treatments and interventions include supportive psychotherapy to assist with stress and coping, genetic counseling, support groups, and psychoeducational programs (Midence et al., 1993). Since no cure exists for SCD, treatments focus on the management of symptoms associated with the disease. One of the most frequent and severe stressors associated with SCD is the experience of pain crises, the uncertainty of when a pain crisis will occur, and the adverse effects the painful episodes have on daily life. While there is no specific means of preventing pain episodes, various therapies for managing pain have been researched and are currently standard practice. The most common medical treatments for pain crises include narcotics, analgesics, warmth and hydration. Unfortunately, many of the analgesics used for the treatment of SCD are the narcotics, such as meperidine (Demerol) or morphine, and concerns regarding use of these medications include adverse effects such as sedation and lethargy, which may impair cognitive performance (Davis, 1995).

Psychological interventions also have proven useful for the management of pain crises in children with SCD. Treatments include cognitive-behavioral techniques, biofeedback, hypnosis, and behavioral techniques. Self-regulatory strategies and patient-controlled anesthetic devices are forms of cognitive-behavioral techniques. However, the use of self-administered anesthetic devices has been found to be of questionable success for those patients who are also suffering from major psychological problems (Lemanek et al., 1995). Cognitive-behavioral programs that train children and adolescents with SCD to modify their negative thinking and passive coping patterns and to take an active approach to coping by using multiple strategies may prove to be effective in assisting in the management of pain (Gil et al., 1993). Biofeedback also has been demonstrated to be effective for managing pain crises. With this technique, children receive precise and immediate information about biological functions by means of electronic measuring devices (Lemanek et al., 1995). Patients are then trained to make changes in biological functions, thereby decreasing pain sensations. Hypnosis also has been demonstrated to be successful in reducing the number of pain crises in two case studies (Zeltzer, Dash, & Holland, 1979). During hypnosis, patients were instructed to visualize their blood cells dilating in order to allow the sickled red blood cells to flow more easily. Finally, self-hypnosis also has been proven to be successful in assisting with pain management (Midence et al., 1993).

Other behavioral techniques used with this population include relaxation methods and pain behavior contracts (Davis, 1995; Tarnowski & Brown, 1995). Progressive muscle relaxation, meditative breathing, autogenics (repeating certain words), and imagery-based techniques are relaxation techniques that have demonstrated success with children and adolescents (Peterson & Harbeck, 1988). Pain behavior contracts involve various levels of behavior and specific dosages and frequency of pain medications. Subsequently, children move onto higher levels, gaining additional responsibilities for the management of their pain. The intent of this strategy is to foster beliefs of control in the patient, rather than feelings of helplessness that may be caused by the unpredictability and uncontrollability of pain crises. Furthermore, Sharpe et al. (1994) have provided data suggesting the importance of active and adaptive coping in caretakers of children with SCD. The implication of this study is that since maternal coping style has been found to be predictive of children's coping style, interventions that include parents may be very beneficial in managing children's pain (Sharpe et al., 1994).

Information obtained during the psychological evaluation examination may inform school-based interventions to assist the child with attentional difficulties and academic difficulties. The focus may be on individual learning techniques, such as memory skills or summarizing strategies, or on developing compensatory skills to compensate for specific learning problems. Children may be at a level where self-instruction may prove successful, or, in some cases, contingency management techniques may be more appropriate, particularly when behavior is a problem. Shapiro (1989) also has stressed the importance of taking into account instructional contextual factors, such as rate of presentation, reinforcement, contingencies, prompting, cuing, and feedback mechanisms that may affect learning. Rourke (1994) was instrumental in advancing an integrated intervention for children with various types of brain injury through the construction of the Developmental Neuropsychological Remediation/Rehabilitation Model (DNRR). Although this model was initially designed to be used with children with learning disabilities, the steps involved may be appropriate for use with children who suffer from other disorders that involve CNS dysfunction, including SCD. Use of the DNRR begins with the assessment of factors that influence learning capacity by examining the interactions of neuropsychological strengths and weaknesses, learning disabilities, academic achievement, and psychosocial adaptive functioning. Demands of the environment in which the child is learning are then taken into account. Such demands may include various types of behavioral, academic, and psychosocial challenges. Short- and long-term behavioral predictions are made regarding those deficits that may be expected to decrease regardless of intervention efforts and the intervention strategies that will be most appropriate to address those deficits that are not expected to decrease spontaneously. Ideal plans are generated and altered as the availability of remedial resources are identified. Finally, Rourke has recommended ongoing assessment in conjunction with treatment.

LIMITATIONS AND FUTURE DIRECTIONS

Unfortunately, a number of limitations exist in the available research on SCD in children and adolescents. Although many of the studies assess disease severity, severity has been conceptualized differently across studies. Some techniques for quantifying severity have included the number of days missed from school, number of pain crises a year, total number of hospital visits, or a compilation of these indices. However, no accepted measure or index has been recognized as the gold standard, and this may explain some of the discrepancies across studies. Another limitation involves the small sample sizes in clinical studies, which may limit statistical power, thereby obscuring significant results that may occur with an otherwise larger sample. Further, the variability of age ranges across studies is also problematic, because it makes comparisons among studies difficult. Longitudinal studies are needed to follow children and adolescents through the lifespan and to evaluate the cumulative effects of the illness over time. Further, problems are inherent in maternal reports of child behavior problems. An association has been found between maternal psychological adjustment, specifically maternal levels of anxiety and depression, and maternal reports of child behavioral problems (Lemanek et al., 1995). This has significant ramifications for the validity of maternal reports of child behavioral problems. Thus, it is recommended that studies evaluate children's functioning across situations. Finally, many of the studies have failed to control for type of hemoglobinopathy (HbSS, HbSC and HbS-beta-thalassemia), an index that is highly associated with disease severity (Sharpe et al., 1994).

SUMMARY

SCD is a genetic disorder that compromises the shape of red blood cells and their oxygen-carrying capacity. These abnormalities lead to multiple physiological pathologies. The ischemia and the subsequent tissue damage caused by this condition leave many children with the burden of managing recurrent painful episodes. Since the symptoms of SCD impact a child's ability to perform routine activities, this disease impacts a child's life on a daily basis. With the decreasing mortality rate among individuals with SCD, concomitant problems, such as neurocognitive impairments, depression, and decreased involvement with peers, are emerging as a result of living with a chronic disease. Although there is a body of research that has investigated the psychosocial impact of SCD on individuals, many questions still remain. The inconsistencies in research findings need to be resolved in order to generate a more cohesive understanding of SCD. Research efforts are emerging that have identified those variables that contribute to the resiliency of children with SCD or their vulnerability to the development of psychosocial problems. More research needs to be conducted in order to facilitate the development of effective interventions that will promote adaptive development in children with SCD, thereby improving the quality of life for these children and their families.

REFERENCES

Adams, R. J. (1994). Neurologic complications. In S. H. Embury, R. P. Hebbel, N. Mohandes, & M. H. Steinberg, (Eds.), *Sickle cell disease: Basic principles and clinical practice* (pp. 599–621). New York: Raven Press.

Armstrong, F. D., Thompson, R. J., Wang, W., Zimmerman, R., Pegelow, C. H., Miller, S., Moser, F., Bello, J., Hurtig, A., & Vass, K. (1996). Cognitive function-

Tarnowski, K., & Brown, R. (1995). Psychological aspects of pediatric disorders. In M. Hersen & R. Ammerman (Eds.), *Advanced abnormal child psychology* (pp. 393–410). Hillsdale, NJ: Erlbaum.

Thompson, R., Gil, K., Keith, B., Gustafson, K., George, L., & Kinney, T. (1994). Psychological adjustment of children with sickle cell disease: Stability and change over a 10-month period. *Journal of Consulting and Clinical Psychology, 62*(4), 856–860.

Wasserman, A.L., Wilimas, J. A., Fairclough, D. L., Mulhern, R. K., & Wang, W. (1991). Subtle neuropsychological deficits in children with sickle cell disease. *American Journal of Pediatric Hematology/Oncology, 13*, 14–20.

Wechsler, D. (1974). *Manual for the Wechsler Intelligence Scale for Children—Revised (WISC-R)*. San Antonio, TX: Psychological Corporation.

Whitten, C. F. & Fischoff, J. (1974). Psychosocial effects of sickle cell disease. *Archives of Internal Medicine, 133*, 681–689.

Zeltzer, L., Dash, J., & Holland, J. (1979). Hypnotically induced pain control in sickle cell anemia. *Pediatrics, 10*, 81–85.

CHAPTER NINE

Cardiac Conditions

ALAN M. DELAMATER
ERIKA U. BRADY
MARC J. BLUMBERG

As a result of advances in the medical and surgical treatment of cardiovascular disease in children, many pediatric patients who would have previously died as a result of their illness are now surviving. Consequently, there has been increased concern regarding the long-term cognitive and psychosocial sequelae of these disorders and their treatments. In recent years a number of studies have begun to examine the cognitive and psychosocial sequelae associated with cardiac conditions in children.

This chapter first focuses on the major types of pediatric cardiac disease and the medical management of each. Cardiac conditions in children include congenital heart disease (CHD), acquired heart disease, and arrhythmias. The effects of cardiac disease on children's cognitive development and behavioral and emotional functioning are then reviewed. The majority of developmental research in this area has been conducted on children with CHD, who comprise the largest single group of children with cardiac problems.

MEDICAL ASPECTS OF PEDIATRIC CARDIAC DISORDERS

Congenital Heart Disease

Approximately 8 children in 1,000 are born with CHD (Gersony, 1987). CHD refers to a variety of disorders involving structural defects to the heart or the coronary blood vessels. Most cases are diagnosed during infancy and are presumed to be due to a combination of genetic and environmental factors. CHD can occur as an isolated birth defect, or it can be associated with various other anomalies. CHD is divided into cyanotic and acyanotic subtypes, each having a distinctive clinical presentation. For example, it is only in the cyanotic type of CHD that oxygenation of the blood is significantly reduced. As reviewed later in the chapter, cyanosis has been implicated as one important factor in deficits in cognitive and psychosocial functioning.

Acyanotic Congenital Heart Disease

In acyanotic CHD the blood is shunted away from the body and to the lungs as a result of holes in the walls of the heart chambers. This is the most common type of CHD and includes ventricular septal defects (about 28% of CHD cases), atrial septal/atrial–ventricular canal defects (about 10% of CHD), patent ductus arteriosus (about 10% of CHD), and coarctation (i.e., constriction) of the aorta (about 5% of CHD). Valvular lesions (which obstruct blood flow at the valves) may result in either pulmonic stenosis (about 10% of CHD) or aortic stenosis (about 7% of CHD). Cardiomyopathy (i.e., disease of the heart muscle) is another type of acyanotic CHD with hypertrophic, congestive, and restrictive subtypes (Gersony, 1987).

Cyanotic Congenital Heart Disease

In cyanotic CHD the blood is also shunted away from the lungs, but as a consequence of a communication between the systemic and pulmonary circulations. The result is a reduction in oxygenation of the blood referred to as cyanosis. Examples of these defects include pulmonary atresia and tetralogy of Fallot (TOF), each of which account for about 10% of CHD cases. Another 5% of CHD cases involve transposition of the great arteries (TGA), in which there is a reversal of the aorta and pulmonary arteries, leading to mixing of oxygenated and deoxygenated blood.

Medical Management

As a result of differences in lesion location and severity, children and adolescents may experience various symptoms, which can include fatigue, dyspnea (shortness of breath), growth failure, cough, cyanosis, and chest pain. With mild versions of the disease no treatment is typically needed other than regular medical follow-up. Patients with mild to moderate disease could be expected to function normally, but those with severe disease will likely have decreased exercise tolerance and restricted physical activity. Due to increased susceptibility to fatigue, headaches, and dizziness, cyanotic patients are advised to avoid high altitudes, abrupt changes in temperature, and situations in which dehydration could occur. Females with severe cyanotic CHD are at increased risk for problems related to pregnancy; with corrective surgery, those with mild or moderate disease can have normal pregnancies.

The most severe defects can now be corrected surgically during infancy. Even though mortality rates are low, the surgery itself may result in adverse changes in functioning in both significant and subtle ways, including mental retardation, language and learning disorders, and movement and seizure disorders (Fallon, Aparicio, Elliott, & Kirkham, 1995; Ferry, 1987, 1990). Neurological problems following cardiac surgery have reported prevalence rates ranging from 2% to 25%. Imaging studies and autopsies of infants who have died have documented acquired brain lesions following open-heart surgery, including evidence of diffuse hypoxic/ischemic injury, areas of focal infarction, and microscopic abnormalities in gray and white matter (Miller, Mamourian, Tesman, Baylen, & Myers, 1994; Muraoka et al., 1981).

In recent years several new trends have developed in the surgical treatment of CHD: primary surgical repair during the neonatal period; use of low-flow cardiopulmonary bypass; and use of extracorporeal membrane oxygenation (ECMO). In a clinical series of 304 neonates who underwent primary surgical repair, a total mortality rate of 11.8% was observed (Castaneda et al., 1989). Low-flow cardiopulmonary bypass rather than hypothermic circulatory arrest as a support technique during cardiac surgery has been shown to be associated with lower postoperative central nervous system (CNS) perturbations and fewer neuropsychological deficits (Newburger et al., 1993; Oates, Simpson, Turnbull, & Cartmill, 1995). ECMO has been successfully used in life-threatening situations for cardiac support and as a bridge to transplantation when children decompensate after open-heart surgery or suffer acute decompensation due to chronic cardiomyopathy or viral myocarditis (del Nido, 1996; Klein, Shaheen, Whittlesey, Pinsky, & Arciniegas, 1990). The neurodevelopmental effects of ECMO are discussed in a later section.

Interventional catheterization has been increasingly used for repair of certain types of CHD, as an alternative to open-heart surgery (Lock, Keane, Mandell, & Perry, 1992). For example, angioplasty has been shown to be efficacious for recurrent coarctation of the aorta and valvuloplasty has been successfully used for pulmonic and aortic stenosis. Interventional catheterization has also been used to treat patent ductus arteriosus and atrial septal defects.

In those cases where neither open-heart repairs nor interventional catheterization are feasible, heart transplantation has become an accepted treatment approach (Addonizio, 1996; Baum & Bernstein, 1993). More than 1,200 pediatric heart transplantations have been conducted through

1994, with 1-year survival of approximately 77% and 5-year survival of 70% (Addonizio, 1996; Hosenpud, Novick, Breen, Keck, & Daily, 1995). The impact of transplantation on child functioning is considered in a later section of this chapter.

Follow-up at regular intervals is an important part of treatment. Depending on the status of the lesion, patients may be seen anywhere from once a week to once a year. Many patients seen by pediatric cardiologists are older children and adolescents whose defects were corrected in early childhood. Routine tests for evaluation and monitoring include chest radiographs, electrocardiograms, echocardiography, exercise testing, radionuclide studies, and cardiac catheterization. Because invasive procedures such as catheterization may be stressful for young patients, routine clinical practice for most patients involves heavy sedation, including medications with amnestic properties. After corrective surgery, some patients and parents may fear recurrence of heart-related problems or have unrealistic perceptions concerning physical activity restrictions, creating distress. Residual problems may exist, requiring further interventions including surgery. Additional information on the medical aspects of CHD can be found in Gersony (1987) and Fyler (1992).

Acquired Heart Disease

Bacterial and/or viral infections in childhood can also damage the heart, resulting in a variety of disorders. These include infective endocarditis, rheumatic heart disease, and diseases of the myocardium and pericardium (Gersony, 1987). Although normal children may acquire these diseases, children with CHD may be particularly susceptible. Another type of acquired heart disease is coronary artery disease secondary to Kawasaki syndrome (Newburger, 1992).

Medical treatment for acquired heart disease includes prophylactic drug regimens, and sometimes cardiac surgery is required to repair the structural damage to the heart. When other treatment options are exhausted in severe cases, for example, when myocarditis progresses to cardiomyopathy, heart transplantation may be undertaken as a last resort.

Although mortality is low with early diagnosis and treatment, acquired heart disease still remains a significant cause of morbidity and mortality among children. Preventive interventions are therefore extremely important in the medical management of acquired heart disease. One of the major problems seen in clinical practice is nonadherence with prophylactic drug regimens. Despite the fact that these diseases pose a considerable health risk for children, empirical studies with this population are lacking. More research addressing cognitive development, psychosocial adjustment, and regimen adherence of children with acquired heart diseases is needed.

Arrhythmias

Childhood arrhythmias or cardiac rhythm disturbances can result from CHD (both acyanotic and cyanotic subtypes), acquired heart diseases, or acquired systemic disorders (Walsh & Saul, 1992). Primarily as a result of improved diagnostic methods with electrocardiogram, arrhythmias in children have been identified more frequently in recent years. Adding to this number are the survivors of cardiac surgery for CHD who may be at increased risk for arrhythmias. Some rhythm disturbances are common in children, such as premature atrial and ventricular beats, but are not associated with significant health risks in the majority of cases. However, severe untreated arrhythmia may lead to sudden death. The primary risk associated with an arrhythmia is severe tachycardia (fast heart rate) or bradycardia (slow heart rate) which leads to decreased cardiac output. The most common significant arrhythmias are bypass tracts such as Wolff–Parkinson–White (pre-excitation) syndrome (a type of supraventricular tachyarrhythmia) and congenital heartblock (a type of bradyarrhythmia) (Gersony, 1987).

Treatments for arrhythmias include pharmacological agents, surgery to remove bypass tracts, and implanted pacemakers and defibrillators. For some extreme cases unresponsive to these methods, heart transplantation may be needed. Problems with dosage of medications, variable responses, adverse side effects, and regimen adherence may be significant in the treatment of pediatric arrhythmias. Relatively little developmental, psychological, or behavioral research has been conducted with these patients.

COGNITIVE DEVELOPMENT
General and Disease-Related Issues

There are a number of factors that influence cognitive development in children with cardiovascular disease. Infancy and early childhood are periods when many chronic diseases can have negative effects on brain development and, therefore, on cognitive functions because the brain develops rapidly during the first several years of life. For example, glial proliferation and myelination in the central nervous system take place most rapidly during the first year of life (Epstein, 1978, 1986). Any interference with the process of brain development or growth, physical or psychosocial, may have a permanent negative effect on development. In children with heart disease, malnutrition may be present, and growth deficits are common.

In addition, there are factors that may impact cognitive development that are specifically the result of the pathophysiology of the disease. There are a number of processes that can interrupt the flow of oxygenated blood to the brain acutely or chronically in children with heart disease. In cyanotic CHD, oxygenation of the blood is reduced, which can interfere with brain development and produce brain injury. For some children with CHD, the risk of cerebrovascular injury is increased. In more severe cases, low cardiac output and cardiac arrhythmias may result in decreased blood flow to the brain. Children with severe heart disease may have cardiac arrests. Although they may be successfully resuscitated, these acute anoxic events could also have a negative impact on cognitive function. Finally, in some instances, CHD occurs in conjunction with other defects, forming a syndrome with associated cognitive deficits such as Down's syndrome.

A second set of factors influencing cognitive development in children with CHD are effects of treatment. Neurological sequelae of cardiac surgery are relatively common. As survival has increased, greater attention has focused on the effects of different procedures with the eventual aim of minimizing neurological damage. Possible pathogenetic mechanisms include microembolization (air and/or particulate matter), inadequate cerebral perfusion, hypoxia, and biochemical disturbances leading to neuronal damage, and hyperperfusion (Fallon et al., 1995; Ferry, 1987; Miller et al., 1994). Low-flow cardiopulmonary bypass and deep hypothermic circulatory arrest are two widely used support techniques, both of which can affect cerebral metabolism and hemodynamics, leading to cerebral ischemia/reperfusion injury in some children (du Plessis et al., 1994). The maximum time of circulatory arrest with hypothermia to protect the brain without neurological sequelae is controversial. However, clinical experience suggests that the "safe period" is approximately 45–60 minutes. Low-flow cardiopulmonary bypass has been advocated as an alternative to complete circulatory arrest because it produces less neurological sequelae. However, this support technique also can produce adverse neurological events due to microembolisms and hypoperfusion.

The use of ECMO for cardiac support also carries specific risks of neurological damage (Mendoza, Shearer, & Cook, 1991). In many cases, ECMO involves permanent ligation of the right common carotid artery and right internal jugular vein; however, if ECMO is required in the immediate time period following cardiotomy, cannulation is performed through the sternotomy. ECMO can affect blood flow rate and velocity, and brain imaging during ECMO or immediately following decannulation has shown evidence of hemorrhage or lesions (Lott, McPherson, Towne, Johnson, & Starr, 1990).

Heart transplantation also confers significant risk of neurological complications, with neurological sequelae reported in approximately 20% of heart transplant patients (Baum et al., 1993). In addition to the risks associated with open-heart surgery and cardiopulmonary bypass discussed earlier, use of drugs such as cyclosporine and steroids can have deleterious developmental consequences (Martin et al., 1992; Stewart, Kenard, Waller, & Fixler, 1994).

Finally, there are psychosocial variables that are common to children in whom significant chronic disease develops in infancy or early childhood. These include physical restriction, parental overprotection, reduced opportunities for peer socialization, frequent and/or prolonged hospitalizations resulting in relative isolation, and absence from school.

Effects of Congenital Heart Disease on Cognitive Development

In the following sections, studies that have investigated the impact of CHD on cognitive development will be reviewed. First, studies that have looked at cognitive outcomes for children with CHD as a whole are discussed, with particular attention to comparisons of cyanotic and acyanotic disease. The impact of different surgical and support techniques, including low-flow cardiopulmonary bypass, ECMO, and heart transplantation, are then discussed.

A number of studies have compared the cognitive status of children with cyanotic heart disease to children with acynotic heart lesions, with most studies demonstrating significantly lower cognitive functioning in the cyanotic group. One of the first was done by Linde, Rasof, and Dunn (1967), who compared preschool-age children with cyanotic CHD, acyanotic CHD, and two control groups of typically developing siblings and children from a well-child clinic. The children with CHD were assessed for intelligence (using either the Cattell, Gesell, or Stanford–Binet scale) prior to corrective cardiac surgery. Results showed significantly lower IQ for cyanotic compared with acyanotic children, and both CHD groups were lower than the control groups. However, the mean IQ for the cyanotic group was in the average range (mean of 96 vs. 104 for acyanotic). Furthermore, physical disability measures were associated with IQ scores, but only for younger patients. In a 5-year follow-up of these same children, Linde, Rasoff, and Dunn (1970) found significant increases in IQ scores only for cyanotic children who had received corrective surgery.

Silbert, Wolff, Mayer, Rosenthal, and Nadas (1969) examined children with cyanotic CHD (most of whom had prior open-heart surgery), children with acyanotic CHD with congestive heart failure, and children with acyanotic mild CHD. Children were tested between the ages of 4 and 8 years with the Stanford–Binet and several standardized tests of perceptual–motor and gross motor coordination skills. Children with cyanotic disease had significantly lower IQ scores and performed more poorly on the perceptual–motor and gross motor tasks. However, scores for the cyanotic group was in the normal range of intelligence (mean of 105 vs. 115 for acyanotic/congestive heart and 118.5 for acyanotic/mild CHD).

Aram, Ekelman, Ben-Shachar, and Levinsohn (1985) studied cognitive development in a sample of children with CHD ranging in age from 3 months to 15 years. A number of standardized intelligence tests (Bayley Scales, McCarthy, Wechsler Preschool and Primary Scales of Intelligence [WPPSI], or Wechsler Intelligence Scale for Children—Revised [WISC-R]) were administered, depending on the age of the child. Children with cyanotic heart disease were compared with children with acyanotic heart disease, and significantly lower IQ scores were observed for the cyanotic children (mean of 104 vs. 113).

DeMaso, Beardslee, Silbert, and Fyler (1990) evaluated children with tetrology of Fallot (TOF), children with transposition of the great arteries (TGA), and a group of children originally diagnosed with acyanotic CHD (ventricular septal defect, atrial septal defect, patent ductus arteriosis, or cardiomyopathy) but who had spontaneous recovery without medical intervention. All children in the study sample were diagnosed prior to 1 year of age and were tested between ages 5 and 6. In most cases the WPPSI was used as the measure of intelligence. The findings revealed that children in both cyanotic groups had significantly lower IQ scores than the controls. Fourteen percent of children with TGA and 22% of those with TOF had IQ scores less than 79, compared with only 3% of the acyanotic children. Moreover, 40% of TGA and 45% of TOF children had clinically significant CNS impairment.

Although these studies indicate that, as a group, children with cyanotic heart disease are more vulnerable with respect to overall cognitive development than children with acyanotic disease, several studies suggest that children with acyanotic heart disease also perform more poorly than typically developing controls. Linde, Rasof, and Dunn (1967) found that acyanotic children, tested prior to corrective surgery, achieved lower scores than the control groups. Yang, Liu, and Townes (1994) compared the test performance of children from China with acyanotic heart disease to a control group and reported that the scores of the acynotic group were lower on tests of intelligence.

For children with cyanotic heart disease there is evidence supporting the notion that surgery conducted at earlier ages is associated with improved cognitive functioning. For example, in a study of cyanotic children (mean age at testing was 5.8 years) who had corrective surgery for TGA prior to testing, Newburger, Silbert, Buckley, and Fyler (1984) found IQ (measured by a short form of the WPPSI) to be in the average range (mean of 102). While there was no difference compared with acyanotic children (all with ventricular septal defect) who had also received corrective surgery, a significant inverse correlation was observed between age at repair (reflecting duration of hypoxia) and IQ for the cyanotic children; there was no relationship between age at repair and IQ for the acyanotic group.

O'Dougherty, Wright, Garmezy, Loewenson, and Torres (1983) evaluated a number of developmental outcomes in a sample of children with TGA, using standardized measures of intelligence, perceptual–motor functioning, and academic achievement. The children had open-heart surgical repair during early childhood (mean age of 2 years) and were tested at a mean age of 9.1 years. Although the mean IQ of the group was in the normal range, the distribution was bimodal, with more children than expected having borderline or lower intelligence (13%) or superior or very superior intelligence (16%). An inverse correlation was observed between age at surgery and IQ, perceptual–motor function, and academic achievement. Forty-two percent of the sample required special education programming at school. Analyses indicated that age at surgical correction, growth failure, congestive heart failure, CNS infection, cerebrovascular stroke, and lower socioeconomic status, and family stress were associated with poorer outcomes. Although the sample size was too small for use of multivariate analyses to refine the risk model, the findings suggest that chronic hypoxia has adverse effects on cognitive development.

Wright and Nolan (1994) examined the impact of cyanotic heart disease on children's school performance. They compared the academic and intellectual performance of 29 children ages 7–12 years with TGA or TOF whose lesions had been corrected before age 2.5 to 36 children with cardiac murmurs that did not require treatment. Children with evidence of major CNS trauma as a result of the cardiac lesion or its treatment were excluded. Children with cyanotic heart disease performed significantly worse on the measure of intelligence (WISC-R) and on all academic measures assessed by the Wide Range Achievement Test—Revised (WRAT-R). However, the mean IQ score fell within the average range, while mean performance on academic measures was within the low-average range. In addition, teacher ratings revealed significant differences between the groups with respect to arithmetic performance, with children in the cyanotic group more likely to rated as below grade level in arithmetic. There was no statistically significant association between cognitive or academic functioning and any of the medical or surgical parameters, including age at surgery.

Several studies have investigated specific cognitive and neuropsychological deficits associated with CHD. A number of studies indicate that perceptual–motor skills are adversely affected by CHD (Linde et al., 1967; Newburger et al., 1984; Silbert, Wolff, Mayer, Rosenthal, & Nadas, 1969). As cyanosis, presumably due to hypoxia, has been linked with greater intellectual impairment, processes presumed to be more sensitive to hypoxia have been investigated. Although the actual effects of chronic hypoxia on the developing CNS are not known, inferences have been made based on findings such as those of adults with chronic obstructive airways disease, a condition associated with hypoxia (Prigatano & Levin, 1988), and those of infants with perinatal hypoxia (Spreen, Risser, & Edgell, 1995). Based on these assumptions, researchers have examined attention, vigilance, and information-processing capacity.

Several studies have shown deficits in attentional processes in children with cyanotic heart disease. O'Dougherty, Wright, Loewenson, and Torres (1985) compared cyanotic children to a sample of control children matched for age, race, and socioeconomic status but with no history of sensory, neurological, or learning problems. The cyanotic CHD group scored significantly lower on the WISC-R Freedom from Distractibility factor than would be expected based on the standardization sample; in addition, 23% of the CHD sample versus only 4% of the WISC-R standardization sample had a 30-point discrepancy between Verbal and Performance IQ. Although 80% of the CHD sample had IQ scores in the average range or above, only 36% of the sample had academic achievement measures at or above grade level. On the continuous performance test (CPT), significant differences were observed between CHD and control children in terms of errors of omission and commission, signal–noise discrimination, and sustained attention.

Similarly, O'Dougherty, Nuechterlein, and Drew (1984) compared the performance of children with CHD to children with a *Diagnostic and Statistical Manual of Mental Disorders*, revised 3rd edition (DSM-III-R; American Psychiatric Association, 1987), diagnosis of attention deficit disorder (ADD) on a test of sustained attention (using the CPT). The two groups performed comparably with regard to overall vigilance. The children with ADD displayed difficulty with inhibitory control, whereas the CHD children had greater difficulty sustaining attention over time.

O'Dougherty, Berntson, Boysen, Wright, and Teske (1988) examined cardiac responses to nonsignal stimuli and to signal stimuli in a vigilance task in children with CHD (cyanotic and acyanotic), children with ADD, and typically developing children. Overall task performance was lower in subjects with heart defects and in the ADD group, but there were no significant differences between children with cyanotic and acyanotic CHD. Cardiac measures revealed that typically developing children displayed significantly larger heart rate deceleration to the target stimuli than did either of the clinical groups. Moreover, exaggerated heart rate deceleration was observed to vibrotactile stimuli in both clinical groups. Regression analyses revealed that the magnitude of the cardiac response to somatosensory stimuli was predictive of task performance (both within and between subject groups), with larger responses associated with higher error rates and lower perceptual sensitivity. For the normal control group, age was significantly related to false alarm rate, but this pattern was much weaker in the CHD and ADD groups, suggesting that typical age-related changes in attentional capacity may be disrupted for children with CHD and ADD. In addition to differences in test performance, parent ratings for the children with CHD and ADD indicated significant problems with attention and hyperactivity.

However, in a more recent study, Wright and Nolan (1994) found no association between medical or surgical parameters and measures of attentional and processing difficulties. The authors comment that the nature of the cognitive and academic difficulties displayed are not fully explained by chronic hypoxia.

Kramer, Awiszus, Sterzel, van Halteren, and Claßen (1989) compared intellectual functioning in 4- to 14-year-old children with CHD to control children who had benign heart murmurs. The CHD group was divided into those with and without significant symptoms with regard to physical capacity. The findings indicated that symptomatic children had significantly lower IQ scores than healthy controls (mean of 103 vs. 114 for older children). Although there were no significant differences between the symptomatic and asymptomatic CHD groups, the latter group had slightly higher scores. However, the study sample was heterogeneous with regard to cyanosis, type of defect, and history of surgery.

In a study of long-term outcome of children with CHD, Utens et al. (1994) examined the functioning of a heterogeneous group of young adults in comparison to a group of normal controls. The CHD group had a significantly higher mean IQ score; however, the mean IQ score was inflated due to missing scores for a significant number, including 15 who could not complete the IQ test due to mental retardation. For the group as a whole, 17% had intellectual performance 1 standard deviation below the mean, a rate comparable to the control group. In comparing specific diagnostic groups, the group with pulmonary stenosis performed significantly better (mean IQ score = 110) than the group with TOF (mean IQ score = 98.8).

Two studies have examined the effects of surviving a cardiac arrest on the functioning of children with CHD. Morris, Krawiecki, Wright, and Walter (1993) examined the neuropsychological functioning of 2- to 14-year-old children, the majority of whom had CHD, who survived cardiac arrest with in-hospital resuscitation. A battery of standardized tests was administered at some unspecified time after resuscitation. Results were compared to the normative mean of the various tests used in the study, rather than to a control group. More children than expected scored less than 1 standard deviation below the normative means for the various tests used in the study. It was not known whether the observed deficits were due to cyanotic CHD or to cardiac arrest. However, a longer duration of cardiac arrest was associated with worse performance. Although this study is limited by the small and heterogeneous sample, the findings suggest that children surviving cardiac arrest may be at increased risk for cognitive and academic difficulties.

Bloom, Wright, Morris, Campbell, and Krawiecki (1997) compared 16 children with CHD who had sustained a cardiac arrest in the hospital to a medically similar group of children with CHD to examine the additive impact of cardiac arrest on the functioning of children with CHD. The children in the cardiac arrest group had significantly lower scores on measures of general cognitive, motor, and adaptive behavior functioning, as well as greater disease severity. Forty-four percent of the cardiac arrest group performed at least 1 standard deviation below the mean on the general cognitive index, as compared to only 6% of the children who had not sustained a cardiac arrest. Although the occurrence of a cardiac arrest alone did not add significantly to the prediction of outcome measures, the interaction of cumulative medical risk and presence of a cardiac arrest was significant. For children who had sustained a cardiac arrest, each unit of increase of the medical risk index was accompanied by a 6.9-unit decrease in predicted cognitive functioning. Duration or number of cardiac arrests did not correlate with any outcome measures.

Impact of Newer Medical Interventions

As noted earlier, several new developments have occurred in the past decade regarding medical and surgical interventions for cardiac disease in children. Surgical repair for CHD is now commonly undertaken during the neonatal period, as studies have demonstrated the advantages of early repair (Castaneda et al., 1989). As survival rates of heart surgery have increased dramatically, and as surgery is routinely being performed during infancy (thereby reducing the impact of chronic hypoxia), increased attention has focused on neurological sequelae related to surgical and support techniques. A number of studies have documented reduced neurological sequelae and better outcome with the use of low-flow cardiopulmonary bypass (Bellinger, Rappaport, Wypij, Wernovsky, & Newburger, 1997; Bellinger et al., 1995; Newburger et al., 1993). In this section, studies evaluating intraoperative variables affecting cognitive development (hypothermic circulatory arrest vs. low-flow cardiopulmonary bypass), neuropsychological effects of ECMO, heart transplantation, and pacemakers are discussed.

Hypothermic Circulatory and Low-Flow Cardiopulmonary Bypass

The effect of cardiovascular surgical support variables was studied by Bellinger et al. (1991) in a sample of 28 children who underwent corrective cardiac surgery in early infancy. The children had developmental evaluations (Bayley Scales for children younger than 30 months of age and McCarthy Scales for older children) after surgery when they were between 7 and 53 months of age to explore whether cardiopulmonary bypass perfusion variables are associated with later cognitive function. The sample was homogenous with respect to diagnosis: All had TGA repaired by the arterial switch operation using deep hypothermic circulatory arrest. The mean duration of deep hypothermic circulatory arrest was 64 ± 10 minutes (mean ± *SD*). Median age at repair was 4 days (range 1–125 days). Overall cognitive development score was 101.2 ± 11.1. Duration of deep hypothermic circulatory arrest was not associated with performance. However, for core cooling periods of less than 20 minutes' duration, shorter cooling periods were associated with significantly lower scores. These data suggest that patients undergoing relatively long periods of deep hypothermic circulatory arrest may require some minimum time of cardiopulmonary bypass cooling to avoid CNS injury.

Bellinger et al. (1995) conducted a randomized clinical trial of 171 children with TGA repaired by an arterial switch operation that used either predominantly total circulatory arrest or predominantly continuous low-flow cardiopulmonary bypass. Developmental and neurological evaluations and magnetic resonance imaging (MRI) were performed at 1 year of age. Approximately one-fourth of the infants had a ventricular septal defect; these children were older at the time of surgery, so statistical analyses adjusted for the presence or absence of a ventricular septal defect. Subsequent analyses revealed that the presence of this defect was an independent risk factor for lower scores on developmental testing. The infants assigned to circulatory arrest, as compared with those assigned to low-flow bypass, had a lower mean score on the Psychomotor Development Index of the Bayley Scales of Infant Development (a 6.5-point deficit) and a higher proportion had scores <80 (27% vs. 12%). The score on the Psychomotor Development Index was inversely related to the duration of circulatory arrest. Neurological abnormalities were more common among the children assigned to circulatory arrest, and the risk of neurological abnormalities increased with the duration of circulatory arrest. The method of support was not associated with the prevalence of abnormalities on MRI scans of the brain, scores on the Mental Development Index of the Bayley Scale, or scores on a test of visual-recognition memory. Perioperative electroencephalographic seizure activity was associated with lower scores on the Psychomotor Development Index and an increased likelihood of abnormalities on MRI scans of the brain.

In a follow-up study of these children, Bellinger et al. (1997) compared the developmental status based on parent-completed questionnaires. Responses to parental questionnaires completed when the children were 2.5 years old indicated that the children in the circulatory arrest group, especially those with a ventricular septal defect, manifested poorer expressive language.

Oates et al. (1995) compared 114 children (51 with TOF, 30 with TGA, and 33 with ventricular septal defect) who had their defects repaired with the use of deep hypothermia and circulatory arrest to 54 children who had atrial septal defects repaired with the use cardiopulmonary bypass. The children were assessed for intellectual and neuropsychological function at an average of 9–10 years after the operation. Children with preoperative intellectual handicaps or postoperative neurological complications were excluded. The only significant difference in the neuropsychological measures was that the bypass group had reaction times 2–3 seconds shorter on average than those of the hypothermic circulatory arrest group. Although there were no significant differences in intelligence scores between the groups, a relationship between IQ scores and arrest time was found. Regression analysis of IQ against duration of arrest showed a significant decrease in IQ with increasing arrest time, indicating a decrease of 3–4 points for each extra 10 minutes of arrest time.

Extracorporeal Membrane Oxygenation

Extracorporeal membrane oxygenation (ECMO) is a relatively new surgical procedure involving cardiopulmonary bypass of blood via cannulation of the right common carotid artery and right internal jugular vein (Klein, 1988). This life-saving technique is used for children whose risk of survival is less than 20% without ECMO (Short, Miller, & Anderson, 1987). ECMO is now considered a standard therapy for neonatal respiratory failure that is unresponsive to other interventions. ECMO has also been applied to children whose cardiopulmonary status deteriorates rapidly following surgery for repair of CHD (Klein et al., 1990). This latter group of patients is generally older, ranging from infants to preschoolers. In addition, increasing numbers of children are being placed on ECMO for acute decompensation of chronic cardiomyopathy or for a viral myocarditis (del Nido, 1996).

Over the past 15 years, as ECMO has been used more, investigators have examined the developmental course of these infants. Results have generally shown that children treated with ECMO during the neonatal period develop at or just below age-expected levels, in terms of growth and intellectual functioning up to 3 years of age (Andrews, Nixon, Ciley, Roloff, & Bartlett, 1986; Taylor, Glass, Fitz, & Miller, 1987). Longer-term follow-up studies into middle childhood similarly have indicated that most children appear to have normal growth and development using global measures, but neurological complications have occurred in nearly 20% of cases (Hofkosh et al., 1991; Schumacher, Palmer, Roloff, LaClaire, & Barlett, 1991).

Less is known, however, about children who have received ECMO after cardiac surgery. Hagerott et al. (1990) examined neurodevelopment in preschool-aged children (mean age of 39 months) who had ECMO after cardiac surgery 2 years previous to the study, compared with cardiac controls (without ECMO) and typically developing children who tested as controls. ECMO patients had significantly more impairment than the other groups, including abstract reasoning and lateralized motor impairment (left hand). These same children were reevaluated 2 years later, at ages 4–6, and exhibited continued deficits in left-hand motor skill, as well as lower visual memory and visual–spatial constructive skills, compared with both cardiac and typically developing controls (Tindall, Rothemel, Delamater, Pinsky, & Klein, in press).

Heart Transplantation

Children with very severe CHD, acquired cardiac disease, or intractable arrhythmias may need heart transplantation. This operation was first performed successfully in children over 20 years ago. Survival rates and quality of life have improved dramatically in recent years as more transplants have been performed and techniques refined. Heart transplantation is now considered an accepted modality for patients whose disease is end-stage and for whom there are no alternative treatments (Addonizio, 1996; Baum & Bernstein, 1993). However, approximately 20% of children may have neurological complications following heart transplantation (Baum et al., 1993; Martin et al., 1992).

Little systematic data are available concerning cognitive development of children after heart transplantation. Clinical descriptive reports suggest that children do not have major abnormalities and that rehabilitation is very good as children return to school and engage in age-appropriate activities (e.g., Backer et al., 1992; Starnes et al., 1989).

Trimm (1991) administered Bayley Scales of Infant Development five times over 30 months to 29 infants who received heart transplants before 4 months of age. During the follow-up period only two children had Mental Development Index scores less than 84, but 12 patients had scores less than 84 on the Psychomotor Development Index. In a more recent report of neurodevelopmental outcomes of children receiving transplants during infancy, Baum et al. (1993) found a mean Bayley Mental Development Index of 87 and a Psychomotor Development Index of 90, with 67% of the sample having scores in the normal range.

Wray and Yacoub (1991) compared children who received heart transplants to children who had corrective open-heart surgery and healthy control children. The transplant group had lower developmental scores than the healthy controls, but mean scores were within normal limits. For children older than 5 years of age, however, the transplant group was significantly lower than both groups on developmental and academic achievement scores. Those with a history of cyanotic CHD did worse regardless of transplant or open-heart surgery.

Wray, Pot-Mees, Zeitlin, Radley-Smith, and Yacoub (1994) compared 65 children who had been given heart ($n = 41$) or heart–lung transplants ($n = 24$) to 52 children who had had other types of cardiac surgery and to 45 healthy children. The children in the transplant group ranged in age from 6 months to 16 years, and the assessments were conducted 3–25 months following transplantation. The children with other types of cardiac surgery had various cyanotic and acyanotic conditions, with 49 having had corrective surgery and 3 palliative surgery. A similar proportion of the transplant and cardiac surgery groups had been chronically ill since birth. Developmental and cognitive measures indicated that children given transplants, particularly those under 4.5 years of age, had significantly lower scores on several developmental parameters . In this younger age group, the transplant and cardiac groups did not differ significantly from each other, but both groups performed significantly below the typically developing controls in all developmental areas. Performance on all tests, however, was within the average range. Among study children in the school-age range (4.5–16 years), the transplant group achieved significantly lower overall IQ than the two comparison groups, and also performed significantly worse than the healthy group on tests of short-term memory, nonverbal reasoning, and speed of information processing. Their performance on the short-term memory subtests also was significantly lower than the cardiac group. There were no significant differences in behavioral ratings between the transplant and reference groups, though the proportion of children with significant problem behavior at home was higher in the transplant and cardiac groups than in the healthy children.

BEHAVIORAL AND EMOTIONAL FUNCTIONING

A number of studies have examined the behavioral and emotional functioning of children with CHD. While early studies suggested a negative impact on behavior and emotions (e.g., Aurer, Senturia, Shopper, & Biddy, 1971; Green & Levitt, 1962) and family functioning (e.g., Apley, Barbour, & Westmacott, 1967), more recent studies have identified some specific problems observed during early childhood, but fairly adaptive functioning later in childhood.

Some studies have focused on factors related to eating because children with CHD may have impaired growth (Baum, Beck, Kodama, & Brown, 1980) and have been described as having difficulty with feeding (Gudermuth, 1975). Lobo (1992) studied interactions of parents and infants during feeding in a sample of infants with various types of CHD compared with healthy controls matched for age and birth weight. Parent–infant dyads were studied at 16–17 weeks of infant age. Dyads were observed during feeding and were rated with the Nursing Child Assessment Feeding Scale (for which adequate reliability was obtained during the study). Results suggested CHD infants had significantly lower scores than controls, particularly for the following subscales: Clarity of Cues, Responsiveness to Parent, and Fostering of Social/Emotional Growth. Although these results are qualified by methodological limitations, they nevertheless suggest that the behavior of CHD infants may make feeding difficult, increasing the risk of growth problems.

One factor known to contribute to behavioral difficulties is temperament. Marino and Lipshitz (1991) studied temperament in a sample of infants and toddlers with CHD (age range 4–36 months). Parent ratings of temperament were made using standardized rating scales. A control group was not studied, but norms from the infant and toddler temperament scales were used as a comparison. Results showed that CHD infants were more withdrawn, more intense in emotional reactions, and had lower thresholds for stimulation. Toddlers were rated as less active, rhythmic, and intense, and more negative in mood. There was no association between severity of CHD (as determined by oxygen saturation levels and physician ratings) and temperament.

In another study related to temperament and parent–child interaction, Bradford (1990) examined factors related to young children's (age range, 1–4 years) distress during diagnostic procedures. Children were observed with their mothers present while they underwent X-ray examination for possible CHD. Observational ratings of distress were made using reliable methods, and parents were interviewed to identify possible psychosocial factors related to child distress. Stranger sociability and parental discipline were also measured using accepted methods. Forty-seven percent of the sample did not exhibit significant distress during the procedure. High child distress was associated with low stranger sociability and negative parenting style (i.e., use of force and reinforcement of dependency).

An early study by Linde, Rasof, Dunn, and Rabb (1966) examined the emotional adjustment of children with cyanotic CHD, children with acyanotic CHD, typically developing siblings, and typically developing control children recruited from a well-child clinic. Psychologists made ratings of children's psychological adjustment and parenting styles. While the overall adjustment was similar in all groups, poorer levels of adjustment were associated with maternal anxiety and pampering. However, these results are qualified by the use of nonblind, subjective ratings.

Myers-Vando, Steward, Folkins, and Hines (1979) studied feelings of vulnerability in a sample of 8- to 16-year-old children with CHD who previously had surgical repair for a variety of defects. The control group consisted of healthy children from the same geographical area. Using projective methods, CHD children were rated as seeming more vulnerable to illness when projecting to adulthood. The small study sample, however, limits the generalizability of this finding.

Kramer et al. (1989) evaluated personality in children with CHD compared with healthy controls. Although no differences were observed in younger children, among older children (9–14 years) there was some evidence suggesting increased anxiety, impulsiveness, and inferiority among CHD patients with physical limitations as compared with healthy controls. However, given the unknown reliability and validity of the measures used, these findings must be considered tentative.

DeMaso et al. (1990) examined global psychological functioning as part of their study of children with cyanotic CHD, described in the section of this chapter on cognitive development. Based on clinical interviews with parents, a behavioral symptom checklist, and observations during the testing protocol, ratings of global psychological functioning were made on a 5-point scale (from no impairment to severe impairment). Excellent interrater reliability was reported. Both groups of children with cyanotic CHD (TGA and TOF) were rated as being lower in psychological functioning than the control group of healthy children who had spontaneous recovery of their heart problem. There was no difference between the cyanotic subgroups. Using multiple regression analysis, psychological functioning was predicted by degree of CNS impairment and IQ.

DeMaso et al. (1991) examined the effects of maternal perceptions and disease severity on the behavioral–emotional adjustment of a sample of 4- to 10-year-old children with CHD. The criterion measure was the Total Behavior Problems score from the Child Behavior Checklist. Predictor variables included measures of parenting stress, parental locus of control, and a measure of disease severity (based on number of hospitalizations, invasive procedures, outpatient visits, and a cardiologist's rating). The mean T-score for total behavior problems for the group was 52.2, indicating good overall functioning. Similarly, the mean scores for parenting stress and locus of control were very close to the means from the norms for these measures. Maternal perceptions accounted for the majority of variance (33%) in child adjustment, with medical severity explaining only 3% of the variance.

Measures of behavioral and emotional functioning (the Child Behavior Checklist and the Vineland Adaptive Behavior Scales) were included by Morris et al. (1993) in their study of children surviving cardiac arrest. Although a significant proportion of the sample scored less than 1 standard deviation below the mean for norms on the Vineland subscales, there was little evidence suggesting significant behavioral problems on the Child Behavior Checklist.

Spurkland, Bjornstad, Lindberg, and Seem (1993) examined behavioral functioning in adolescents (mean age of 16 years) with "complex" (i.e., cyanotic) CHD, compared with a group who had repaired atrial septal defects and were in good health. Measures included the Child Behavior Checklist, standardized clinical interviews for diagnosis of psychiatric disorders (Child Assessment Schedule and Children's Global Assessment Scale), and parent interviews to assess family dysfunction. Physical capacity of patients was measured by standardized bicycle ergometer stress test. Results showed those with complex CHD had significantly lower physical capacity and more psychiatric diagnoses (42% vs. 27% of controls), with overanxious disorder and dysthymic disorder being the most common diagnoses. Only one-third of youths with complex CHD were functioning normally, with one-third having minor to moderate problems, and another third having serious dysfunction. In the acyanotic group, only 4% had a major psychiatric disorder, with 54% functioning normally and 42% having minor to moderate problems. Greater psychopathology was associated with more severe physical impairment. Behavior ratings by mothers revealed clinically significant problems in 19% of the complex group compared with only 4% in the acyanotic group. Similar levels (about 50%) of chronic family problems were apparent in both groups.

Casey, Sykes, Craig, Power, and Mulholland (1996) examined the behavioral adjustment of 26 children with surgically palliated complex CHD compared to 26 children with innocent heart murmurs. Behavior ratings by teachers indicated that children with CHD were more withdrawn than control children. Parent ratings indicated that children with CHD were more withdrawn, had more social problems, and engaged in fewer activities. Degree of family strain and exercise tolerance were significant predictors of teacher-rated school performance. Measures of intellectual functioning were not available, but teacher reports indicated that significantly more students with CHD were performing academically in the borderline or clinical range.

Few studies are available on the longer-term behavioral and emotional adjustment of children with CHD. Using the Cattell 16 PF Personality Inventory, Garson, Williams, and Redford (1974) evaluated personality factors in a study of patients with TOF whose mean age was 19 years. Compared to test norms (based on college students), the study sample was more neurotic, with greater dependency, overprotection, weaker superego, more impulsivity, and less ambition. These findings are limited, however, by the reliance on self-report and lack of an appropriate control group.

Baer, Freedman, and Garson (1984) examined psychological functioning in a sample of young adults (representing 50% of available patients) who had surgical correction for TOF during childhood. Patients were divided into two groups based on age at surgery: Mean age at time of surgery for the two groups was 6.5 versus 12.5 years. The Cattell 16 PF was used to measure personality. Patients also completed an instrument measuring family conditions around the time of surgery and the Children's Report of Parental Behavior Inventory (yielding scores for Acceptance, Autonomy, and Control). Parents completed a survey of family interaction style. Results suggested that patients who had surgery later in childhood described their current personality as more timid and reserved, less venturesome, and more apprehensive than those who had surgery earlier in childhood. The retrospective ratings indicated that those with later surgery recalled their parents as being more involved but less controlling and strict than those who received surgery at an earlier age. No significant findings were observed from parental reports.

Utens et al. (1994) investigated the long-term psychosocial outcome of young adults who had had surgical correction for CHD in childhood. The young adults obtained better scores than the control group on a self-report measure of emotional functioning. No significant differences were found with respect to occupational attainment and overall social functioning. However, the young adults with CHD were more likely to be living with their parents.

Psychosocial Adjustment after Heart Transplantation

Uzark et al. (1992) examined psychosocial adjustment following transplant in a group of children who had a mean age of 10 years at the time of study; the mean time after transplantation was almost 2 years. Parent behavior ratings (using the Child Behavior Checklist) indicated that these children had significantly lower levels of social competence and more behavior problems than the normative population. In particular, depressive symptoms were noted to be the most common psychological problem among these patients. Psychosocial problems of children were associated with greater family stress and fewer family resources for coping effectively with stress.

Significant stress may be associated with the posttransplantation regimen, including daily doses of immunosuppressive medications that may have considerable side effects, as well as extensive medical follow-up, including right ventricular endomyocardial biopsy. Regimen adherence problems may become an issue, yet few studies have addressed this. One report of pediatric patients indicated 20% had significant nonadherence, increasing the chances of graft rejection (Douglas, Hsu, & Addonizio, 1993). In a study of adult patients, those who did not adhere well to the regimen had a higher incidence of hospital readmission and higher total medical costs (Paris, Muchmore, Pribil, Zuhdi, & Cooper, 1994).

Mai, McKenzie, and Kostuk (1990) studied the psychosocial adjustment of adult survivors of heart transplantation. Evaluations were conducted prior to transplantation and 12 months later. The age range of patients was 15–56 years, with a mean age of 38 years. Before transplantation, 14 patients had a psychiatric diagnosis, but at follow-up only 5 received a psychiatric diagnosis. Preoperative psychiatric status predicted postoperative regimen adherence. Quality of life was significantly improved for the group at follow-up.

Pacemakers

Alpern, Uzark, and Dick (1989) used standardized measures of trait anxiety, self-competence, and locus of control in a study of CHD patients requiring pacemakers. The mean age of the study sample was 13 years, and 33% had cyanotic CHD. The control groups included CHD patients without pacemakers (50% with cyanotic CHD) and healthy children. There were no group differences in anxiety and self-competence, but children with pacemakers reported a more external locus of control. Content analysis of interviews with the children indicated that those with pacemakers had heightened fears of pacemaker failure and social rejection. While the nonpacemaker group and healthy controls viewed children with pacemakers as having significant emotional and social differences, children with pacemakers perceived themselves as no different than their peers. These findings indicate relatively healthy psychological adaptation in CHD children with pacemakers, possibly through the effective utilization of denial. However, the findings suggest that such children may be at risk for difficulties with autonomy, social isolation, and rejection.

SUMMARY AND IMPLICATIONS

Studies of cognitive development in children with heart disease indicate that, in general, overall cognitive functioning for these children falls within the average range, but often is lower than the cognitive functioning in control groups. There are a number of factors that are associated with poorer cognitive outcome, including type of CHD (cyanotic or acyanotic), age at surgical repair, type of surgical support technique, use of ECMO, and episodes of cardiac arrest.

Children with cyanotic CHD are at risk for lower intelligence than children with acyanotic CHD, particularly if their disease is severe and their corrective surgery is not done within the first few years of life. Lower IQ scores have been associated with significant CNS involvement. It appears that corrective surgery confers significant benefits on IQ, especially when conducted at younger ages, presumably due to better oxygenation of the brain during early development. Currently, surgery is usually performed during infancy, minimizing the impact of chronic hypoxia.

However, the surgical support techniques used also can contribute to risk of adverse cognitive functioning. Thus, after surgery, children may still be at risk for subtle deficits in cognitive functioning and learning problems. Use of deep hypothermic circulatory arrest, particularly for arrest times longer than 45 minutes, is associated with lower cognitive functioning as compared to low-flow cardiopulmonary bypass.

The focus of many studies has been on overall cognitive functioning, possibly obscuring impairment in specific areas of functioning. Research findings suggest that children with CHD may be at increased risk for learning problems, with some evidence of attentional problems and lower levels of academic achievement. When achievement and classroom placement are included, increased rates of need for specialized services and academic weaknesses are often reported. However, more studies are needed to identify specific areas of cognitive impairment. Such research must account for the effects of school absence on academic achievement and classroom performance, as lower achievement may be secondary to history of school absences related to illness and treatment rather than impaired learning ability.

In studies comparing cyanotic to acyanotic children, the latter had significantly higher IQ scores, on average about 10 points higher. With the cyanotic mean being around 102, it is surprising that the acyanotic groups generally average above 112. This raises the possibility of sampling bias in the control groups. Without specification of participation rates, however, it remains an open question.

Few controlled studies have been reported with respect to the developmental outcomes of children receiving ECMO or cardiac transplantation. Available findings suggest that children treated with ECMO after cardiac surgery have a general cognitive impairment as well as lateralized deficits of functions performed by the right hemisphere, but more studies with larger samples and longer follow up intervals are needed. After heart transplantation, children's cognitive development appears to be comparable to children with CHD who have not undergone transplantation. As a group, overall cognitive functioning falls within normal limits, although subtle cognitive deficits and lowered academic achievement may be observed. There is some indication that children receiving transplantation at older ages do less well than those treated earlier. While the development and psychosocial adjustment of children after heart transplantation appears to be normal based on clinical reports, there is some evidence of increased depression and lower social competence among older children. This remains an important issue for future studies. Further studies with posttransplant samples are needed, particularly studies of medication adherence, as predictions of adherence are critical in clinical decision making regarding whether or not a patient will receive a transplant.

Available research on behavioral and emotional functioning suggests that infants with CHD have temperamental characteristics that may make feeding difficult. This could in part explain the tendency for children with CHD to have abnormal growth. While there is some evidence of parent–infant interaction problems during feeding, more controlled research is needed in this area.

Regarding psychosocial adjustment later in childhood, there are some reports of adjustment difficulties in the more severe, cyanotic children. Older children may have concerns with social anxiety, autonomy, and feelings of vulnerability. However, mean scores are within the normal range when standardized behavioral ratings are reported. In general, the data suggest that the risk of adjustment problems increases when corrective surgery occurs later in childhood or when physical capacity remains limited and cyanosis persists.

The research literature on CHD has several methodological problems.

Many study samples are small, raising concerns about sampling bias. Gender differences have not been well evaluated. This is particularly problematic when study groups are not equated for gender, as is often the case in the studies reviewed in this chapter. Certain cardiac defects are more likely in boys than girls. When sociodemographic characteristics of the sample are reported, in most cases the sample is predominantly white and in at least the middle range of socioeconomic status. Additionally, samples are often heterogeneous with regard to type of cardiac defect, age of surgical correction, type of surgical procedure, and preoperative health and developmental functioning. A number of studies did not use control groups, relying instead on comparisons to test norms. This approach is problematic because if group differences are observed they cannot necessarily be attributed to CHD per se; rather, differences can be due to having a chronic disease or having frequent contact with health care professionals.

Very little intervention research has been reported. Areas for intervention research could include distress associated with medical procedures, psychosocial adjustment, regimen adherence, and academic functioning. Interventions to reduce distress associated with diagnostic and evaluative procedures such as catheterization or biopsies are needed. Descriptive studies have documented the high rates of distress commonly seen among young patients, but few studies have been reported in this area. Cassell (1965) reported that children who were prepared for catheterization with puppet play exhibited less behavioral distress during the procedure than children who received no special preparation. A recent clinical report suggests that relaxation and imagery techniques without sedation are helpful for pediatric heart transplant patients during endomyocardial biopsy (Bullock & Shaddy, 1993).

Intervention research targeting social anxiety and social skills is also needed, particularly for those children who appear different than their peers (e.g., those who are cyanotic, those with pacemakers, or those who are cushingoid due to antirejection medications). If, as the available findings suggest, older children with more severe disease experience feelings of vulnerability and fears of social rejection, they might benefit from interventions to increase their social competence and decrease their fears.

Clinically, the research findings point to several concerns. Parents should be counseled while their child is still an infant regarding the risk of temperamental difficulties and associated feeding problems during infancy and early childhood, and how to deal effectively with such difficulties. For example, training in feeding skills could be initiated early and may help prevent growth problems commonly observed among CHD children. In addition, counseling regarding potential academic difficulties or learning disabilities may be useful, particularly for school-age children with more severe disease. Considering the potential risk for learning delays, psychoeducational strategies should be planned to facilitate optimal academic performance.

Many parents and patients may have unrealistic beliefs about the risk of sudden death, leading to unnecessary restrictions for the child and greater distress for all. With the frequently disabling effects of cyanotic CHD in particular, however, counseling about reasonable expectations for age-appropriate activities, such as participation in sports, is needed. For older girls anticipating parenthood, counseling is also indicated regarding the significant risks associated with pregnancy.

Very little systematic developmental research has been reported in the area of acquired heart disease of childhood. This is an area needing more research attention. Studies should especially target adherence with prophylactic drug regimens, as this is a significant clinical issue related to morbidity of children and clinical decisions regarding transplantation.

CONCLUSIONS

Developmental research in cardiac disorders of childhood has for the most part focused on congential heart disease. Whereas most children with CHD can be expected to function in the normal range, a number of developmental assessment studies have shown that children with severe forms of CHD are at risk for lower levels of intellectual functioning and academic achievement. To the extent there is more neurological involvement and cyanosis, and surgical repair is done later in childhood, more serious deficits in cognitive development could be expected. Further studies are needed of specific areas of cognitive functioning that may be impacted by cardiac disorders.

Similarly, children with CHD have generally been rated within the normal range on measures of behavioral and emotional functioning. However, if surgical repair is made later in childhood, there seems to be a greater risk for behavioral or emotional difficulties. Future studies should focus on social competence, social anxiety, feelings of vulnerability, and autonomy issues, as these psychological factors may play an important role in the behavioral and emotional adjustment of children with CHD.

There is a particular need for more intervention research. Significant contributions could be made by developing and evaluating interventions to target feeding difficulties in infants, distress associated with medical procedures, academic functioning, social competence, autonomy, and regimen adherence problems for patients after heart transplantation. Furthermore, few developmental or behavioral studies have addressed the issue of acquired heart disease in children. Studies addressing developmental outcomes and adherence with prophylactic medical regimens are needed, particularly intervention studies targeting regimen adherence.

While advances in medical management and surgical approaches have increased longevity and improved quality of life for youngsters with cardiac disorders, more studies of the developmental effects of such approaches are needed, particularly for children receiving ECMO, heart transplants, and pacemakers.

REFERENCES

Addonizio, L. J. (1996). Current status of cardiac transplantation in children. *Current Opinions in Pediatrics, 8,* 520–526.

Alpern, D., Uzark, K., & Dick, M., II (1989). Psychosocial responses of children to cardiac pacemakers. *Journal of Pediatrics, 114,* 494–501.

American Psychiatric Association. (1987). *Diagnostic and statistical manual of mental disorders* (3rd ed., rev.). Washington, DC: Author.

Andrews, A. F., Nixon, C. A., Cilley, R. E., Roloff, D. W., & Bartlett, R. H. (1986). One-to three-year outcome for 14 neonatal survivors of extracorporeal membrane oxygenation. *Pediatrics, 78,* 692–698.

Apley, J., Barbour, R. F., & Westmacott, F. (1967). Impact of congenital heart disease on the family: A preliminary report. *British Medical Journal, 1,* 103–105.

Aram, D. M., Ekelman, B. L., Ben-Shachar, G., & Levinsohn, M. W. (1985). Intelligence and hypoxemia in children with congenital heart disease: Fact or artifact? *Journal of the American College of Cardiology, 6,* 889–893.

Aurer, E. T., Senturia, A. G., Shopper, M., & Biddy, R. (1971). Congenital heart disease and child adjustment. *Psychiatric Medicine, 2,* 210–219.

Backer, C. L., Zales, V. R., Idriss, F. S., Lynch, P., Crawford, S., Benson, D. W., Jr., & Mavroudis, C. (1992). Heart transplantation in neonates and children. *Journal of Heart and Lung Transplantation, 11,* 311–319.

Baer, P. E., Freedman, D. A., & Garson, A., Jr. (1984). Long-term psychological follow-up of patients after corrective surgery for tetralogy of Fallot. *Journal of the American Academy of Child Psychiatry, 23,* 622–625.

Bailey, L., Gundry, S., Razzouk, A., & Wang, N. (1992). Pediatric heart transplantation: Issues relating to outcome and results. *Journal of Heart and Lung Transplantation, 11,* 267–271.

Baum, D., Beck, R., Kodama, A., & Brown, B. (1980). Early heart failure as a cause of growth and tissue disorders in children with congenital heart disease. *Circulation, 62,* 1145–1151.

Baum, D., & Bernstein, D. (1993). Heart and lung transplantation in children. In I. H. Gessner & B. E. Victoria (Eds.), *Pediatric cardiology: A problem oriented approach* (pp. 245–252). Philadelphia: Saunders.

Baum, M., Chinnock, R., Ashwal, S., Peverini, R., Trimm, F., & Bailey, L. (1993). Growth and neurodevelopmental outcome of infants undergoing heart transplantation. *Journal of Heart and Lung Transplantation, 12,* S211–S217.

Bellinger, D. C., Jonas, R. A., Rappaport, L. A., Wypij, D., Wernovsky, G., Kuban, K. C., Barnes, P. D., Holmes, G. L, Hickey, P. R., Strand, R. D., Walsh, A. Z., Helmers, S. L., Constantinou, J. E., Carranzana, E. J., Mayer, J. E., Hanley, F. L., Castaneda, A. R., Ware, J. H., & Newburger, J. W. (1995). Developmental and neurologic status of children after heart surgery with hypothermic circulatory arrest or low-flow cardiopulmonary bypass. *New England Journal of Medicine, 332,* 549–555.

Bellinger, D. C., Rappaport, L. A., Wypij, D., Wernovsky, G., & Newburger, J. W. (1997). Patterns of developmental dysfunction after surgery during infancy to correct transposition of the great arteries. *Journal of Developmental and Behavioral Pediatrics, 18,* 75–83.

Bellinger, D. C., Wernovsky, G., Rappaport, L. A., Mayer, J. E., Castaneda, A. R.,

Farrell, D. M., Wessel, D. L., Lang, P., Hickey, P. R., Jonas, R. A., & Newburger, J. W. (1991). Cognitive development of children following early repair of transposition of the great arteries using deep hypothermic circulatory arrest. *Pediatrics, 87,* 701–707.

Bloom, A. A., Wright, J. A., Morris, R. D., Campbell, R. M., & Krawiecki, N. S. (1997). Additive impact of in-hospital cardiac arrest on the functioning of children with heart disease. *Pediatrics, 99,* 390–398.

Bradford, R. (1990). Short communication: The importance of psychosocial factors in understanding child distress during routine X-ray procedures. *Journal of Child Psychology and Psychiatry, 31,* 973–982.

Bullock, E. A., & Shaddy, R. E. (1993). Relaxation and imagery techniques without sedation during right ventricular endomyocardial biopsy in pediatric heart transplant patients. *Journal of Heart and Lung Transplantation, 12,* 59–62.

Casey, F. A., Sykes, D. H., Craig, B. G., Power, R., & Mulholland, H. C. (1996). Behavioral adjustment of children with surgically palliated complex congenital heart disease. *Journal of Pediatric Psychology, 21,* 335–352.

Cassell, S. (1965). Effect of brief psychotherapy upon the emotional responses of children undergoing cardiac catherization. *Journal of Consulting and Clinical Psychology, 29,* 1–8.

Castaneda, A. R., Mayer, J. E., Jonas, R. A., Lock, J. E., Wessel, D. L., & Hickey, P. R. (1989). The neonate with critical congenital heart disease: Repair—A surgical challenge. *Journal of Thoracic and Cardiovascular Surgery, 98,* 869–875.

del Nido, P. J. (1996). Extracorporeal membrane oxygenation for cardiac support in children. *Annals of Thoracic Surgery, 61,* 336–339.

DeMaso, D. R., Beardslee, W. R., Silbert, A. R., & Fyler, D. C. (1990). Psychological functioning in children with cyanotic heart defects. *Developmental and Behavioral Pediatrics, 11,* 289–293.

DeMaso, D. R., Campis, L. K., Wypij, D., Bertram, S., Lipshitz, M., & Freed, M. (1991). The impact of maternal perceptions and medical severity on the adjustment of children with congenital heart disease. *Journal of Pediatric Psychology, 16,* 137–149.

Douglas, J. F., Hsu, D. T., & Addonizio, L. J. (1993). Noncompliance in pediatric heart transplant patients. *Journal of Heart and Lung Transplantation, 12,* S92.

du Plessis, A. J., Newburger, J., Jonas, R. A., Hickey, P., Naruse, H., Tsuji, M., Walsh, A., Walter, G., Wypij, D., & Volpe, J. J. (1995). Cerebral oxygen supply and utilization during infant cardiac surgery. *Annals of Neurology, 37,* 488–497.

Epstein, H. T. (1978). Growth spurts during brain development: Implications for educational policy and practice. In J. S. Chall & A. F. Mirsky (Eds.), *Education and the brain* (pp. 37–46). Chicago: University of Chicago Press.

Epstein, H. T. (1986). Stages of human brain development. *Developmental Brain Research, 30,* 114–119.

Fallon, P., Aparicio, J. M., Elliott, M. J., & Kirkham, F. J. (1995). Incidence of neurological complications of surgery for congenital heart disease. *Archives of Diseases in Childhood, 72,* 418–422.

Ferry, P. C. (1987). Neurological sequelae of cardiac surgery in children. *American Journal of Diseases of Children, 141,* 309–312.

Ferry, P. C. (1990). Neurologic sequelae of open-heart surgery in children. An "irritating question." *American Journal of Diseases of Children, 144,* 369–373.

Fyler, D. C. (Ed.). (1992). *Nadas' pediatric cardiology.* Philadelphia: Hanley & Belfus.

Garson, A., Williams, R. B., & Redford, T. (1974). Long term follow up of patients with tetralogy of Fallot: Physical health and psychopathology. *Journal of Pediatrics, 85,* 429–433.

Gersony, W. M. (1987). The cardiovascular system. In R. E. Behrman & V. C. Vaughan (Eds.), *Nelson textbook of pediatrics* (13th ed., pp. 943–1026). Philadelphia: Saunders.

Green, M., & Levitt, E. (1962). Constriction of body image in children with congenital heart diseases. *Pediatrics, 29,* 438–443.

Gudermuth, S. (1975). Mothers' reports of early experiences of infants with congenital heart disease. *Maternal Child Nursing Journal, 4,* 155–164.

Hagerott, K. P., Delamater, A., Tindall, S., Rothermel, R., Jr., Pinsky, W., & Klein, M. (1990). *Neuropsychological functioning in preschool aged cardiac patients treated with ECMO.* Paper presented at Florida Conference on Child Health Psychology, Gainesville, FL.

Hofkosh, D., Thompson, A. E., Nozza, R. J., Kemp, S. S., Bowen, A., & Feldman, H. M. (1991). Ten years of extracorporeal membrane oxygenation: Neurodevelopmental outcome. *Pediatrics, 87,* 549–555.

Hosenpud, J. D., Novick, R. J., Breen, T. J., Keck, B., & Daily, P. (1995). The registry of the International Society for Heart and Lung Transplantation: Twelfth official report—1995. *Journal of Heart and Lung Transplantation, 14,* 805–815.

Klein, M. D. (1988). Neonatal ECMO. *TransAmerican Society of Artificial Internal Organs, 34,* 39–42.

Klein, M. D., Shaheen, K. W., Whittlesey, G. C., Pinsky, W. W., & Arciniegas, E. (1990). Extracorporeal membrane oxygenation (ECMO) for the circulatory support of children after repair of congenital heart disease. *Journal of Thoracic and Cardiovascular Surgery, 100,* 498–505.

Kramer, H. H., Awiszus, D., Sterzel, U., van Halteren, A., & Claßen, R. (1989). Development of personality and intelligence in children with congenital heart disease. *Journal of Child Psychology and Psychiatry, 30,* 299–308.

Linde, L. M., Rasof, B., & Dunn, O. J. (1967). Mental development in congenital heart disease. *Journal of Pediatrics, 71,* 198–203.

Linde, L. M., Rasof, B., & Dunn, O. J. (1970). Longitudinal studies of intellectual and behavioral development in children with congenital heart disease. *Acta Paediatrica Scandinavica, 59,* 169–176.

Linde, L. M., Rasof, B., Dunn, O. J., & Rabb, E. (1966). Attitudinal factors in congenital heart disease. *Pediatrics, 38,* 92–101.

Lobo, M. L. (1992). Parent–infant interaction during feeding when the infant has congenital heart disease. *Journal of Pediatric Nursing, 7,* 97–105.

Lock, J. E., Keane, J. F., Mandell, V. S., & Perry, S. B. (1992). Cardiac catheterization. In D. C. Fyler (Ed.), *Nadas' pediatric cardiology* (pp. 187–224). Philadelphia: Hanley & Belfus.

Lott, I. T., McPherson, D., Towne, B., Johnson, D., & Starr, A. (1990). Long-term neurophysiologic outcome after neonatal extracorporeal membrane oxygenation. *Pediatrics, 116,* 343–349.

Mai, F. M., McKenzie, F. N., & Kostuk, W. J. (1990). Psychosocial adjustment and quality of life following heart transplantation. *Canadian Journal of Psychiatry, 35,* 223–227.

Marino, B. L., & Lipshitz, M. (1991). Temperament in infants and toddlers with cardiac disease. *Pediatric Nursing, 17,* 445–448.

Martin, A. B., Bricker, J. T., Fishman, M., Frazier, O. H., Price, J. K., Radovancevic, B., Louis, P. T., Cabalka, A. K., Gelb, B. D., & Towbin, J. A. (1992). Neurologic complications of heart transplantation in children. *Journal of Heart and Lung Transplantation, 11,* 933–942.

Mendoza, J. C., Shearer, L. L., & Cook, L. N. (1991). Lateralization of brain lesions following extracorporeal membrane oxygenation. *Pediatrics, 88,* 1004–1009.

Miller, G., Mamourian, A. C., Tesman, J. R., Baylen, B. G., & Myers, J. L. (1994). Long-term MRI changes in brain after pediatric open heart surgery. *Journal of Child Neurology, 9,* 390–397.

Morris, R. D., Krawiecki, N. S., Wright, J. A., & Walter, L. W. (1993). Neuropsychological, academic, and adaptive functioning in children who survive inhospital cardiac arrest and resuscitation. *Journal of Learning Disabilities, 26,* 46–51.

Muraoka, R., Yokota, M., Aoshima, M., Kyoku, I., Nomoto, S., Kobayashi, A., Nakano, H., Ueda, K., Saito, A., & Hojo, H. (1981). Subclinical changes in brain morphology following cardiac operations as reflected by computed tomographic scans of the brain. *Journal of Thoracic and Cardiovascular Surgery, 81,* 364–369.

Myers-Vando, R., Steward, M. S., Folkins, C. H., & Hines, P. (1979). The effects of congenital heart disease on cognitive development, illness causality concepts, and vulnerability. *American Journal of Orthopsychiatry, 49,* 617–625.

Newburger, J. W., Jonas, R. A., Wernovsky, G., Wypij, D., Hickey, P. R., Kuban, C. K., Farrell, D. M., Holmes, G. L., Helmers, S. L., Constantinou, J., Carrazana, E., Barlow, J. K., Walsh, A. Z., Lucius, K. C., Share, J. C., Wessel, D. L., Hanley, F. L., Mayer, J. E., Castaneda, A. R., & Ware, J. H. (1993). A comparison of the perioperative neurologic effects of hypothermic circulatory arrest versus low-flow cardiopulmonary bypass in infant heart surgery. *New England Journal of Medicine, 329,* 1057–1064.

Newburger, J. W., Silbert, A. R., Buckley, L. P., & Fyler, D. C. (1984). Cognitive function and age at repair of transportation of the great arteries in children. *New England Journal of Medicine, 310,* 1495–1499.

Newburger, J. W. (1992). Kawasaki syndrome. In D. C. Fyler (Ed.), *Nadas' pediatric cardiology* (pp. 319–328). Philadelphia: Hanley & Belfus.

Oates, R. K., Simpson, J. M., Turnbull, J. A., & Cartmill, T. B. (1995). The relationship between intelligence and duration of circulatory arrest with deep hypothermia. *Journal of Thoracic and Cardiovascular Surgery, 110,* 786–792.

O'Dougherty, M., Berntson, G. G., Boysen, S. T., Wright, F. S., & Teske, D. (1988). Psychophysiological predictors of attentional dysfunction in children with congenital heart defects. *Psychophysiology, 25,* 305–315.

O'Dougherty, M., Nuechterlein, K. H., & Drew, B. (1984). Hyperactive and hypoxic children: Signal detection, sustained attention, and behavior. *Journal of Abnormal Psychology, 93,* 178–191.

O'Dougherty, M., Wright, F. S., Garmezy, N., Loewenson, R. B., & Torres, F. (1983).

Later competence and adaptation in infants who survive severe heart defects. *Child Development, 54,* 1129–1142.

O'Dougherty, M., Wright, F. S., Loewenson, R. B., & Torres, F. (1985). Cerebral dysfunction after chronic hypoxia in children. *Neurology, 35,* 42–46.

Paris, W., Muchmore, J., Pribil, A., Zuhdi, N., & Cooper, D. K. C. (1994). Study of the relative incidences of psychosocial factors before and after heart transplantation and the influence of posttransplantation psychosocial factors on heart transplantation outcome. *Journal of Heart and Lung Transplantation, 13,* 424–432.

Prigatano, G. P., & Levin, D. C. (1988). Pulmonary system. In R. E. Tarter, D. H. Van Thiel, & K. L. Edwards (Eds.), *Medical neuropsychology* (pp. 11–26). New York: Plenum Press.

Schumacher, R. E., Palmer, T. W., Roloff, D. W., LaClaire, P. A., & Bartlett, R. H. (1991). Follow-up of infants treated with extracorporeal membrane oxygenation for newborn respiratory failure. *Pediatrics, 87,* 451–457.

Short, B. L., Miller, M. K., & Anderson, K. D. (1987). Extracorporeal membrane oxygenation in the management of respiratory failure in the newborn. *Clinics in Perinatology, 14,* 737–749.

Silbert, A., Wolff, P. H., Mayer, B., Rosenthal, A., & Nadas, A. S. (1969). Cyanotic heart disease and psychological development. *Pediatrics, 43,* 192–200.

Spreen, O., Risser, AT., & Edgell, D. (1995). *Developmental neuropsychology.* New York: Oxford University Press.

Spurkland, I., Bjornstad, P. G., Lindberg, H., & Seem, E. (1993). Mental health and psychosocial functioning in adolescents with congenital heart disease. A comparison between adolescents born with severe heart defect and atrial septal defect. *Acta Paediatrica, 82,* 71–76.

Starnes, V. A., Bernstein, D., Oyer, P. E., Gamberg, P. L., Miller, J. L., Baum, D., & Shunway, N. E. (1989). Heart transplantation in children. *Journal of Heart and Lung Transplantation, 8,* 20–26.

Stewart, S. M., Kennard, B. D., Waller, D. A., & Fixler, D. (1994). Cognitive function in children who receive organ transplantation. *Health Psychology, 13,* 3–13.

Taylor, G. A., Glass, P., Fitz, C. R., & Miller, M. K. (1987). Neurologic status in infants treated with extracorporeal membrane oxygenation: Correlation of imaging findings with developmental outcome. *Radiology, 165,* 679–682.

Tindall, S., Rothemel, R. R., Delamater, A., Pinsky, W. W., & Klein, M. D. (in press). Neuropsychological abilities of children with cardiac disease treated with extracorporeal membrane oxygenation. *Developmental Neuropsychology.*

Trimm, F. (1991). Physiologic and psychological growth and development in pediatric heart transplant recipients. *Journal of Heart and Lung Transplantation, 10,* 848–855.

Utens, E. M., Verhulst, F. C., Erdman, R. A., Meijboom, F. J., Duivenvoorden, H. J., Bos, E., Roelandt, J. R., & Hess, J. (1994). Psychosocial functioning of young adults after surgical correction for congenital heart disease in childhood: A follow-up study. *Journal of Psychosomatic Research, 38,* 745–758.

Uzark, K. C., Sauer, S. N., Lawrence, K. S., Miller, J., Addonizio, L., & Crowley, D. C. (1992). The psychosocial impact of pediatric heart transplantation. *Journal of Heart and Lung Tranplantation, 11,* 1160–1167.

Walsh, E. P., & Saul, J. P. (1992). Cardiac arrhythmias. In D. C. Fyler (Ed.), *Nadas' pediatric cardiology* (pp. 377–434). Philadelphia: Hanley & Belfus.

Wray, J., Pot-Mees, C., Zeitlin, H., Radley-Smith, R., & Yacoub, M. (1994). Cognitive function and behavioral status in paediatric heart and heart–lung transplant recipients: The Harefield experience. *British Medical Journal, 309*, 837–841.

Wray, J., & Yacoub, M. (1991). Psychosocial evaluation of children after open heart surgery versus cardiac transplantation. In M. Yacoub & J. R. Pepper (Eds.), *Annals of cardiac surgery, 90–91* (pp. 50–55). London: Current Science Publications.

Wright, M., & Nolan, T. (1994). Impact of cyanotic heart disease on school performance. *Archives of Disease in Childhood, 71*, 64–70.

Yang, L, Liu, M., & Townes, B. (1994). Neuropsychological and behavioral status of Chinese children with acyanotic congenital heart disease. *International Journal of Neuroscience, 74*, 109–115.

CHAPTER TEN

Organ Transplantation

SUNITA MAHTANI STEWART
BETSY D. KENNARD

The first organ transplants took place in the early 1950s when Murray and his colleagues (Murray, Merrill, & Harrison, 1955) transplanted a related donor kidney. The public's awareness of organ transplantation increased in 1967, when Christian Barnard transplanted the first human heart. Organ transplantation has now become a widely available and accepted procedure in adults and children who suffer from end-stage organ disease (Levenson & Olbrisch, 1996). Improved surgical techniques and treatments, the development of effective immunosuppressants, and careful selection of transplant recipients have greatly improved survival following transplantation (English, Cooper, & Cory-Pearce, 1980; Weiss & Edelmann, 1984). More types of organs are being transplanted, and multiple organ transplants within a single patient are not uncommon. The availability of donor organs limits the rate at which centers can perform transplants on patients on waiting lists for this procedure; however, the development of techniques that bridge patients until an organ becomes available and of organ partitioning procedures means that increasing numbers of patients await transplants and will receive them. Progress in these life-saving techniques has not been matched by similar progress in understanding how disease and transplantation affects cognitive function. While there is a growing body of information on deficits recorded in children with end-stage organ disease and those who have received transplantation, an absence of careful, large-scale, prospective studies significantly limits the clarity of the picture that has emerged.

This chapter will review information related to cognitive function in children who have received heart, kidney, and liver transplantation, as these are the most commonly transplanted solid organs. There have been three recent reviews of the literature on organ transplantation in children (Hobbs & Sexson, 1993; Rodrigue, Greene, & Boggs, 1994; Stewart, Kennard, Waller, & Fixler, 1994), and this chapter will briefly summarize findings from the literature covered in detail in those reviews, highlight specific findings in relation to posttransplant function inasmuch as they would be most relevant to the clinician encountering a child who has received organ transplantation, and describe in detail recent studies that were not covered in those reviews. Finally, a tentative model will be presented, organizing influences on cognitive function in children who have received organ transplantation. The purpose of this model is to serve as a heuristic for future "theory-driven" investigations.

EMPIRICAL STUDIES OF COGNITIVE FUNCTION IN CHILDREN WHO RECEIVE ORGAN TRANSPLANTATION

Heart, Kidney, and Liver Pathology, and the Brain

A very brief description follows of the nature of the deficits for each of the organ systems (see Farmer, 1994, for a more complete review of the effect of organ failure on the brain). However, it should be kept in mind that the effects of end-stage organ disease can be quite widespread. The human body functions as an integrated whole, and advanced disease in heart, kidney, or liver affects other organ systems, including the brain.

Heart Disease

Children who receive heart transplantation have structural or functional defects resulting in low cardiac output. Cardiac arrhythmias resulting in decreased blood flow to the brain, and, less frequently, acute anoxic events as a result of cardiac arrest are part of the medical history of many transplant candidates, and would be expected to have some effect on cognitive function. Some transplant candidates may have congenital heart disease, and may have had previous unsuccessful surgeries to correct structural defects. These surgeries themselves may increase the risk of cerebral damage (Nussbaum & Goldstein, 1992).

Kidney Disease

When the kidneys malfunction, toxins that would normally be excreted in urine remain in the body. Build-up of urea can lead to encephalopathy, with reduced alertness, concentration, memory, and perceptuomotor coordination (Marshall, 1979). Growth failure in congenital renal disease is usual (So et al., 1987). When the disease progresses, dialysis becomes necessary. Dialysis is a temporizing procedure in that it does not replace the malfunctioning kidney, but acts to reduce urea build-up in the system. It also takes a very significant toll on the quality of the lives of the children sustained through this procedure as dialysis requires frequent, long hospital visits. Renal transplantation is usually seen as inevitable upon progression to end-stage renal disease (So et al., 1987).

Liver Disease

The normally functioning liver also serves to degrade substances that are potentially toxic. Obstructions preventing blood flow through the organ and functional deficiencies interfering with metabolism are the most common kinds of defects leading to the need for transplantation. Biliary atresia, a congenital disorder results in obstruction of the ducts that drain bile from the liver into the intestinal tract, is the most common diagnosis of children who receive liver transplantation. Progressive liver disease can result in hepatic encephalopathy. Unlike renal disease, there are no widely used mechanical alternatives to the functioning liver, and donors are primarily cadaveric. Patients who go into liver failure and do not have an organ available for transplantation face the life-threatening condition of elevated intracranial pressure. However, the bioartificial liver, a mechanical device that removes toxins from the blood, is beginning to be used on selected patients to bridge the time gap until an appropriate donor liver is found (Coffman, Hoffman, Rosenthal, Demetriou, & Makowka, 1996).

Children who suffer from end-stage organ disease carry various diagnoses reflecting a variety of etiologies. There is also great variation in disease-related parameters. These children show differences, for example, in age of onset of disease, duration and severity of the disease, time between symptom onset and correction, and the like, all of which could influence the nature and extent of their cognitive deficits.

Cognitive Function in End-Stage Heart, Kidney, and Liver Disease

Heart Disease

The cognitive function of children with acquired heart disease has not been systematically investigated. However the evidence (Linde, Rasof, & Dunn, 1967) is quite strong that children with acyanotic conditions as a group have lower scores on tests of intellectual function than do their siblings and age-matched well children; children with cyanotic conditions have even lower scores. These relative standings persist following corrective surgery

(Silbert, Wolff, Mayer, Rosenthal, & Nadas, 1969). Various correlates of deficit have been examined, including early hypoxia, physical activity restrictions, duration of hospitalization following surgery, age at corrective surgery, documented central nervous system insult, and growth deficits, but none of these factors have been conclusively linked to mental abilities in a large sample of children with extent of deficit (see Stewart et al., 1994 for detailed findings).

Kidney Disease

Renal disease in early life, unless quickly contained through dialysis, results in gross cognitive deficits (McGraw & Haka-Ikse, 1985). Even with dialysis, there is some cognitive delay in some infants (Bock et al., 1989). In school-age children followed longitudinally (Fennell et al., 1990b), deficits were noted in verbal and nonverbal reasoning, visual–motor integration, and memory. Disease indices that correlated with extent of cognitive deficits were duration and level of renal dysfunction (Fennell et al., 1990a). In a recent investigation assessing school performance in 11 children with end-stage renal disease undergoing dialysis (Lawry, Brouhard, & Cunningham, 1994), intelligence test scores were in the average range (Full Scale IQ: mean [*SD*] = 92.9 [16.9]). However, school performance as assessed by the Woodcock–Johnson scales was significantly below grade and age level in Mathematics and Written Language. There was a significant association between age of onset of chronic renal failure and mental abilities. No relationships were reported between intelligence and academic test scores.

Liver Disease

Liver disease predisposes toward developmental delay, especially when it begins in the first year of life (Stewart et al., 1988). In infancy, physical growth, particularly height and head circumference, correlates with cognitive development. In comparison to children with cystic fibrosis matched on a number of demographic variables (Stewart et al., 1992), children with early onset of liver disease show significant deficits in a broad range of cognitive functions. In contrast, children with later onset show deficits in verbal intelligence and tests of acquired knowledge. Tests of specific functions have sometimes yielded contradictory information (Stewart et al., 1994) because of the great heterogeneity of the samples across studies and the relatively small sample sizes, which make subanalyses difficult.

It is quite clear that some children with end-stage organ disease have cognitive deficits both before and after transplantation. It is notable that in the majority of the studies, with the possible exception of infants with end-stage renal disease who do not receive dialysis early in life, there is considerable variation in function, so that many children are functioning in the average and higher ranges even though the mean scores might be lower than a control or normative population. In the case of children with early onset of disease, their vulnerability appears particularly high. Other correlates are poorly understood.

Cognitive Functioning Following
Organ Transplantation

Heart Transplant

Studies on children who have received cardiac transplant are few. In a summary of conference proceedings, Baum, Cutler, Fricker, and Trimm (1991) report on studies assessing infants who have received cardiac transplantation. The conclusions are that neurological examinations and ultrasound reveal no abnormalities in these children in four serial evaluations between 6 and 48 months following transplantation. In addition, the children were found to have normal scores on the Bayley Scales of development. Wray and associates have compared children following transplantation to those who received only cardiac surgery (without transplant) and a healthy control group (Wray, Pot-Mees, Zeitlin, Radley-Smith, & Yacoub, 1994; Wray & Yacoub, 1991). In the more recent investigation they reported on 65 children who had received heart or heart–lung transplants. Children with transplants had intellectual scores in the average range (mean [SD] for overall IQ = 95.2 [12.9]), but scored significantly below both a cardiac surgery (without transplant) group and a healthy control group. Children with cyanotic conditions, regardless of whether or not they had received transplantation, had lower scores. On the Spelling subtests of educational achievement tests, the children who had received transplantation fell significantly below the healthy controls, but were equivalent to the cardiac surgery group. The absence of information from more specific tests of cognitive function leaves a large gap in the literature. Studies in adults (Nussbaum & Goldstein, 1992) show that while there is a small clinically insignificant improvement following transplantation, presurgical deficits in executive functions, memory, sustained concentration, and psychomotor slowing largely persist following transplantation.

Kidney Transplant

In children who have received renal transplantation, some studies report improvement in cognitive function following transplant. Davis, Chang, and Nevins (1990) reported that half of the children who had Bayley or Stanford–Binet scores below 60 before transplant obtained scores above 80 following transplantation. The transplant group as a whole had mean scores in the average range after transplantation, an overall improvement of 10 points. Fennell, Rasbury, Fennell, and Morris (1984) reported on 20 children they had followed longitudinally before and after transplantation. The children showed a gain at 1 month posttransplant evaluation, and no further gain 1 year later. The gains 1 year later were no greater than control children retested at the same time interval. Crittenden, Holliday, Piel, and Potter (1985) reported a statistically significant gain in IQ of 6 points for children tested before and after transplantation; children maintained on dialysis improved by 5 points, which was not a statistically significant improvement. In a recent study, Lawry et al. (1994) reported on the cognitive and academic function of 11 dialysis and 13 kidney transplant patients. Transplant patients had mean scores in the average range on cognitive tests; scores of dialysis patients were lower but the difference was not statistically significant. They found that age of onset correlated positively with IQ. Academic scores were ahead of expectation for transplant patients but not for dialysis patients, who were comparatively delayed in math and written language. No information was provided on whether IQ test scores related to academic achievement.

Liver Transplant

In a study of 29 patients who were all 1 year post-liver transplant, Stewart et al. (1989) found that the group as a whole performed at mean-average to low-average range before as well as after transplant. For the children in the mentally delayed range (IQ < 80) before transplant, there was a mean (statistically nonsignificant) improvement of 8 points. Development of disease in the first year of life predisposed the children to persistent delays. On tests of neuropsychological function in a group of 28 children of mixed duration since transplantation (Stewart et al., 1991), deficits in learning and memory, motor function, visuospatial skills, and abstract reasoning skills were found in comparison to children with cystic fibrosis.

In our review in 1994 (Stewart et al., 1994), we concluded that the literature with regard to end-stage organ disease showed consistency in that children with cyanotic heart disease, infants with end-stage renal disease who did not receive dialysis before they were 4 weeks old, and children with end-stage liver disease symptomatic in the first year of life and with growth delays demonstrated higher vulnerabilities to the development of gross cognitive deficits. The picture following transplantation was not so clear. There continues to be an absence of long-term information, especially with relation to subtle deficits. This summary of the literature continues to hold, by and large; however, there have been some recent studies reported that have not been covered in the previous reviews, to which we now turn.

Long-Term Findings. Bannister et al. (1995) reported on the intellectual status, academic development, social functioning, and physical growth of a group of 37 children who were 5 years or more post-liver transplantation. This was a longitudinal study in which pretransplant evaluation cognitive and growth data were compared with follow-up data. This group partly overlapped with the group on whom 1 year posttransplant data were previously reported (Stewart et al., 1989). Subjects in this study were administered intellectual measures at pre- and posttransplant, which included the Bayley Scales of Infant Development, the Stanford–Binet Intelligence Scale, and the Wechsler Scales, depending on the age of the child at testing. Mental development scores or intellectual quotients were converted to z scores, with the group having a mean (SD) z score of $-.77$ (1.39) before transplant and $-.88$ (1.13) after transplant. Intellectual scores did not change significantly $(p > .05)$ over time. Eleven of the 37 children were mentally delayed prior to transplant, and 9 of these children remained in the delayed range at posttransplant evaluation. Age of onset and diagnostic group were related to mental delay prior to transplant, with children who had early onset of liver disease (defined as diagnosis of liver disease prior to 12 months of age) found to be more at risk for having mental delay at pretransplant. In addition, regression analyses found that age of onset of liver disease and mental delay status prior to transplantation were the most important predictors of IQ scores at the 5-year or more follow-up evaluation. Thus, the 5-year posttransplant picture is not much different than the 1 year findings, and there is little evidence that general cognitive function, as measured by IQ scores, improves for the group of children who receive liver transplantation.

Adaptation. There has been one recent study assessing adaptation, specifically academic functioning, of children who have received liver transplantation. Kennard and associates (1999) considered the academic outcome of 50 children (including the group reported on in the Bannister et al., 1995, study) who were 3 or more years post liver transplantation. Cognitive function was measured by intellectual (Wechsler scales) and academic achievement tests (Woodcock–Johnson—Revised). In addition, information about special education services, and whether the child had repeated a grade, was obtained.

Nine of the children were functioning in the mentally deficient range. For some analyses they were separated from the children with IQ scores above 70, as one aim of the study was to assess the presence of more subtle deficits in children with "normal" levels of intellectual function. The children with IQ scores above 70 ($n = 41$) as a group scored below normative means, using grade norms, on academic achievement in the areas of math and written language. However, on examination of individual scores, two-thirds of this group had scores at or above the low-average range for their grade in each academic area. When IQ–academic discrepancy scores were examined, 26% of the children had learning disabilities. Of those functioning within the normal ranges, 60% of them were actually achieving above expected levels based on intellectual ability. Academic function was not related to diagnosis, time between diagnosis and transplant, or age at time of transplant. With regard to academic experiences, 48% of the 50 subjects had received special education services at some time at follow-up, and 48% had a history of repeating a grade. All children with IQ scores below 70 were receiving special education services and four had repeated a grade. Of those children who were above 70 on IQ measures, 37% were in special education, and 40% had repeated a grade. Almost two-thirds of the children with IQ scores above 70 who showed learning disabilities had *not* received special education services.

This study supports existing literature which indicates that intellectual and academic deficits are present in this population. While as a group these children perform below the normative population on academic measures of achievement, two-thirds are at least low average range. Of clinical import is that the majority of children with subtle deficits were not receiving special services. Evidence for three categories of academic outcome were found: those who function at or above expected levels based on intelligence (56%), those who function below their ability level (26%), and those who function within the mentally deficient range of intelligence (18%). Of note is that many children were actually achieving above their intellectual levels, suggesting that additional environmental factors may be heavily influencing achievement.

Unfortunately, there are few such studies relating findings on measures of cognitive ability to actual adaptive functioning of these children in "real world" settings. This is particularly problematic for clinicians working with this population, who are frequently asked by the caretakers of these children about what they might expect in the follow-up period with respect to cognitive, academic, and social functioning. Furthermore, such studies are particularly needed as they provide information regarding the manifestations of cognitive deficits, and form the base for considering remedial interventions.

The Effect of Immunosuppressants

An additional area that is emerging in the medical literature, with less attention paid to it at this point in the psychological literature, is the effects of immunosuppressants. Immunosuppression is part of the expected lifelong regimen for transplant candidates. Cyclosporine has been the primary immunosuppressive agent for almost 15 years, and improved survival rates following transplantation have been attributed directly to its advent (Miller, 1996). Neurotoxicity is a recognized complication of this agent, reported in individuals receiving heart (McManus, O'Hair, & Schweiger, 1992), kidney (Wilczek, Ringden, & Tyden, 1985), and liver (Wijdicks, Wiesner, & Krom, 1995) transplantation. Its use has been associated with evoked potential changes as well as deficits on the Trail Making Test and mental state examination (Grimm et al., 1996). Cumulative levels showed significant correlations with P300 evoked potential 4 and 12 months after transplantation in adult cardiac transplant patients. The precise cognitive manifestations of high levels and neurotoxicity have not been comprehensively investigated in adults. Except in a single investigation in which cyclosporine levels were incidentally included (description follows), the neurotoxic effects of immunosuppresants have not been investigated at all in children.

Kennard et al. (1999) in an investigation with a central interest in academic achievement in the posttransplant population, assessed whether immunosuppressant levels related to cognitive measures. They found that cyclosporine levels obtained within 1 month of the follow-up evaluation were negatively associated with nonverbal and spatial measures. They also correlated negatively with the academic achievement measures of reading and written language. These data are preliminary, as a comprehensive assessment should also include cyclosporine cumulative dosage; however, the findings should stimulate more studies investigating the relationships between cognitive function and cyclosporine levels.

Recent developments in transplant technology include the increasing use of tacrolimus (also known as FK506) as an immunosuppressant following surgery. A recent randomized trial (Fung et al., 1996) showed that use of FK506 was less likely to result in acute rejection of the transplanted organ than was cyclosporine, and overall it resulted in equivalent survival rates. There are several additional benefits of FK506 over cyclosporine: FK506 can be taken orally, reducing hospital stays and costs following transplantation (Cox & Freese, 1996). Furthermore, FK506 does not cause hirsutism or gingival hyperplasia (Cox & Freese, 1996), which are troubling physical disfiguring side effects of cyclosporine. Patients on FK506 (unlike those on cyclosporine) can be taken off prednisone, resulting in significant improvement in growth indices following transplantation (Shapiro et al., 1994). Options that optimize growth and normalize physical appearance are particularly attractive, as they allow for an improved quality of life. However, neurotoxicity is a more frequent complication of FK506 (Mueller et al., 1994). The effects of FK506 on cognitive function have not yet been investigated.

FUTURE DIRECTIONS AND A MODEL

Starfield (1985) describes research as progressing through several stages, from exploratory to descriptive to analytic and finally to experimental research. The first two stages involve progressively better specification of variables to be observed. At the analytic level, research includes specific hypotheses about the relationships among these variables, which are again observed rather than manipulated. At the level of experimental research, variables are manipulated and participants are randomly assigned to the conditions. In many situations involving chronic illness, random assignment to conditions is either not possible or unethical, and studies where there are systematic differences in measurements from participants who are in different conditions are classified as quasi-experimental research. The field of investigation of cognitive function in children who have received organ transplantation is largely at the descriptive and very occasionally at the analytic level.

While it is quite apparent that this population of children have a high probability of having cognitive deficits, many questions still remain. These questions relate to the *specific characteristics* of those children who have the deficits, and the *extent* of the deficits. We propose a theoretical framework that reflects some of current findings in the field, and some additional hypotheses. This model is presented visually in Figure 10.1. We have borrowed the framework proposed by Wallander and associates (Wallander, Varni, Babani, Banis, & Wilcox, 1989) to guide research on psychological adaptation of chronically ill children, and are grateful to this group for stimulating our thinking in this area. We have employed the term "cognitive function" in a general fashion, as the model could be used in considering studies of both specific and general functions. This model is necessarily limited, with no claim for comprehensiveness, and should be seen primarily as a discussion point and a heuristic to support "theory-driven research" (Wallander, 1992).

Children who receive organ transplantation vary along the dimensions proposed within the model as influencing cognitive development. We propose that this variation accounts for a significant amount of the variability in cognitive function that is observed in these children.

Influences on cognitive function include both "risk" and "facilitative" factors. Among the risk variables, first, there are the effects *specific to the pathophysiology of the disease*. These vary from disease to disease but also within each disease, from child to child. For example, malnutrition is common to end-stage organ disease, and in early life affects brain growth. Chronic hypoxia in early childhood in early childhood is associated with cognitive functioning in later years. Some of the influence from these factors may be permanent (as might be expected in significant early malnutrition), and other influences may be transitory and even reversible (as in the case of encephalopathy in end-stage liver disease).

A second set of "risk" factors we propose are those described as *iatrogenic effects*. Treatment of end-stage organ disease, and its cure, organ transplantation, carries risks to cognitive development. Prior to transplantation, interventions such as dialysis or open-heart surgery might affect cognitive functions. Organ transplantation is major invasive surgery and

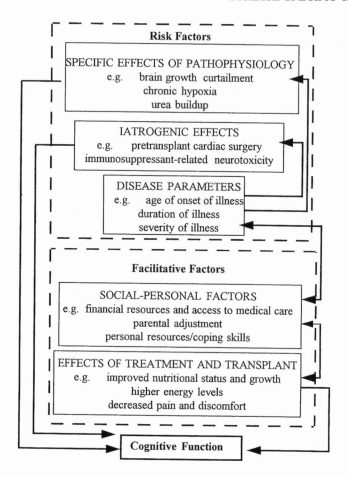

FIGURE 10.1. A conceptual model for research on cognitive function in children who receive organ transplantation. Adapted from Wallander, Varni, Babani, Banis, and Wilcox (1989). Copyright 1989 by Plenum Publishing Corp. Adapted by permission.

carries the risk of short-term as well as long-term cognitive compromise. For example, cardiac surgery in general results in increased neurological risk (Nussbaum & Goldstein, 1992). Immunosuppressants are known to be neurotoxic, although their effects on subtle cognitive functioning have yet to be systematically examined. Organ rejection episodes usually follow transplantation and need containment with high doses of immunosuppressants and steroids, which may also have negative effects on cognitive function. Again, there may be great variability in the recovery from the surgery, number of rejection episodes, frequency of rehospitalization, and level of immunosuppressants required to contain rejection, all of which may also affect levels of cognitive function in the child who has received organ transplantation.

A third set of variables that has been examined in past studies relates to *disease parameters*. These include duration of the disease and severity of illness, which are inversely associated with cognitive functioning. Age of onset of disease is a known risk variable, with earlier onset carrying greater risk. Time since transplant also has been investigated as a variable that affects cognitive function, with the expectation that the greater stability that comes with distance from transplantation would result in improvements in cognitive functioning.

The major facilitative variable investigated has been *the effect of treatment and transplantation*. The cognitive functioning of certain groups of children (e.g., infants with end-stage renal disease) benefits from transplantation. While empirical studies using standardized testing in other groups have not demonstrated a clear benefit of transplantation on cognitive function, this may be due to methodological issues in the investigations reviewed earlier in this chapter.

Less investigated in the transplantation literature have been the variables that in most models of adaptation in chronic illness are given a significant role. These variables relate to social–ecological and personal–intrapersonal influences. They would include socioeconomic status, parental education level, life stress, maternal and paternal adjustment, family adjustment, and the level of conflict versus levels of support provided to each other by family members. In a meta-analysis reported by Lavigne and Faier-Routman (1993), many of these variables were found to relate to psychological adjustment in pediatric illness. Wallander et al. (1989) describe these variables as "resistance" factors and suggest that these variables may play an important role in counterbalancing the deleterious effects of risk factors. In studies of cognitive function in children who have received organ transplantation, to date these variables are rarely studied.

There are undoubtedly complex interrelationships between these variables. For example, while *disease parameters* such as duration and age of onset of disease have been investigated as they influence cognitive function, in this model we hypothesize that these relationships are mediated through the other two groups of "risk" variables: *pathophysiological effects* of the disease and *iatrogenic effects of treatment*. Age of onset may play an important role because the developing brain is most vulnerable to the effects of malnutrition and toxicity during infancy and early childhood (Epstein, 1978). Children with more severe liver and kidney disease are likely to have higher levels of circulating toxins that are ultimately harmful to cognitive development. More aggressive treatment may be necessary for children with greater disease severity, and may also include greater iatrogenic cognitive risks.

Within the facilitative factors, additional relationships are hypothesized. Families with greater *social and personal* resources are more likely to be able to maximize *treatment* access opportunities. Their compliance with medical treatment, for example, may be better than that of the overburdened and chaotic family. Similarly, with improved nutritional status and growth as a result of better treatment, children may develop better personal resources as they have access to more age-typical opportunities.

Risk factors and facilitative factors also may influence each other. For example, *disease parameters* may affect *social and personal* resources. Families with severely ill children, whose illness has continued for a long time, may become more financially and personally stressed. The interaction between risk and facilitative factors may therefore be bidirectional. Families with greater financial resources may be in a better position to obtain timely medical treatment and minimize the risk from poorly managed disease.

The development of such a model and its usefulness in the long term requires that more explicit hypotheses be made about the mechanisms of the effects of disease. More discussion is needed about this issue than has so far appeared in the literature. For example, we have found that while there is an assumption by medical personnel, parents, and researchers that the child will function more "normally" following transplantation, the pathway between transplant and improved functioning has not been clearly delineated. Hypotheses about the mechanisms underlying successful adaptation to transplantation guide the choice of variables examined in future research. Ultimately, such studies will point the way for the design of interventions influencing outcomes.

Some nonspecific improvement would be expected for the child on most evaluations simply because he or she is feeling better. However, would change be expected also in "underlying ability"? Undoubtedly, this would depend upon the specific abilities measured. In certain cases one might expect that there have been brain-based structural changes that might be irreversible as a result of damage from the disease. For example, deficits that result from curtailed brain growth secondary to malnutrition in infancy might fall into this category. In very young children receiving organ transplantation, restored nutrition to the brain may result in increased brain growth. Improved nutrition in later life, however, does not have major impact on the brain. On the other hand, some cognitive functions may be improved. Those, for example, that depend upon exposure for their level of function might show improvement, assuming that these opportunities are provided following transplantation for the children. After a period of time following transplantation the life of these patients in many cases is closer to that of their healthy age peers than it was prior to transplantation (Zitelli et al., 1988). As an example, following transplantation children might be more likely to engage with objects in their environment such as jigsaw puzzles and household tools. Consequently, their visual reasoning and fine motor skills might improve. They may have the energy and attention span to read more, ultimately improving their verbal skills and vocabulary. They may have opportunities to be exposed on a systematic basis to concepts taught in school. Certainly these experiences would not be expected to dramatically change the cognitive function (and test scores) of basically healthy children. However, it is not known whether exposure to these learning experiences, which medically well children receive routinely, would enhance the development of cognitive skills in children who have undergone transplantation and have lacked such experiences in the past.

CONCLUSIONS

In summary, there is evidence from multiple studies that children who receive organ transplantation can show deficits in a broad range of cognitive function. The literature does not suggest that there are universal benefits on cognitive functions as a result of organ transplantation. However, several large gaps remain in our information base. First it is unclear as to *which* children are most vulnerable to developing cognitive delays and difficulties. Information is lacking about correlates of the compromises found before and after transplantation, so that relative risk can be assessed for individual children. Second, the adaptive manifestations of cognitive abilities have been much less investigated. There is more information in the published literature about the disease-related characteristics of children who do poorly on certain aspects of neuropsychological batteries than about how they manage academically at school.

From a research viewpoint, the problems in the empirical literature, outlined in 1994 (Stewart et al., 1994), still persist. Few studies include control groups, and the appropriate control group that does not have unknown deficits specific to a different disease would be difficult to obtain. The highly heterogeneous population makes questionable the conclusions that are drawn from small samples. The interaction between development and disease is particularly difficult to capture, and the state of the art does not allow for reliable prediction of later deficits through measurements in early life. Global measures such as IQ continue to be the primary assessment instruments. Long-term findings are significantly limited.

Some additional issues have recently emerged, or were not clearly highlighted in the previous review. First, while serial assessments are necessary in accounting for the large variability in the population in functioning prior to transplantation, there needs to be greater awareness of practice effects. A control group that receives identical testing at the same intervals is necessary. Second, there is growing evidence of the neurotoxic effects of immunosuppressants. While there have been some studies in the adult population examining the association between cyclosporine levels and cognitive functions, there is an absence of such studies in the pediatric population. As there is some suggestion that FK506 has greater neurotoxic effects than cyclosporine, and as its use is becoming more prevalent, it is important that future studies examine the effect of this drug on cognitive function.

What are the implications of these findings for practitioners? First, there is enough evidence from various studies to show that the chances of compromises in cognitive function are high in children with end-stage organ disease who receive transplantation. As transplant programs identify children who will eventually need transplantation, frequently well before their disease has progressed to end-stage, monitoring their cognitive function is clinically justified. There are no empirical grounds for the belief held by some medical practitioners that cognitive deficits observed prior to transplantation are transient. Early identification of children with deficits translates into greater opportunities for remediation and stimulation efforts. Second, the few studies that have been conducted with regard to the academic function of these children suggest that their deficits are frequently unrecognized in their school environment. Many children are in fact not severely impaired, and their deficits may be easy to miss without a careful assessment. There is strong justification for routine comprehensive psychoeducational assessments for children who are candidates for, or recipients of, organ transplantation.

Surprisingly, there have been few new studies in the medical or psychological literature on cognitive functioning in the pediatric organ transplant population, despite the fact that there are increasing numbers of potential participants and many more centers that offer organ transplantation than there were several years ago. This dearth of studies may reflect the prioritization of medical research resources with the focus on biomedical investigations, as well as the shrinking of behavioral research dollars. Future studies need to be clearly theory driven, and more discussion is needed about the mechanisms of the effects of disease and transplantation on cognitive function. The technology to support the lives of children with end-stage organ disease continues to become more sophisticated; our understanding of their broader psychosocial functioning needs to keep pace with this improved technology.

REFERENCES

Bannister, M., Stewart, S. M., Kennard, B. D., Benser, M., Andrews, W. S., & Moore, P. E. (1995, September). *Developmental and physical growth status of pediatric liver transplantation patients at least 5 years after surgery.* Paper presented at the meeting of the Joint Congress on Liver Transplantation, London.

Baum, M. F., Cutler, D. C., Fricker, F. J., & Trimm, R. F. (1991). Physiologic and psychological growth and development in pediatric heart transplant recipients. *Journal of Heart and Lung Transplantation, 10,* 848–855.

Bock, G. H., Conners, C. K., Ruley, J., Samango-Sprouse, C. A., Conry, J. A., Weiss, I., Eng, G., Johnson, E. L., & David, C. T. (1989). Disturbances of brain maturation and neurodevelopment during chronic renal failure in infancy. *Journal of Pediatrics, 114,* 231–238.

Coffman, K. L., Hoffman, A., Rosenthal, P., Demetriou, A., & Makowka, L. (1996). Neurological and psychological sequelae in transplant recipients after bridging with bioartificial liver. *General Hospital Psychiatry, 18,* 20S–24S.

Cox, K. L., & Freese, D. K. (1996). Tacrolimus (FK506): The pros and cons of its use as an immunosuppressant in pediatric liver transplantation. *Clinical and Investigative Medicine, 19,* 389–392.

Crittenden, M. R., Holliday, M. A., Piel, C. F., & Potter, D. E. (1985). Intellectual development of children with renal insufficiency and end-stage disease. *International Journal of Pediatric Nephrology, 6,* 275–280.

Davis, J. D., Chang, P., & Nevins, T. E. (1990). Successful renal transplantation accelerates development in young uremic children. *Pediatrics, 86,* 594–600.

English, T., Cooper, D., & Cory-Pearce, R. (1980). Recent experience with heart transplantation. *British Medical Journal, 281,* 699–702.

Epstein, H. T. (1978). Growth spurts during brain development: Implications for educational policy and practice. In J. S. Chall & A. F. Mirsky (Eds.), *Education and the brain* (pp. 343–370). Chicago: University of Chicago Press.

Farmer, M. E. (1994). Cognitive deficits related to major organ failure: The potential role of neuropsychological testing. *Neuropsychology Review, 4,* 117–160.

Fennell, R. S., Fennell, E. B., Carter, R. L., Mings, E. L., Klausner, A. B., & Hurst, J. R. (1990a). Association between renal function and cognition in childhood chronic renal failure. *Pediatric Nephrology, 4,* 16–20.

Fennell, R. S., Fennell, E. B., Carter, R. L., Mings, E. L., Klausner, A. B., & Hurst, J. R. (1990b). A longitudinal study of the cognitive function of children with renal failure. *Pediatric Nephrology, 4,* 11–14.

Fennell, R. S., Rasbury, W. C., Fennell, E. B., & Morris, M. K. (1984). The effects of kidney transplantation on cognitive performance in a pediatric population. *Pediatrics, 74,* 273–278.

Fung, J. J., Eliasziw, M., Todo, S., Jain, A., Demetris, A. J., McMichael, J. P., Starzl, T. E., Meier, P., & Donner, A. (1996). The Pittsburgh randomized trial of tacrolimus compared to cyclosporine for hepatic transplantation. *Journal of the American College of Surgeons, 183,* 117–125.

Grimm, M., Yeganehfar, W., Laufer, G., Madi, C., Kramer, L., Eisenhuber, E., Simon, P., Kupilik, N., Schreiner, W., Pacher, R., Bunzel, B., Wolner, E., & Grimm, G. (1996). Cyclosporine may affect improvement of cognitive brain function after successful cardiac transplantation. *Circulation, 94,* 1339–1345.

Hobbs, S. A., & Sexon, S. B. (1993). Cognitive development and learning in the pediatric organ transplant recipient. *Journal of Learning Disabilities, 26,* 104–113.

Kennard, B. D., Stewart, S. M., Phelan-McAuliffe, D., Waller, D. A., Bannister, M., Fiorvani, M., & Andrews, W. S. (1999). Academic outcome in long term survivors of pediatric liver transplantation. *Journal of Developmental and Behavioral Pediatrics, 20,* 17–23.

Lavigne, J. V., & Faier-Routman, J. (1993). Psychological adjustment to pediatric physical disorders: A meta-analytic review and comparison with existing models. *Journal of Developmental and Behavioral Pediatrics, 14,* 117–123.

Lawry, K. W., Brouhard, B. H., & Cunningham, R. J. (1994). Cognitive functioning and school performance in children with renal failure. *Pediatric Nephrology, 8,* 326–329.

Levenson, J. L., & Olbrisch, M. E. (1996). Introduction. *General Hospital Psychiatry, 18,* 2S–4S.

Linde, L. M., Rasof, B., & Dunn, O. J. (1967). Mental development in congenital heart disease. *Journal of Pediatrics, 71,* 198–203.

Marshall, J. R. (1979). Neuropsychiatric aspects of renal failure. *Journal of Clinical Psychiatry, 40,* 81–85.

McGraw, M. E., & Haka-Ikse, K. (1985). Neurologic–developmental sequelae of chronic renal failure in infancy. *Journal of Pediatrics, 106,* 579–583.

McManus, R. P., O'Hair, D. P., & Schweiger, J. (1992). Cyclosporine-associated central neurotoxicity after heart transplantation. *Annals of Thoracic Surgery, 53,* 326–328.

Miller, L. W. (1996). Cyclosporine-associated neurotoxicity: The need for a better guide for immunosuppressive therapy. *Circulation, 94,* 1209–1211.

Mueller, A. R., Platz, K. P., Bechstein, W. O., Scattenfroh, N., Stoltenburg-Didinger, G., Blumhardt, G., Christe, W., & Neuhaus, P. (1994). Neurotoxicity after orthotopic liver transplantation: A comparison between cyclosporine and FK506. *Transplantation, 58,* 155–170.

Murray, J. E., Merrill, J. P., & Harrison, J. H. (1955). Renal homotransplantation in identical twins. *Surgery Forum, 6,* 432–436.

Nussbaum, P. D., & Goldstein, G. (1992). Neuropsychological sequelae of heart transplantation: A preliminary review. *Clinical Psychology Review, 12,* 475–483.

Rodrigue, J. R., Greene, A. F., & Boggs, S. R. (1994). *Journal of Clinical Psychology in Medical Settings, 1,* 41–70.

Shapiro, R., Tzakis, A., Scantlebury, V., Jordan, M., Vivas, C., Ellis, D., Gilboa, N., Irish, W., Hopp, L., & Reyes, J. (1994). Improving results of pediatric renal transplantation. *Journal of the American College of Surgeons, 179,* 424–432.

Silbert, A., Wolff, P. H., Mayer, B., Rosenthal, A., & Nadas, A. S. (1969). Cyanotic heart disease and psychological development. *Pediatrics, 43,* 192–200.

So, S. K. S., Chang, P., Najarian, J. S., Mauer, S. M., Simons, R. L., & Nevins, T. E. (1987). Growth and development in infants after renal transplantation. *Journal of Pediatrics, 110,* 343–350.

Starfield, B. (1985). The state of research on chronically ill children. In N. Hobbs & J. M. Perrin (Eds.), *Issues in the care of children with chronic illness* (pp. 109–131). San Francisco: Jossey-Bass.

Stewart, S. M., Campbell, R., McCallon, D., Waller, D. A., & Andrews, W. S. (1992). Cognitive patterns in school-age children with end-stage liver disease. *Journal of Developmental and Behavioral Pediatrics, 13,* 331–338.

Stewart, S. M., Hiltebeitel, C., Nici, J., Waller, D. A., Uauy, R., & Andrews, W. S. (1991). Neuropsychological outcome of pediatric liver transplantation. *Pediatrics, 87,* 367–376.

Stewart, S. M., Kennard, B. D., Waller, D. A., & Fixler, D. (1994). Cognitive function in children who receive organ transplantation. *Health Psychology, 13,* 3–13.

Stewart, S. M., Uauy, R., Kennard, B. D., Benser, M., Waller, D., & Andrews, W. S. (1988). Mental development and growth in children with chronic liver disease of early and late onset. *Pediatrics, 82,* 167–172.

Stewart, S. M., Uauy, R., Waller, D. A., Kennard, B. D., Benser, M., & Andrews, W. S. (1989). One year follow-up of mental and motor development and social competence in pediatric patients receiving successful liver transplantation. *Journal of Pediatrics, 114,* 574–581.

Wallander, J. L. (1992). Theory-driven research in pediatric psychology: A little bit on why and how. *Journal of Pediatric Psychology, 17,* 521–535.

Wallander, J. L., Varni, J. W., Babani, L., Banis, H. T., & Wilcox, K. T. (1989). Family resources as resistance factors for psychological maladjustment in chronically ill and handicapped children. *Journal of Pediatric Psychology, 14,* 157–173.

Weiss, R. A., & Edelmann, C. M. (1984). End-stage renal disease in children. *Pediatrics in Review, 5,* 294–303.

Wijdicks, E. F. M., Wiesner, R. H., & Krom, R. A. F. (1995). Neurotoxicity in liver transplant recipients with cyclosporine immunosuppression. *Neurology, 45,* 1962–1964.

Wilczek, H., Ringden, O., & Tyden, G. (1985). Cyclosporine associated central nervous system toxicity after renal transplantation. *Transplantation, 39,* 110–115.

Wray, J., Pot-Mees, C., Zeitlin, H. Radley-Smith, R., & Yacoub, M. (1994). Cognitive function and behavioural status in paediatric heart and heart–lung transplant recipients: The Harefield experience. *British Medical Journal, 309,* 837–841.

Wray, J., & Yacoub, M. (1991). Psychosocial evaluation of children after open heart surgery versus cardiac transplantation. In M. Yacoub & J. R. Pepper (Eds.), *Annals of cardiac surgery 90–91* (pp. 50–55). London: Current Science Publications.

Zitelli, B. J., Miller, J. W., Gartner, J. C., Malatack, J. J., Urbach, A. H., Belle, S. H., Williams, L., Kirkpatrick, B., & Starzl, T. E. (1988). Changes in life-style after liver transplantation. *Pediatrics, 82,* 173–180.

CHAPTER ELEVEN

Seizure Disorders

JENNIFER R. HIEMENZ
GEORGE W. HYND
MARTA JIMENEZ

Epilepsy is considered by many to the be the most prevalent chronic neurological disorder in children (Bolter, 1986), and prevalence estimates have ranged from as low as 4–8 children in 1,000 (Blom, Heijbel, & Bergfors, 1978) to as high as 1% of all children (Zupanc, 1996). Children with epilepsy frequently display cognitive sequelae that may adversely impact academic performance and social interactions. This chapter reviews the common cognitive, neuropsychological, and behavioral characteristics of children with epilepsy, the typical effects of common antiepileptic medications on cognition and behavior, and various other seizure-related phenomena and their relative impact on cognitive functioning and academic achievement.

Epilepsy is commonly implicated as a cause of impaired behavioral, emotional, cognitive, and academic functioning in seizure-prone children, and some authors have even postulated that some forms of learning disability may be viewed as a manifestation of subclinical seizure activity (Hynd & Willis, 1988). Recently a large body of research has examined the effects of antiepileptic drugs (AEDs) on cognitive function and the relationship between cognitive impairment and side or site of epileptic focus (e.g., Chaudhry, Najam, De Mahieu, Raza, & Ahmad, 1992; Zupanc, 1996). As epilepsy has a relatively early onset and often lasts over the course of a lifetime, the possibility that epilepsy will impact a child's development, school performance, and life adjustment is quite large (Black & Hynd, 1995; Bolter, 1986). The presence of recurrent seizures can interfere with normal development through a number of means, including negative social reactions, parental anxieties and apprehensions, learning difficulties, and altered neurological functions (Bolter, 1986). An understanding of the cognitive and behavioral features of epilepsy and its treatment is essential to all professionals who assist in the assessment and remediation of children with epilepsy.

It must be noted that children with epilepsy represent a heterogeneous group that varies along several dimensions including etiology, seizure variables (including type, frequency, age of onset, and duration of the seizure disorder), observed electroencephalographic (EEG) activity, antiepileptic medication, gender, and environment. The relationship among these variables, intellectual ability, and scholastic performance has received considerable attention. Epilepsy is also often unique in that the clinical presentation, progression, and underlying etiology may vary considerably from case to case.

SEIZURE CLASSIFICATION AND DEFINITIONS

Epilepsy may be defined as two or more unprovoked epileptic seizures (Henrikson, 1990) and is therefore not the same as a single seizure (e.g., febrile seizure), or numerous seizures that are attributable to an identified pathological brain state. A seizure can be defined as a behavioral event that results from a sudden electrical discharge of neurons in the brain. The specific type of seizure is defined by the behavior during the event, in which different types and locations of electrical discharge within the brain will lead to different behavioral outcomes. Seizures themselves can typically last from a few seconds to 20–30 minutes (Sachs & Barrett, 1995), may occur occasionally to many times a day (e.g., absence seizures), and are usually followed by a period of confusion and somnolence known as the postictal ("after-seizure") state. One study examining prevalence and incidence of epilepsy found that 50–70% of individuals who suffer from recurrent seizures will manifest their first attack during childhood and adolescence (Hauser & Nelson, 1989). The two peak ages for onset for epilepsy seem to be during the first 2 years of life and at the age of puberty (Glaser, 1979). Although some researchers have called for a more clinical approach to classification due to the heterogeneity of seizure disorders as a whole (Mosewich & So, 1996; Murphy & Dehkharghani, 1994), the International Classification of Epileptic Seizures (Commission on Classification and Terminology of the International League Against Epilepsy, 1989) is the most widely accepted classification scheme of seizures in use today. According to this classification system, epilepsy can arise either as the result of a variety of pathological brain states, referred to as symptomatic epilepsy, or from unidentifiable causes, in which case it is called idiopathic epilepsy. Whether seizures arise from known or unidentifiable causes, they are generally divided into two general categories depending on location of the seizure activity within the brain: partial and generalized.

Partial Seizures versus Generalized Seizures

Seizures are referred to as partial if epileptic discharges are localized and restricted to a circumscribed area of the brain. In partial, or focal, seizures the observed abnormal EEG activity is restricted to a discrete cortical region. The symptomatology of a partial seizure may be limited to elementary sensory or motor processes, or it may include more complex disturbances of consciousness, behavior, cognition, or affect. Partial seizures are classified primarily on the basis of whether or not consciousness is impaired during the attack. Simple partial seizures involve no loss of consciousness, whereas complex partial seizures involve loss of consciousness (Pellock, 1989). Complex partial seizures may begin as simple partial seizures or as complex partial ones from the beginning, but all involve loss of consciousness combined with localization of seizure activity. The term "temporal lobe epilepsy" was commonly used in the past to describe one subset of complex partial seizures, but its limited diagnostic and treatment utility have decreased its clinical use as a diagnostic category (Sachs & Barrett, 1995). Simple partial and complex partial seizures are more often difficult to treat than generalized seizures, and children with partial seizures are more likely to have substantial learning problems, which may be related to the site of epileptic focus (Henrikson, 1990). In addition, one or more medications, usually in high doses, may be employed, which may further contribute to learning problems.

The electrical discharge of generalized seizures simultaneously involves both cerebral hemispheres and their subcortical connections and structures. Children with generalized seizures commonly present with impaired consciousness that is frequently accompanied by abnormal bilateral motor activity. Generalized seizures may be convulsive or nonconvulsive (Pellock, 1989) and can either begin as generalized seizures or can evolve from partial to generalized. They can be further divided on the basis of the presence or absence of major motor disturbances (e.g., tonic, clonic, and tonic–clonic) ranging from typical absence (the classic petit mal) to generalized tonic–clonic convulsions (grand mal) (Pellock, 1989). Absence seizures are characterized by a loss of consciousness, sometimes without any accompanying motor symptoms, and can resemble staring spells or daydreaming. However, often there may be subtle mouth or finger movements. They typically last only about 5–10 seconds, and can therefore be difficult to detect (Sachs & Barnett, 1995). They may also repeat several times during the day. Tonic seizures are generalized seizures which present as violent contractions of the large muscle groups. Clonic seizures are characterized by rhythmic, repetitive jerking movements. Atonic seizures involve the sudden and complete loss of muscle tone throughout the body, and often present as a drop attack. Finally, myoclonic seizures are generalized seizures in which small muscle groups show sudden brief, repetitive contractions or "twitches" (Sachs & Barnett, 1995).

Age-Dependent Seizure Disorders

Seizures are reported to be the most common neurological event in newborn infants, most likely because the threshold for all provoked seizure activity is much lower in neonates. Lombroso (1996) describes this mechanism as an "overexpression" of receptors for excitatory amino acids within the brain, which leads to rapid and easy onset and offset of seizure activity in the neonatal brain. Like seizures of older children, infantile seizures also are categorized by etiology into idiopathic and symptomatic seizures. Although some infantile seizures are termed idiopathic, it is difficult to determine whether recurrent "idiopathic" seizure activity is due to the deleterious effects of prior seizures or to underlying damage or dysfunction (Dulac, 1995).

Febrile seizures, considered to be a benign epilepsy, fall into the symptomatic category, and are usually provoked by high fever that is not associated with intracranial infection. They are the most common seizure type in children, affecting 2–4% of all children (Wyllie, 1994), with a peak incidence in the second year of life (Hauser, 1994). They are age dependent, occurring in very young children, have a genetic component, and are outgrown (Holmes, 1987). Simple febrile seizures last less than 15 minutes and are not localized, whereas complex febrile seizures last longer, can recur, and have focal features (Duchowny & Harvey, 1996). Febrile seizures are considered to be a risk factor for the later development of other epilepsies (e.g., partial complex) only if they are prolonged, recur within one illness, or have focal features (e.g., complex febrile seizures) (Nelson & Ellenberg, 1984), which suggests some underlying pathology. Nelson and Ellenberg (1976) reported the results of the National Collaborative Perinatal Project, a large population-based study of 50,000 pregnancies in which 1,706 children with febrile seizures were followed up to 7 years of age, and found that the overall incidence of later afebrile seizures was not increased, compared to children with no history of febrile seizures and who were neurologically normal. However, when Annegars, Hauser, and Shirts (1987) followed children for an average of 18 years, they did find an increased incidence of afebrile seizures (7%) among 687 patients with a history of febrile seizures. Further, Monetti et al. (1995) found a history of febrile seizures in 20% of patients with idiopathic generalized epilepsy, compared with 1.8% of control subjects. The general consensus regarding the role of febrile complex seizures in future epilepsy is that rather than playing a direct causal role in the subsequent development of idiopathic generalized epilepsy, febrile complex seizures may actually represent an early expression of a low seizure threshold that could be expressed later in life by the development of idiopathic generalized seizures.

Other age-dependent seizure disorders that are not attributable to symptomatic causes such as fevers include the Ohtahara, West, and Lennox–Gastaut syndromes (Donat, 1992), which some have argued are manifestations of a developmental progression of the same seizure disorder. Ohtahara syndrome was originally named "early infantile epileptic encephalopathy"; usually appears within the first 3 months of life, particularly within the first 10 days (Donat, 1992), and is considered to be the most severe form of the age-dependent epilepsies due to its early onset and severity. Etiology is most often congenital brain malformations, and therefore the prognosis is quite poor. Four of Ohtahara's original 14 patients died in their first year, and all of the surviving patients had severe disabilities. West syndrome, characterized by infantile spasms and developmental delay, seems to be related to Ohtahara syndrome, in that Ohtahara's surviving patients all met diagnostic criteria for West syndrome at the appropriate age, which is between 3 and 10 months. However, not all infants with West syndrome have previously demonstrated Ohtahara syndrome, so it is unclear whether this demonstrates a different developmental manifestation of the same disorder (Donat, 1992). Lennox–Gastaut syndrome, unlike the earlier-appearing West and Ohtahara syndromes, appears after age 1 or 2, and is characterized by tonic seizures and mental retardation. Approximately 30% of children with West syndrome later develop Lennox–Gastaut syndrome, but not all children with Lennox–Gastaut syndrome have previously had either West or Ohtahara syndrome (Donat, 1992; Lombroso, 1996). In general, however, the incidence of severe cognitive deficits is quite high (up to 80%) in children with these early-onset seizure disorders, and it appears that the earlier the onset appears, the worse the prognosis is for the child. The prognosis is particularly dismal if the seizure disorder is symptomatic, or linked to an underlying brain pathology, since outcomes are generally worse for symptomatic epilepsies than for idiopathic (Donat, 1992; Dulac, 1995; Lombroso, 1996; Talwar, Baldwin, Hutzler, & Griesemer, 1995).

Etiology and Prognosis of Seizure Disorders

The two broad categories that divide the etiology of epilepsy—symptomatic (also known as secondary or acquired) and idiopathic (also known as primary or essential)—have differential prognoses for future seizure activity. In symptomatic epilepsy, which is associated with organic pathology or complicated by other neurological problems, the onset of seizures is directly attributable to an acquired cerebral or general systemic disease. Symptomatic epilepsies appear to reveal age-specific patterns in terms of underlying pathological processes. In particular, during school years, high fevers, infectious diseases, and cerebral trauma constitute the major etiological factors underlying seizures (Bolter, 1986). Symptomatic epilepsy syndromes are more frequently associated with unfavorable outcomes with respect to intellectual ability and scholastic performance, with the underlying etiology as the determining factor for future intellectual development (Dam, 1990).

In approximately two-thirds of epileptic cases, no evidence can be found for an underlying cause. Such seizures have been termed idiopathic (Hynd & Willis, 1988). The preponderance of these seizures are generalized, and include absence (petit mal), tonic–clonic (grand mal), and myoclonic seizures, which may occur alone or in various combinations (Bourgeois, 1992). Patients with idiopathic epilepsy more often report a positive family history of seizures than patients suffering from symptomatic seizures (Monetti et al., 1995), which suggests a genetic predisposition for epilepsy in these patients. Other risk factors found to be associated with idiopathic generalized epilepsy (IGE) include a history of febrile seizures, a family history of febrile seizures, continued physical stress during pregnancy, advanced maternal age, and birth order greater than three. Bourgeois (1992) and Monetti et al. (1995) found no association between complications of pregnancy or delivery and subsequent development of IGA, supporting the earlier findings of Nelson and Ellenberg (1984). It appears that in the absence of neurological impairment, epilepsy is not associated with perinatal factors, and individual predisposition may play a major role in the development of IGE (Monetti et al., 1995). Children with the highest risk of seizure recurrence (80–90%) are those with a single complex partial seizure, abnormal neurological findings, or epileptiform discharges on EEG. Those with the lowest risk (30%) after an unprovoked seizure are those who experienced a generalized tonic–clonic seizure, have normal neurological findings, and have a normal electroencephalogram (Wyllie, 1994). Children who begin having generalized seizures at or later than 5–7 years of age without evidence of a brain lesion usually have a good prognosis (Monetti et al., 1995).

Following the classification of epileptic seizures, a syndrome-driven approach has received increasing attention. Epileptic syndromes are most often defined by specific clusters of behavioral signs and symptoms that customarily co-occur (Vassella, 1994). They are based on clinical features (e.g., predominant seizure type(s), neurological manifestations), EEG (ictal and interictal), evolutional features (e.g., etiology, family history, age of onset, development over time, prognosis), and response to AED treatment (Bolter, 1986). The findings that different syndromes may involve similar genetic factors, and conversely, that the same syndrome may be related to different underlying causes, emphasize the heterogeneous nature of these syndromes (Vasella, 1994).

Seizure-Related Phenomena

"Aura" is a term that in the past was used to describe phenomena experienced prior to the onset of a seizure. However, this term, aura, is not preferred today as seizures may begin with partial simple or partial complex features, and may consist of any of the manifestations of a simple partial seizure. The particular sensation experienced is determined by the cortical location of the electrical discharge and may include somatosensory, auditory, visual, olfactory, or gustatory sensations, as well as complex subjective experiences such as fear, embarrassment, dizziness, déjà vu, or jamais vu (Engel, 1989).

A prodrome is an awareness of an impending seizure that may be detected by some patients and their parents hours or days prior to seizure onset. It is distinguished from a partial simple seizure in that the prodrome is not part of the ictal event. The physiological basis of prodromes has not yet been established, but they are known to occur more commonly in generalized tonic–clonic (GTC) seizures and to a lesser extent in patients with complex partial seizures. A prodrome might be experienced as headaches, irritability, insomnia, changes in personality, or activity level or a feeling of impending doom (Engel, 1989). Thus, in those cases where an aura or prodrome is known to exist, the classroom teacher and other school personnel who work closely with the student must be aware of the typical preseizure behaviors exhibited or perceptions experienced by the child and need to be sensitive to their occurrence.

There are two types of temporary disturbances in mental function that may occur during or immediately after epileptic discharges. Brief lapses in consciousness may be seen in childhood absence and in complex partial epilepsy. Temporary, isolated cognitive or behavioral deficits may also be seen resulting from epileptic discharges originating in focal cortical areas responsible for higher-order functions. For example, when language areas are affected, various types of language impairment may result, including word-finding problems, paraphasias, or articulation problems (Thierry, 1993). Postictal deficits may occur over hours, days, or weeks. The duration is variable and is not related to the duration of the seizure (Thierry, 1993).

ACADEMIC ACHIEVEMENT
IN CHILDREN WITH EPILEPSY

Learning problems in particular seem to occur in children with epilepsy, and referrals for evaluation for special education eligibility are quite common. Academic difficulties are greatest in arithmetic, spelling, reading comprehension, and word recognition (Gourley, 1990), and boys with epilepsy may be more likely to underachieve at school and to be more impaired with respect to reading skills (Stedman, Van Heyningen, & Lindsey, 1982; Stores & Hart, 1976). Mahapatra (1990) employed a process-oriented approach to the study of reading performance in children with generalized seizure disorder and found that compared with normal children who were matched on age, gender, and level of education, children with epilepsy were found to perform at significantly lower levels in reading. Performance was more impaired for comprehension of a paragraph than for reading words in isolation. In contrast to normal controls, significant weaknesses were also found in patients with respect to the processes of coding and planning, even when attention was intact.

It is well established that children with epilepsy are at greater risk than other children of experiencing difficulties in school, even when cognitive ability is taken into account. Impairments are most frequently seen on tests of reading, spelling, arithmetic, and word recognition, but not on design copying or on tests of creative, rather than academic, ability (Cull, 1988). Holdsworth and Whitmore (1974) found in a study of 85 school children with recurrent seizures that 16% were regarded as falling seriously behind and 53% were functioning at a below average educational level. It was also noted that 42% of the children were described as inattentive by their teachers and that their inattentiveness was associated with decreased school performance. In the famous Isle of Wight study, Rutter, Tizard, and Whitmore (1970) reported that more than twice as many children with epilepsy revealed serious reading comprehension problems when compared to age-matched children without a diagnosis of epilepsy, and reading problems in these children were unrelated to their level of intelligence.

There is also evidence suggesting that arithmetic skills are particularly at risk in children with epilepsy (Bagley, 1970; Green & Hartlage, 1971). Bolter (1986) found impaired performance (defined as a standard score 1 or more standard deviations below an expected level based on the child's Full Scale IQ) in 3% of the children for word recognition, 13% for spelling, and 26% for arithmetic calculation using the Wide Range Achievement Test.

Bennett-Levy and Stores (1984), using a teacher-completed questionnaire, found that teachers perceived children with epilepsy as having significantly more problems than their nonepileptic peers with respect to overall achievement, concentration, and the mental processing of information. When level of academic achievement was controlled for, children with epilepsy were still perceived by their teachers as being significantly less alert (Cull, 1988).

Mitchell, Chavez, Lee, and Guzman (1991) investigated the relative roles of epilepsy-related factors and sociocultural factors as determinants of academic achievement and IQ in 44 children, ages 5–13, with generalized, partial, and absence seizures and found that underachievement was more common among these children than among controls. After adjusting for measured levels of cognitive ability, 38% of the children were determined to be underachieving in reading comprehension, 31% in mathematics, and 32% in spelling. Along with level of parent education, subscales of the Home Observation for Measurement of the Environment (HOME) that assess educational materials in the household and family participation in developmentally stimulating activities were found to be the best predictors of IQ. Academic performance levels on the Peabody Individual Achievement Test (PIAT) in Reading Recognition, Reading Comprehension, General Knowledge, and Spelling were unrelated to seizure and medication variables. Underachievement in mathematics was, however, found to be significantly related to duration of seizure disorder (Mitchell et al., 1991). Severity, duration, and treatment of epilepsy appeared to play a minor role in underachievement relative to family setting, parent attitude, and underlying neurological abnormalities. The authors emphasize the potential role of cultural and socioeconomic variables as confounds in the studies of children with epilepsy and with other physical illnesses. Further, they recommend caution in the interpretation of studies investigating the role of seizure variables drawn from biased samples of patients attending teaching centers or other facilities that serve disadvantaged populations to a disproportionate degree. Mitchell and colleagues (1991) conclude that parents of children who are performing well academically at the time of initial diagnosis can probably be reassured that their child will continue to perform well in the future.

EFFECTS OF SEIZURES ON COGNITIVE AND PERCEPTUAL FUNCTIONING

While individuals with epilepsy as a group tend to fall within the normal range of intelligence, the distribution of their scores is skewed toward the lower end of functioning (Hynd & Willis, 1988). While the common stereotype is that all children with epilepsy fall into a lower cognitive ability range by virtue of the diagnosis, it is vital that a distinction be drawn between state-dependent intellectual deficits brought about by AED therapy or postictal recovery states, and permanent intellectual deficits that result from neurological damage or pathology (Besag, 1995). Chaudhry et al. (1992) demonstrated cognitive impairment in patients with epilepsy prior to initiation of AED therapy. In a controlled study of patients with epilepsy, ages 10–50, and 15 volunteers in which scores were obtained on four Wechsler Intelligence Scale for Children—3rd edition (WISC-III; Wechsler, 1991) or Wechsler Adult Intelligence Scale—Revised (WAIS-R; Wechsler, 1981) subtests (Picture Completion, Picture Arrangement, Block Design, and Object Assembly), the mean intellectual scores obtained by untreated epilepsy patients were significantly lower than those of age-matched controls. Bolter (1986), in a study of epileptic children, found that as a group the children fell within the average range of intelligence on the WISC-R

(Full Scale IQ: $\overline{X}$ = 92.74, *SD* = 14.21). However, only 13% earned scores in the above-average range (Full Scale IQ > 110), while 48% earned scores that were in the below-average range (Full Scale IQ < 90), indicating a more negatively skewed distribution than would be expected.

The majority of children with epilepsy maintain the same level of IQ over the years, and cognitive ability is generally within average ranges or above in idiopathic epilepsies (Thierry, 1993). The IQ scores of children with symptomatic epilepsy are significantly lower than those of children with idiopathic epilepsy, and there is a greater percentage of IQ scores within the handicapped range. However, as symptomatic epilepsy is related to some specific causal agent, such as neurological damage, children in this group seem to be much more heterogeneous and their deficits could be explained by the damage itself, rather than by the resulting seizure activity. This pattern of lower performance for children with symptomatic epilepsy also seems to be reflected in academic achievement. It is important to note as well that performance levels in IQ can fluctuate significantly within an individual with epilepsy, simply due to state effects of medication or postictal events (Besag, 1995). Consequently, the results of a single assessment at one point in time could lead to an inaccurate estimate of the child's actual abilities (Cull, 1988). Because some children show marked deterioration while others show gradual decline, neurological status within the first year of life, prior to the first seizure, may be an important prognostic indicator of intellectual ability at 7 years of age, when used as a reference point (Cull, 1988).

Aldenkamp, Gutter, and Beun (1992) found that age at onset correlates well with intellectual level, a finding which confirms earlier studies suggesting that patients with a younger age at onset are more likely to have lower cognitive abilities (Dodrill, 1986; Farwell, Dodrill, & Batzel, 1985). Similarly, Czochanska, Langner-Tyszka, Eosiowski, and Schmidt-Sidor (1994) found that in children with epilepsy onset during the first year of life, including those with West syndrome, the degree and type of existing central nervous system damage are decisive in determining outcome. Since children with an earlier onset of epilepsy are more likely to have a more severe form and a greater degree of damage, this finding makes a great deal of sense. Children with a greater degree of damage or pathology will naturally have a poorer predicted outcome. However, age at onset may be a better descriptor of number of years with seizures. Aldenkamp et al. (1992) found that number of seizures during lifetime is a concomitant factor, and Czochanska et al. (1994) found that cessation of seizures may also have some influence on improving developmental outcome. These findings support a relationship between impaired IQ and seizure activity. However, they may also be interpreted as support for the hypothesis that excessive seizure activity can actually cause or be related to some neurological damage, which in turn can be seen as subtle deficits in overall performance.

In addition to deficits in general intellectual abilities, there is also evidence of impairments in more specific cognitive functions. Given the evidence for nonspecific difficulties such as poor memory, lower IQ scores, behavior problems, and academic delays, and the contradictory nature of the evidence regarding the impact of seizure type, seizure severity, duration of the disorder, and the effects of medication on these phenomena, Mitchell, Zhou, Chavez, and Gutman (1992) investigated whether children with seizures differ from normal children on specific cognitive abilities and processes. They addressed reaction time, attention, and impulsivity, and examined the relation of these processes, if any, to general cognitive delays, seizure variables, and AED therapy. Mitchell et al. (1992) found that despite normal intelligence, children with epilepsy performed significantly worse than normal children in reaction time and attention, but not on measures of impulsivity. Patients who were considered cognitively impaired (IQ between 65 and 90) evidenced even greater slowing on reaction time measures, which is a confounding factor. The severity and duration of seizure disorder had little impact on performance; however, the sample size was too small to examine possible differences among seizure types. Mitchell et al. concluded that slowed reaction times and inattention were not primarily the result of seizures or treatment, but resulted from similar or coexisting neurological abnormality. Their findings also indicate that slowed reaction times do not necessarily reflect cognitive impairment, but may contribute to relatively lower performance scores on timed tasks on commonly administered IQ tests (Mitchell et al., 1992). This study is one of the few to address the issue of slowed reaction time, which may be due to various causes, including AED therapy, in measuring cognitive ability.

On tests of visual–motor coordination, normal control groups made significantly fewer errors than children with epilepsy (Cull, 1988) and performed more quickly than those with idiopathic epilepsy. Poor performances were reported on tests of psychomotor function, even in the presence of average cognitive abilities. Parents in this study reported attention and coordination problems more frequently in children who are underachieveing in reading, spelling, and general knowledge. Moreover, parents of patients who were found to be underachieving in reading reported more overactivity in their children, and parents of patients who were found to be underachieving in spelling reported more attention and activity problems in their children (Mitchell et al., 1991). However, these data parallel the general findings regarding comorbidity of learning disabilities and attention-deficit/hyperactivity disorder quite well, and it is not clear that these findings are specific to children with epilepsy.

ELECTROENCEPHALOGRAPHY

EEG measurement of epileptic activity in the brain is likely the most widely used assessment technique in seizure disorders. However, epileptic discharges are variable events and are subject to many internal and external influences. A "normal" EEG does not exclude the diagnosis of epilepsy since the child may not be having a seizure at that particular time, nor do epileptic discharges on EEG necessarily prove epilepsy because they may be clinically observed in otherwise healthy young children (Thierry, 1993). Although not necessary for the diagnosis of epilepsy, EEG often assists in the classification of the seizure or the syndrome. In particular, EEG has been shown to be especially useful in differentially diagnosing neonatal epileptic seizures from other spasms, which present as clinically quite similar (Clancy, 1996). Correct classification is necessary in order to choose the correct treatment options, which has a vital influence on the child's educational development (Henrikson, 1990).

In addition to diagnosing the type of seizure, EEG is also useful in quantifying the waveform and amplitude of the electrical discharge and in roughly locating the focus of epileptic activity. Most children with epilepsy have interictal (between seizures) discharges in the EEG. However, these discharges are highly variable within a given child, and the consequences of the same epileptiform discharges vary from patient to patient (Henrikson, 1990). Further, the normal variations in EEG patterns that are seen as a result of the child's own physical and neurological development must be taken into account when evaluating the EEG results (Mizrahi, 1996). The frequency of both manifest seizures and interictal discharges are also influenced by environmental factors, stress, time of day, wakefulness, psychological testing, and school activities. In addition, there has long been evidence that subclinical electrical paroxysms, which are not always picked up on EEG measurements, can impair ongoing performance (Davidhoff & Johnson, 1964; Hutt, 1972). The Holmfrid study (Aldenkamp et al., 1993) found that of children who were seizure free for 1 year and were subsequently withdrawn from medication, a subgroup of children with a former diagnosis of absence seizures showed poorer performance on several cognitive tasks after withdrawal of AED, which these authors attributed to an increase in subclinical wave activity. Research has shown that the relationship between ictal EEG discharges and cognitive impairment is dependent on the type of discharge, the type of cognitive task, and possibly the duration of performance (Aarts, Binnie, Smit, & Wilkins, 1984; Mirsky & Van Buren, 1965).

EFFECTS OF ANTIEPILEPTIC DRUGS ON COGNITIVE FUNCTIONS

While many of the cognitive and behavioral effects of seizure disorders are attributable to the disorder itself, a significant number of behavioral and cognitive changes can result from the use of antiepileptic medications, particularly when more than one AED is used at a time. Much of the past research on the effects of AED use on children's cognitive and academic performance has been flawed by poor experimental design and no control for polypharmacy (Penry, 1986). However, some current studies have more carefully examined the psychological effects of AEDs when used alone in controlling seizures.

AEDs do not differ greatly with respect to efficacy in a general sense, but different AEDs have been found to be more effective in controlling different types of seizures, making appropriate classification of seizure type the most important variable in predicting AED efficacy. For example, carbamazepine (CBZ) has been found to be most effective with simple and complex partial seizures, whereas valproic acid or ethosuxamide is used primarily with absence seizures, and gabapentin can provoke absence seizures in children whose seizures are not of the absence type (Zupanc, 1996). The relative efficacy of AED with respect to seizure control is determined primarily by seizure type, and complete seizure control varies between approximately 10% and 90% (Bourgeois, 1992).

AEDs also produce different types and degrees of toxicity and side effects on cognitive functioning (Bourgeois, 1992). Toxic effects of AEDs can be divided into two types, with 95% of them being relatively infrequent and benign, and usually related to either the dosage or the combination of AEDs, and the remaining 5% being potentially severe or irreversible, and generally consisting of "mental and behavioral changes, impaired coordination and balance, gastrointestinal disturbance, and skin changes" (Bourgeois, 1992, p. 25). Cognitive impairment may go unnoticed, particularly in young children who are less aware and possibly less concerned about their performance than adolescents and adults and for whom parents and teachers may lower expectations when they become aware of a diagnosis of epilepsy (Bourgeois, 1992). Table 11.1 summarizes the indications and side effects for use of the most common AEDs and for those that have been introduced more recently.

Carbamazepine

Carbamazepine, or Tegretol, is most commonly indicated as a first-line agent for use with simple and complex partial seizures in children (Penry, 1986). The side effects are usually most pronounced early in treatment and at high levels of the drug, and may include ataxia, allergic rash, impaired motor coordination, and nausea, as well as an overall calming effect, which makes it popular for use with children who may have comorbid attention-deficit/hyperactivity disorder. At extremely high levels of dosage, or when combined with other AEDs, severe impairment of cognitive function has been noted (Zupanc, 1996). A study by Trimble (1990) noted that CBZ appears to improve hand–eye coordination and manual dexterity in a dose-dependent way, and increases speed of performance on certain tasks. Additionally, more rapid memory scanning was found at lower drug levels, but the error rate

TABLE 11.1. Common Side Effects and Indications for AEDs Most Often Used in Children

Generic name	Brand name	Indications	Side effects
Carbamazepine	Tegretol	Simple and complex partial seizures	Ataxia, impaired motor coordination, nausea; overall calming effect; allergic rash; fewer effects on cognition than other AEDs
Phenobarbital	Phenobarbital	Simple and complex partial seizures; generalized tonic–clonic seizures; all types of seizures in neonates	General sedative; slowed processing and reaction time; hyperactivity
Valproic acid	Depakote	Combination of absence and tonic–clonic or myoclonic seizures; tonic–clonic or myoclonic seizures alone; complex partial seizures	Liver toxicity at high levels; nausea; weight gain; similar to carbamazepine (fewer cognitive side effects than other AEDs)
Phenytoin	Dilantin	Partial and generalized seizures	Physical dysmorphic side effects such as coarsening of facial features, increase in facial hair, gingival hyperplasia; higher incidence of mental retardation
Ethosuxamide	Zarontin	Absence seizures	Lack of research documenting side effects
Felbamate	Felbatol	Lennox–Gastaut syndrome or medically refractory seizures only	Aplastic anemia, liver failure; insomnia; anorexia; vomiting; headache; somnolence
Lamotrigine	Lamictal	Age 16 years and older with partial seizures	Allergic rash; headaches; somnolence; vomiting
Gabapentin	Neurontin	Partial seizures with and without secondary generalization in age 12 years and older; not for use with absence seizures	Minimal cognitive side effects; dizziness, fatigue, headache, somnolence; irritability, agitation
Vigabatrin	Sabril	Infantile spasms; Lennox–Gastaut syndrome	Lack of research; possible hyperactivity

increased with an increased dosage. CBZ appears to have fewer effects on cognitive function than do other AEDs, but the side effects worsen with polypharmacy or dosage above therapeutic levels. One study by Coenen, Konings, Aldenkamp, Renier, and van Luijtelaar (1995) compared CBZ with valproic acid (VPA) on cognitive processes, and found that while CBZ users demonstrated better motor performance, VPA users showed better attention and memory performance than CBZ users. Both AEDs showed much milder side effects than either phenytoin or phenobarbital.

Forsythe, Butler, Berg, and McGuire (1991), in a well-controlled study, compared the effects of carbamazepine (CBZ), phenytoin (PHY), and valproic acid (VPA) on cognitive functioning in 64 children newly diagnosed with tonic–clonic, complex partial, or partial seizures with secondary generalization. The assessment battery included tests of visual memory (immediate and delayed), auditory memory (digits forward and backward), visual scanning (vigilance), Stroop Test (concentration), and speed of information processing. Although the three AEDs proved to be equally effective with respect to seizure control, in general, CBZ had the most side effects, whereas VPA had the fewest. The sum of the five memory tests was found to be the most sensitive measure of the effects of medication. Impaired recent recall on CBZ was apparent at 6 months of treatment and was more pronounced at 1 year. Speed of information processing was impaired after only 1 month with both CBZ and PHY.

Phenobarbital

Phenobarbital is an AED that has been primarily used with children presenting with simple and complex partial seizures, as well as generalized tonic–clonic seizures (Penry, 1986). Common side effects are primarily sedating in nature, and it tends to lower concentration and motor speed. Other effects noted have included slower reaction time, decreased memory, cognitive dysfunction, paradoxical hyperactivity, aggression, and sleep disturbances. In one study by Holmes (1987), phenobarbital adversely affected attention span, short-term memory, and performance on WISC-R Full Scale IQ and Vocabulary, Block Design, and Picture Completion subtests. However, these side effects seemed to be reversible, as improvements were noted on cognitive, perceptual, and memory assessments after the withdrawal of barbiturates. Vining et al. (1987) compared phenobarbital and VPA use in children and found that children taking phenobarbital performed worse on neuropsychological measures, and also received more severe parental behavior ratings of hyperactivity. Despite the abundance of negative side effects, however, phenobarbital remains the AED of choice for treating all types of seizures in neonates (Zupanc, 1996).

Valproic Acid (Sodium Valproate)

Valproic acid (VPA), or Depakote, has been traditionally used with children presenting with a combination of absence and tonic–clonic or myoclonic seizures, or with tonic–clonic or myoclonic seizures alone, and is considered the best choice for treating myoclonic seizures. Although some early studies reported that it made children "bright and lively," higher doses may impair performance on cognitive tasks (Trimble, 1990). Physical side effects may include liver toxicity at high dosage levels, ataxia and impaired motor coordination, and nausea and weight gain. Like CBZ, VPA tends to have fewer physical and cognitive side effects than drugs such as phenytoin and phenobarbital, but at higher doses and when used in combination with other AEDs, side effects are more common and more intense (Holmes, 1987).

Phenytoin

Phenytoin (PHY), or Dilantin, has been shown to be effective in treating both partial and generalized seizures, but it tends to have many more physical and cognitive side effects than other, equally effective AEDs such as CBZ and VPA. Common physical side effects include a coarsening of facial features and an increase in facial hair, which make it an unpopular choice for either young adults or women (Zupanc, 1996). It may also produce gingival hyperplasia. Cognitive side effects can include progressive encephalopathy and mental retardation (in relation to toxic doxage) (Trimble, 1990), and most studies have concluded that these effects are more common and intense than those of other AEDs, such as VPA and CBZ (Coenen et al., 1995; Holmes, 1987; Penry, 1986; Trimble, 1990).

Ethosuxamide

Ethosuxamide, or Zarontin, is most often prescribed for treating absence seizures that present without accompanying tonic–clonic or myoclonic seizures (Penry, 1986). Research has been limited regarding its side effects, and the results have been conflicting, with some studies noting improvement in cognitive performance and others noting deterioration (Trimble, 1990). Physical side effects are the same as those of most other AEDs at high doses and can include nausea, vomiting, ataxia, and impaired motor coordination (Zupanc, 1996).

Felbamate

Felbamate, or Felbatol, is an AED that has only recently been reapproved by the Food and Drug Administration (FDA) for treatment of Lennox–Gastaut syndrome or medically refractory seizures only. It has been banned for use with all other epileptic conditions. Serious side effects including aplastic anemia and liver failure limit its use with children. Less serious side effects have included anorexia, vomiting, insomnia, headache, and somnolence, but these were all decreased when felbamate was used as monotherapy or was initiated gradually (Pellock, 1996).

Lamotrigine

Lamotrigine, or Lamictal, has been recently proven effective and safe for use with children age 16 or older, but it can be used with younger children if other AEDs are ineffective. Allergic rash, dizziness, headaches, ataxia, somnolence, and vomiting are the most common side effects (Zupanc, 1996).

Gabapentin

Gabapentin, or Neurontin, has been recently approved as adjunctive treatment of partial seizures with and without secondary generalization in children age 12 and older. Gabapentin is contraindicated in treating absence seizures, and can induce absence seizures in children who do not present with them. No drug interactions have been noted, and studies have shown that it is generally safe and well tolerated, with minimal cognitive side effects. Physical side effects can include dizziness, fatigue, headache, and somnolence in older patients, and agitation and irritability in children (Zupanc, 1996).

Investigational Antiepileptic Drugs

Recently, a number of new AEDs have been under investigation regarding their utility and safety in treating seizure disorders in children. Although these are rarely prescribed as first-line agents, their use has increased in the past few years. Vigabatrin, or Sabril, has been shown to be quite effective in the treatment of infantile spasms, particularly those associated with tuberous sclerosis, Lennox–Gastaut syndrome, or other intractable, localization-related epilepsies. This AED is currently being researched to determine its efficacy and undesirable effects of its use (Zupanc, 1996). The ketogenic diet has also reemerged in popularity in the past few years for treatment of intractable epilepsy, particularly in Lennox–Gastaut syndrome or intractable primary generalized seizures. In the 1920s, Haddow M. Keith of the Mayo Clinic noted that patients stopped seizing when they became ketotic. Based on this observation, Keith popularized the ketogenic diet for the treatment of intractable seizures, but this approach became much less popular with the advent of AED treatment.

The dosage of AEDs varies greatly in children, much more so than in adults. On a weight basis, children may require doses two to four times greater than adult doses, and their functioning may therefore be more impacted by side effects than that of adults. Due to the extreme diversity in the capacity to eliminate drugs in children, the relationship between AED dose and its action is not linearly related to weight in children, as it is in adults (Dodson, 1987). Further, the effects of polypharmacy are much more variable in children, as the kinetics of drug absorption are affected differently when a second or third drug is added. Relative drug clearance declines progressively until age 10–15, when adult values are achieved (Guelen, Van der Kleijn, & Woudstra, 1974). This diversity in drug response among children may necessitate an extended period of trials with different medications at varying doses in order to attain seizure control. In addition to monitoring blood levels, Henrikson (1990) recommends that using EEG plus video monitoring and computer testing, as well as using cognitive activities, be considered in determining therapeutic levels of AEDs.

In one review of recent trends in the treatment of childhood epilepsy, Bourgeois (1992) notes that the use of medication has become more judicious and more systematic. A shift has occurred in the general philosophy of epilepsy treatment from emphasis on strict seizure control toward a recognition of the importance of the overall quality of life for the patient, such that children with epilepsy are now treated with a smaller number of drugs, resulting in a concomitant reduction in sedative and cognitive side effects (Bourgeois, 1992). The majority of the cognitive and physical side effects historically associated with AED treatment have been due to polypharmacy and excessive dosages. Monotherapy seems to be quite effective in most patients, avoids undesirable drug interactions, and greatly improves patient compliance with the AED treatment regimen. Earlier studies have shown improvement in alertness and cognitive functioning following reductions in drug levels (Bennett, Dunlop, & Zirling, 1983; Theodore & Porter, 1983) or using monotherapy rather than polypharmacy. The efficacy of increased drug dose or polypharmacy must always be weighed against side effects, reduced epileptiform activity demonstrated, and adverse cognitive effects to be avoided (Henrikson, 1990). Overall, the most important variable in predicting the efficacy of any one AED is appropriate seizure classification in the first place, as most AEDs are indicated for specific types of seizures and not for others. It is also difficult to determine when seizures require treatment beyond pharmocological intervention, such as surgery, and this area has been debated in the literature (Camfield & Camfield, 1996).

Additionally, in uniquely difficult cases, or with specific syndromes (e.g., Rasmussen's syndrome), ablative surgery may be a reasonable course of action in enhancing seizure control. Neuropsychological evaluations must be conducted prior to and after surgery.

ASSESSMENT AND REMEDIATION

Many children with epilepsy do not fit neatly into general categories or syndromes. Therefore, each child must be evaluated individually (Henrikson, 1990). Assessment of these students is best accomplished by a multidisciplinary team that represents all areas of concern, including pediatricians, parents, teachers, psychologists, speech–language pathologists, and occupational and physical therapists. Neuropsychological evaluation is helpful in detecting subtle changes in alertness and cognition caused by medication and in identifying specific cognitive and/or perceptual deficits that may be obscured by behavioral disturbances (Black & Hynd, 1995). Specific functions assessed might include concentration, immediate memory and delayed recall (with verbal and visual–spatial material), verbal fluency, verbal comprehension (oral and written), visual–spatial perception, visual–motor integration, and planning and cognitive flexibility, in addition to academic performance in reading, math, spelling, and written expression. The goal of such an assessment would be to construct a diagnostic profile of well-developed capacities as well as weaknesses and functional deficits (Wehrli, 1987). Environmental demands should be adjusted to the child's abilities in order to optimize self-esteem, academic performance, and psychosocial functioning. Students with epilepsy could have any form of learning disorder (e. g., reading, arithmetic, written expression), and a variety of remedial measures may need to be considered (Henrikson, 1990).

Teachers, parents, and other caregivers need to be familiar with the specific features of the child's seizures (including auras or prodromes if they are known to occur), how to recognize and manage a seizure, the student's medication regimen and how it might affect school performance and behavior, and what restrictions on activity, if any, are necessary (Engel, 1989). The multidisciplinary team is also in an ideal position to educate teachers and classmates about epilepsy and to correct any negative misconceptions and prejudices. Teachers might also assist with socialization, encourage confidence and initiative, and provide opportunities for the child to earn the respect of peers (Engel, 1989).

CONCLUSION

The psychological consequences of epilepsy can include neuropsychological impairments, accompanying altered brain functions, the possibility of recurrent seizures, and the effects of prolonged treatment with one or more anticonvulsive medications. All may contribute to the development of cognitive-behavioral difficulties, although in most cases a causal link has not been identified due to the heterogeneous nature of the population. However, epilepsy is not synonymous with diminished intellectual capacity in children (Bolter, 1986). As a group, these children exhibit mild and nonspecific impairments, although the great amount of variability in the population as a whole makes it impossible to predict any individual's cognitive abilities simply by nature of the diagnosis. Measures of overall cognitive abilities, such as the Wechsler scales, provide little information regarding the specific nature of cognitive deficits or educational needs, and IQ tests do not reveal characteristic profiles of children with epilepsy. Assessment of academic achievement and psychosocial functioning, appropriate intervention, and, when necessary, attention to school placement are important aspects of the comprehensive treatment of children with epilepsy (Mitchell et al., 1991).

In general, the diagnosis of epilepsy is made based on behavioral symptoms and EEG findings. Although the IQ distribution is negatively skewed among patients with epilepsy, these children do exhibit the full range of intellectual ability, and lowered cognitive performance may result, in many cases, from slowed reaction time. The course of epilepsy is highly variable, initial seizure types may later evolve into other types of seizures, and it is important to follow these children throughout their academic careers, documenting any changes in symptoms and/or educational needs. Underlying pathology must be taken into account when predicting future function of a child with epilepsy, as the seizures can be as much a symptom as an etiology of problems. Finally, response to medication in children is different from that in adults, and school personnel should work closely with medical providers regarding management of a child's seizure activity and possible side effects of AEDs. Finally, to facilitate the most positive outcome for children with epilepsy, it is absolutely essential that the diagnosis be accurate and that compliance with medication regimens be monitored carefully.

REFERENCES

Aarts, J. H. P., Binnie, C. D., Smit, A. M., & Wilkins, A. J. (1984). Selective cognitive impairment during focal and generalized epileptiform EEG activity. *Brain, 107*, 293–308.

Aldenkamp, A. P., Alpherts, W. P. C., Blenow, G., Elmqvist, D., Heifbel, J., Nilsson, H. L., Sandstedt, P., Tonnby, B., Wahlander, L., & Wosse, E. (1993). Withdrawal of antiepileptic medication in children: Effects on cognitive function. The multicenter Holmfrid study. *Neurology, 43*, 41–50.

Aldenkamp, A. P., Gutter, T., & Beun, A. M. (1992). The effect of seizure activity and paroxysmal electroencephalographic discharges on cognition. *Acta Neurologica, 86*(Suppl. 140), 111–121.

Annegers, J. F., Hauser, W. A., & Shirts, S. B. (1987). Factors prognostic of unprovoked seizures after febrile convulsions. *New England Journal of Medicine, 316*, 493–498.

Bagley, C. (1970). The educational performance of children with epilepsy. *British Journal of Educational Psychology, 40*, 82–83.

Bennett, H. S., Dunlop, T., & Zirling, P. (1983). Reduction of polypharmacy for epilepsy in an institution for the retarded. *Developmental Medicine and Child Neurology, 25*, 735–737.

Bennet-Levy, J., & Stores, G. (1984). The nature of cognitive dysfunction in school-children with epilepsy. *Acta Neurologica Scandinavica, 69*(Suppl. 99), 79–82.

Besag, F. M. C. (1995). Epilepsy, learning, and behavior in childhood. *Epilepsia, 36*(Suppl. 1), S58–S63.

Black, K. C., & Hynd, G. W. (1995). Epilepsy in the school aged child: Cognitive-behavioral characteristics and effects on academic performance. *School Psychology Quarterly, 10*(4), 345–358.

Blom, S., Heijbel, J., & Bergfors, P. G. (1978). Incidence of epilepsy in children. *Epilepsia, 19*, 343–350.

Bolter, J. F. (1986). Epilepsy in children: Neuropsychological effects. In J. B. Obrzut & G. W. Hynd (Eds.), *Child neuropsychology: Vol. 2. Clinical practice* (pp. 59–81). New York: Academic Press.

Bourgeois, B. F. D. (1992). Childhood epilepsy: Pharmacological considerations. *Acta Neurologica Scandinavica, 86*(Suppl. 140), 23–27.

Camfield, P. R., & Camfield, C. S. (1996). Antiepileptic drug therapy: When is epilepsy truly intractable? *Epilepsia, 37*(Suppl. 1), S60–S65.

Chaudhry, H. R., Najam, N., De Mahieu, C., Raza, A., & Ahmad, N. (1992). Clinical use of Piracetam in epileptic patients. *Current Therapeutic Research, 52*(3), 355–360.

Clancy, R. R. (1996). The contribution of EEG to the understanding of neonatal seizures. *Epilepsia, 37*(Suppl. 1), S52–S59.

Coenen, A. M. L., Konings, G. M. L. G., Aldenkamp, A. P., Renier, W. O., & van Luijtelaar, E. L. J. M. (1995). Effects of chronic use of carbamazepine and valproate on cognitive processes. *Journal of Epilepsy, 8*, 250–254.

Commission on Classification and Terminology of the International League Against Epilepsy (1989). Proposal for revised classification of epilepsies and epileptic syndromes. *Epilepsia, 30*, 389–399.

Cull, C. A. (1988). Cognitive function and behavior in children. In M. R. Trimble & E. H. Reynolds (Eds.)., *Epilepsy, behavior and cognitive function* (pp. 97–111). New York: Wiley.

Czochanska, J., Langner-Tyszka, B., Eosiowski, Z., & Schmidt-Sidor, D. (1994). Children who develop epilepsy in the first year of life: A prospective study. *Developmental Medicine and Child Neurology, 36*, 344–350.

Dam, M. (1990). Children with epilepsy: The effect of seizures, syndromes, and etiological factors on cognitive functioning. *Epilepsia, 31*(Suppl. 4), S26–S29.

Davidhoff, R. A., & Johnson, L. C. (1964). Paroxysmal EEG activity and cognitive motor performance. *Electroencephalography and Clinical Neurophysiology, 16*, 343–354.

Dodrill, C. B. (1986). Correlates of generalized tonic–clonic seizures with intellectual, neuropsychological, emotional, and social function in patients with epilepsy. *Epilepsia, 27*, 399–411.

Dodson, W. E. (1987). Special pharmacokinetic considerations in children. *Epilepsia, 28*(Suppl. 1), S56–S70.

Donat, J. F. (1992). The age-dependent epileptic encephalopathies. *Journal of Child Neurology, 7*, 7–21.

Duchowny, M., & Harvey, A. S. (1996). Pediatric epilepsy syndromes: An update and critical review. *Epilepsia, 37*(Suppl. 1), S26–S40.

Dulac, O. (1995). Epileptic syndromes in infancy and childhood: Recent advances. *Epilepsia, 36*(Suppl. 1), S51–S57.

Engel, J., Jr. (1989). *Seizures and epilepsy.* Philadelphia: Davis.

Farwell, J. R., Dodrill, C. B., & Batzel, L. W. (1985). Neuropsychological abilities of children with epilepsy. *Epilepsia, 26*(5), 395–400.

Forsythe, I., Butler, R., Berg, I., & McGuire, R. (1991). Cognitive impairment in new cases of epilepsy randomly assigned to carbamazepine, phenytoin, and sodium valproate. *Developmental Medicine and Child Neurology, 33*, 525–534.

Glaser, G. H. (1979). The epilepsies. In P. Beeson, W. McDermott, & J. B. Wyngaarden (Eds.), *Cecil textbook of medicine* (pp. 851–862). Philadelphia: Saunders.

Gourley, R. (1990). Educational policies. *Epilepsia, 31*(Suppl. 4), S59–S60.

Green, J. B., & Hartlage, L. C. (1971). Comparative performance of epileptic and nonepileptic children and adolescents. *Diseases of the Nervous System, 32*, 418–421.

Guelen, P. J. M., Van der Kleijn, E., & Woudstra, U. (1974). Statistical analysis of pharmacokinetic parameters in epileptic patients chronically treated with antiepileptic drugs. In J. Shneider, D. Janz, C. Gardner-Thorpe, H. Meinardi, & A. L. Sherwin (Eds.), *Clinical pharmacology of anti-epileptic drugs* (pp. 2–10). New York: Springer-Verlag.

Hauser, W. A. (1994). The prevalence and incidence of convulsive disorders in children. *Epilepsia, 35*(Suppl. 2), S1–S6.

Hauser, W. A., & Nelson, K. B. (1989). Epidemiology of epilepsy in children. *Cleveland Clinic Journal of Medicine, 56*(Suppl., Part 2), S185–S194.

Henrikson, O. (1990). Education and epilepsy: Assessment and remediation. *Epilepsia, 31*(Suppl. 4), S21–S25.

Holdsworth, L., & Whitmore, K. (1974). A study of children with epilepsy attending ordinary schools: I. Their seizure patterns, prognosis, and behavior in school. *Developmental Medicine and Child Neurology, 16*, 746–758.

Holmes, G. L. (1987). *Diagnosis and management of seizures in children.* Philadelphia: Saunders.

Hutt, S. J. (1972). Experimental analysis of brain activity and behavior in children with "minor" seizures. *Epilepsia, 13*, 520–534.

Hynd, G. W., & Willis, W. G. (1988). *Pediatric neuropsychology.* Boston: Allyn & Bacon.

Lombroso, C. T. (1996). Neonatal seizures: A clinician's overview. *Brain and Development, 18*, 1–28.

Mahapatra, S. (1990). Reading behavior in children with epilepsy. *Psychological Studies, 35*(3), 170–178.

Mirsky, A. F., & Van Buren, J. M. (1965). On the nature of the absence in centrocephalic epilepsy: A study of some behavioral, electroencephalographic and autonomic factors. *Electroencephalography and Clinical Neurophysiology, 18*, 334–338.

Mitchell, W. G., Chavez, J. M., Lee, H., & Guzman, B. L. (1991). Academic underachievement in children with epilepsy. *Journal of Child Neurology, 6*, 65–72.

Mitchell, W. G., Zhou, Y., Chavez, J. M., & Guzman, B. L. (1992). Reaction time, attention, and impulsivity in epilepsy. *Pediatric Neurology, 8*(1), 19–24.

Mizrahi, E. M. (1996). Avoiding the pitfalls of EEG interpretation in childhood epilepsy. *Epilepsia, 37*(Suppl. 1), S41–S51.

Monetti, V. C., Graneiri, E., Casetta, I., Tola, M. R., Paolino, E., Malagu, S., Govoni,

V., & Quatrale, R. (1995). Risk factors for idiopathis generalized seizures: A population-based case control study in Copparo, Italy. *Epilepsia, 36*(3), 224–229.

Mosewich, R. K., & So, E. L. (1996). A clinical approach to the classification of seizures and epileptic syndromes. *Mayo Clinic Proceedings, 71,* 405–414.

Murphy, J. V., & Dehkharghani, F. (1994). Diagnosis of childhood seizure disorders. *Epilepsia, 35*(Suppl. 2), S7–S17.

Nelson, K. B., & Ellenberg, J. H. (1984) Obstetric complications as risk factors for cerebral palsy or seizure disorders. *Journal of the American Medical Association, 251,* 1843–1848.

Pellock, J. M. (1989). Syndromes of chronic epilepsy in children. In M. R. Trimble (Ed.), *Chronic epilepsy, its prognosis and management* (pp. 73–85). New York: Wiley.

Pellock, J. M. (1996). Utilization of new antiepileptic drugs in children. *Epilepsia, 37*(Suppl. 1), S66–S73.

Penry, J. K. (1986). *Epilepsy: Diagnosis, management, quality of life.* New York: Raven Press.

Rutter, M., Tizard, J., & Whitmore, K. (1970). *Education health and behavior.* London: Longman.

Sachs, H., & Barrett, R. P. (1995). Seizure disorders: A review for school psychologists. *School Psychology Review, 24*(2), 131–145.

Stedman, J., Van Heyningen, R., & Lindsey, J. (1982). Educational underachievement and epilepsy. A study of children from normal schools admitted to a special hospital for epilepsy. *Early Childhood Development Care, 9,* 65–82.

Stores, G., & Hart, J. (1976). Reading skills of children with generalized or focal epilepsy attending ordinary schools. *Developmental Medicine and Child Neurology, 18,* 705–716.

Talwar, D., Baldwin, M. A., Hutzler, R., & Griesemer, D. A. (1995). Epileptic spasms in older children: Persistence beyond infancy. *Epilepsia, 36*(2), 151–155.

Theodore, W. H., & Porter, R. J. (1983). Removal of sedative–hypnotic antiepileptic drugs from the regimen of patients with intractable epilepsy. *Annals of Neurology, 13,* 320–324.

Thierry, D. (1993). Annotation: Cognitive and behavioral correlates of epileptic activity in children. *Journal of Child Psychology and Psychiatry, 34*(5), 611–620.

Trimble, M. R. (1990). Antiepileptic drugs, cognitive function, and behavior in children: Evidence from recent studies. *Epilepsia, 31*(Suppl. 4), S30–S34.

Vassella, F. (1994). Seizure types and epileptic syndromes. *European Neurology, 34*(Suppl. 1), 3–12.

Vining, E. P. G., Mellits, E. D., Dorsen, M. M., Cataldo, M. F., Quaskey, S. A., Spielberg, S. P., & Freeman, J. M. (1987). Psychologic and behavioral effects of antiepileptic drugs in children: A double-blind comparison between phenobarbital and valproic acid. *Pediatrics, 80*(2), 165–174.

Wechsler, D. (1981). *Manual for the Wechsler Adult Intelligence Scale—Revised (WAIS-R).* New York: Psychological Corporation.

Wechsler, D. (1991). *Wechsler Intelligence Scale for Children—Third Edition: Manual.* New York: Psychological Corporation.

Wehrli, A. (1987). Function deficits and remediating techniques. In A. P. Aldenkamp, W. C. J. Alpherts, H. Meinardi, & G. Stores (Eds.), *Education and epilepsy* (pp. 110–117). Amsterdam: Swets & Zeitlinger.

Wyllie, E. (1994). Children with seizures: When can treatment be deferred? *Journal of Child Neurology, 9*(Suppl. 2), 2S8–2S13.

Zupanc, M. L. (1996). Update on epilepsy in pediatric patients. *Mayo Clinic Proceedings, 71,* 899–916.

CHAPTER TWELVE

Traumatic Brain Injury

LINDA EWING-COBBS
DOUGLAS R. BLOOM

Pediatric traumatic brain injury (TBI) represents a major public health problem and contributes to the spectrum of disability that occurs in relation to acquired brain injury. In this chapter, we will briefly highlight major epidemiological and neuropathological findings as they bear on outcome studies. Chronic neuropsychological, academic, and psychosocial sequelae of TBI will be discussed, with emphasis on newer areas of research, including injury in young children, language and discourse studies, and executive functions.

EPIDEMIOLOGY OF TRAUMATIC BRAIN INJURY

Epidemiological studies identified a fatality rate of 10 per 100,000 and a prevalence rate of 180–220 per 100,000 children (Annegers, Grabow, Kurland, & Laws, 1980; Kraus, 1995). The mortality rate is 5 times the mortality rate of childhood leukemia, which is the next leading cause of death in childhood (Klauber, Barrett-Connor, Marshall, & Bowers, 1981). Major causes of pediatric brain injury included falls (35%), recreational activities (29%), and motor vehicle accidents (24%) (Kraus, Fife, Cox, Ramstein, & Conroy, 1986). The quality of outcome after TBI varies with the severity of the initial injury, yielding outcomes ranging from death to persistent vegetative state to variable cognitive and physical sequelae. The severity of injury is most frequently based on the Glasgow Coma Scale score (GCS; Teasdale & Jennett, 1974), which ranges from 3 to 15 and evaluates three components of consciousness: eye opening, motor response, and verbal response. Scores from 3 to 8 reflect a severe injury producing coma, operationally defined as the absence of eye opening, inability to follow one-stage commands, and failure to utter recognizable words. Moderate TBI is defined by GCS scores from 9 to 12; mild TBI is defined by scores from 13 to 15, indicating that patients are alert, have spontaneous eye opening, and have verbal responses ranging from confused to oriented. The duration of coma and posttraumatic amnesia (confusion and failure to encode new information in ongoing memory) are also commonly used to estimate the severity of TBI and show strong relationships with long-term outcome measures. Although the majority of hospitalized pediatric TBI cases involve mild injuries, approximately 7% are moderate and 5% are severe (Kraus et al., 1986). Although few injuries are categorized as severe, children surviving severe TBI commonly have significant chronic cognitive, motor, and psychosocial sequelae that complicate adaptation at home, at school, and in the community. The remainder of this chapter will discuss neuropsychological, academic, and psychosocial consequences of TBI.

NEUROPATHOLOGICAL AND NEUROIMAGING FINDINGS

Neuroimaging and neuropathology studies have clarified the mechanisms of injury and frequent abnormalities. Most severe TBI cases involve a combination of diffuse and focal injury. Neuropathological studies identified diffuse cerebral injury occurring at the time of impact as the primary cause of brain injury in patients with closed head injury (Adams, Mitchell, Graham, & Doyle, 1977; Strich, 1956). Subsequent degeneration of white matter, particularly in the corpus callosum, parasagital areas of the cerebral hemispheres, the internal capsule, and the pons, was a common finding (Strich, 1970). Secondary brain injury occurs as a consequence of cerebral edema, increased intracranial pressure, hypoxia, and pressure effects from expanding mass lesions (Levin, Benton, & Grossman, 1982). Severe TBI initiates release of a cascade of excitotoxic neurotransmitters that can cause additional widespread neuronal injury (Hayes & Dixon, 1994). Magnetic resonance imaging (MRI) scans visualized frequent mass lesions in children and adolescents with moderate to severe TBI. Mendelsohn and colleagues (1992) identified hemispheric lesions in 71% of a series of pediatric patients consecutively admitted to an acute pediatric trauma unit. In a subsequent study, Levin and colleagues (1993) reported focal areas of abnormal signal intensity in 75% of the sample; lesions occurred most frequently in the dorsolateral frontal, orbito-frontal, and frontal lobe white matter.

NEUROPSYCHOLOGICAL OUTCOMES
Intelligence

Prospective longitudinal studies of intellectual recovery after severe TBI in children ages 5–15 at the time of injury typically report initial reduction in both Verbal and Performance IQ scores in comparison to children with orthopedic injuries or matched controls when evaluated 1–3 months after the injury; by 6 months to 1 year, the Performance IQ score remains impaired relative to the Verbal IQ score and a relatively stable pattern of intellectual functioning is obtained (Chadwick, Rutter, Brown, Shaffer, & Traub, 1981; Jaffe et al., 1992). By 1 year after TBI, the mean IQ scores for mild, moderate, and severe TBI groups were in the average range (Chadwick, Rutter, Brown, Shaffer, & Traub, 1981; Jaffe et al., 1993). Jaffe and colleagues (1993) estimated respective mean losses of 2, 9, and 13 Full Scale IQ points 1 year after mild, moderate, and severe TBI.

All studies of intellectual recovery from TBI in school-age children and adolescents are based on the Wechsler scales. The frequent finding of lower Performance IQ than Verbal IQ scores following severe TBI may be a function of the subtest format of the Verbal and Performance scales. While the Verbal scale largely evaluates previously learned information such as vocabulary, fund of knowledge, and social reasoning, the Performance IQ scale contains 5 timed subtests requiring problem solving with novel materials, with bonus points for rapid responses. Therefore, when lower Performance IQ than Verbal IQ scores are obtained, additional evaluation is needed to determine whether performance deficits are based on task demands for visual–spatial analysis, planning and problem solving, attention, motor skills, and/or motor speed.

Using cluster analytic techniques, Donders (1993) identified four distinct profiles of Wechsler Intelligence Scale for Children—Revised (WISC-R) subtest scores obtained within 12 months of TBI in children and adolescents with loss of consciousness. The four clusters contained (1) subtest scores uniformly in the average range, (2) relatively better Verbal than Performance scores, (3) globally depressed scores, and (4) reduced efficiency on several Verbal subtests and the Coding subtest. Given the heterogeneity of scores, Donders (1993) inferred that it is important to use additional measures to assess sequelae of TBI. Moreover, there is great variability in intellectual outcome, with strong interrelationships between indices of preinjury IQ, socioeconomic status, family functioning, and injury severity.

Visual–Spatial, Motor, and Somatosensory Outcomes

Visual–spatial and visual motor areas have often been described as areas of specific vulnerability following severe TBI. Relative to patients with mild to moderate TBI or to orthopedic controls, patients with severe TBI show persisting deficits on measures of motor speed, manual dexterity, visual–motor integration, and complex visual–spatial problem solving (Bawden, Knights, & Winogron, 1985; Chadwick, Rutter, Shaffer, & Shrout,1981; Jaffe et al., 1993; Winogron, Knights, & Bawden, 1984). Speeded motor performance is particularly affected after severe TBI. Bawden et al. (1985) divided the tests from the Halstead–Reitan Neuropsychological Test Battery into those requiring high speed, moderate speed, and low to no speed. Children with severe TBI did not sustain global deficits in motor or visual–spatial areas. Although they had disproportionate deficits on tasks with high requirements for motor speed, such as finger and foot tapping tasks, pegboards, and the WISC-R Coding subtest, they were not deficient on tasks with low requirements for motor speed, such as motor strength, motor control, or visual–spatial abilities.

Using analysis of individual growth curves, Thompson et al. (1994) assessed change in motor, visual–spatial, and somatosensory skills in children ages 6–15 who sustained TBI of varying severity. Over a 1-year recovery period, slower rates of change were obtained for younger than for older children on measures of visual–motor integration, timed pegboard, and a timed tactile recognition task. Younger children who sustained severe TBI had slower recovery rates than young children with less severe TBI. Recovery curves were similar in older patients regardless of injury severity.

Persistent neurological deficits were noted by Massagli et al. (1996), who identified normal neurological evaluations in only 2 of 25 children 1 year following severe TBI. Neurological deficits were typically mild; the most frequent abnormalities were aphasia, dysdiadochokinesia (difficulty alternately flexing and extending a limb) and other coordination problems, and agraphesthesia. The pattern of neurological findings varied across children; most abnormalities occurred in only one child.

Attention and Memory

Intact attention and memory are essential for successful completion of both cognitive and socially based tasks. Attention and memory deficits occur frequently after pediatric TBI. As attention is a multidimensional construct, studies of attentional outcome after pediatric TBI have yielded inconsistent findings depending on the dimension of attention evaluated, differences in measures employed, interval between the injury and assessment, and the characteristics of the samples. Although attentional deficits are common during the early stages of recovery from TBI (Chadwick, Rutter, Shaffer, & Shrout, 1981; Jaffe et al., 1992), some investigators have not identified persisting injury severity group differences at least 1 year after the injury (Chadwick, Rutter, Shaffer, & Shrout, 1981; Kinsella et al., 1995; Perrott, Taylor, & Montes, 1991). Long-term follow-up studies ranging from 6 months to 8 years after TBI have noted persisting impairment on measures of psychomotor speed and accuracy, divided attention, focused attention, shifting attention, and sustained attention (Dennis, Wilkinson, Koski, & Humphries, 1995; Ewing-Cobbs, Prasad et al., 1998; Jaffe et al., 1993; Kaufmann, Fletcher, Levin, Miner, Ewing-Cobbs, 1993; Knights et al., 1991, Levin et al., 1993; Murray, Shum, & McFarland, 1992). In contrast, severity group differences are not consistently identified on attentional indices reflecting the encoding of verbal information, such as on the Wechsler (1974) Digit Span subtest or Freedom from Distractibility index (Donders, 1993; Kaufmann et al., 1993; Warschausky, Keuman, & Selim, 1996).

Memory is the most significant area of neuropsychological deficiency after pediatric TBI (Levin & Eisenberg, 1979). On verbal list learning tests, children with severe TBI consistently showed a significantly slower rate of learning and a reduction in the amount of information acquired over trials than children with lesser injuries (Jaffe et al., 1993; Kinsella et al., 1997; Levin et al., 1988, 1993; Yeates, Blumenstein, Patterson, & Delis, 1995). Patients with severe TBI did not consistently show differences in learning characteristics such as semantic clustering or consistency in recall over trials (Jaffe et al., 1993; Yeates et al., 1995). Anderson et al. (1997) identified impairments persisting for 1 year after severe TBI on a story recall task but not on a test of everyday memory. Visual memory has been studied infrequently. Levin and colleagues (1988, 1994) described impairment in visual recognition memory after severe TBI; patients had difficulty discriminating between newly presented and previously presented pictures. Anderson et al. (1997) described lower performance after severe TBI on a spatial tapping test but not on a spatial learning task.

Language and Discourse

Although children infrequently show persisting aphasia after severe TBI, they often have difficulties using language to communicate effectively. Language has been examined at the level of specific abilities and discourse. Studies of specific language skills conducted at least 1 year after TBI revealed that performance was lower in patients with severe TBI in comparison to patients with mild to moderate TBI on tests of general language functions as well as on several lexical and comprehension measures, including verbal fluency, object naming latency, confrontation naming, and auditory comprehension of grammatically complex sentences (Chadwick, Rutter, Shaffer, & Shrout, 1981; Jordan & Murdoch, 1990; Jordan, Ozanne, & Murdoch, 1988; Winogron et al., 1984).

Discourse refers to the communicative use of language in context (Dennis & Lovett, 1990). Discourse may be evaluated at the level of text microstructure or macrostructure (Kintsch & van Dijk, 1978). Microstructure encompasses information corresponding to individual words and sentences and their relationship to the text, while macrostructure refers to relationships between large units of text such as the theme or gist. As discourse tasks tap many other cognitive abilities, such as planning, sequencing, word retrieval, working memory, and goal regulation, they may provide sensitive indices of actual information-processing abilities.

Dennis and Barnes (1990) reported long-term discourse deficits characterized by difficulty interpreting ambiguous sentences and metaphors, drawing inferences, and developing sentences using specific parts of speech. Story retelling tasks disclosed few persisting deficits after TBI at the level of text microstructure but very significant deficits in macrostructure. Although children with severe TBI produced shorter narratives containing fewer words and sentences than children with lesser injuries, severity group differences were not apparent on measures of the length or syntactic complexity of sentences, speech fluency, or the rate of speech production (Chapman et al., 1992; Chapman, Levin, Wanek, Weyrauch, & Kufera, 1998; Ewing-Cobbs, Brookshire, Scott, & Fletcher, 1998). Variable findings have been reported regarding the use of cohesive devices that connect parts of the text. Cohesion occurs when the meaning of the text is related across sentences by the use of specific cohesive items such as personal and demonstrative pronouns and conjunctions. Although some investigators did not find differences in cohesion (Chapman et al., 1992; Jordan, Murdoch, & Buttsworth 1991), Ewing-Cobbs, Brookshire, et al. (1998) reported fewer correct uses of cohesive ties and more cohesive errors, indicating difficulty relating meaning across sentences. Text macrostructure is markedly affected by severe TBI. Narratives produced after severe TBI are characterized by a significant loss of information, difficulties correctly sequencing the narrative, and loss of story structure, yielding impoverished and disjointed content (Chapman et al., 1992, 1998; Ewing-Cobbs, Brookshire, et al., 1998).

Executive Functions

Executive functions refer to a group of related but separable higher-order cognitive abilities including planning, impulse control, working memory, mental-set maintenance, attentional control (Roberts & Pennington, 1996), metacognition, and development and implementation of strategies for problem solving (Pennington, 1994). The prefrontal lobes are generally regarded as the neuroanatomical basis for executive functions (Levin et al., 1996). As previously noted, recent neuroimaging research using MRI scans has shown the frontal lobes to be selectively vulnerable to focal brain lesion following moderate to severe TBI in children (Levin et al., 1993; Mendelsohn et al., 1992).

Some researchers have focused primarily on the relationship of neuropsychological outcome measures, including executive functions, with severity of TBI. For example, Jaffe and his associates (Jaffe et al., 1992, 1993; Jaffe, Polissar, Fay, & Liao, 1995) conducted a 3-year longitudinal study in which they evaluated a variety of cognitive abilities, including adaptive problem solving (i.e., logical reasoning, speed of information processing, cognitive flexibility). In general, Jaffe et al. (1995) found that relative to mildly injured children, severely injured children demonstrated significant deficiencies in adaptive problem solving skills at 3 months following injury, made significant recovery by 1 year postinjury, but showed plateauing of performance over the following 2 years. Even though moderately and severely injured children obtained adaptive problem-solving scores within normal limits by 3 years postinjury, their performance remained significantly below that of noninjured matched control children.

Dennis and colleagues (Dennis, Barnes, Donnelly, Wilkinson, & Humphreys, 1996) investigated metacognitive skills in a cross-sectional study involving knowledge appraisal and knowledge management with normal and TBI children at least 6 months following injury. The performance of TBI children was impaired on a knowledge appraisal task requiring that they analyze statements for semantic–pragmatic or grammatical anomalies and then attempt to repair the anomalous statements. Younger TBI children (less than 7 years) were deficient on a knowledge management task where they were to monitor the adequacy of two-step map directions that were either ambiguous or unambiguous. In general, poor performance by TBI children on the metacognitive tasks was associated with younger age at injury and at testing, lower GCS score, frontal lobe contusions with coma, bilateral brain contusions, and left-sided brain contusions.

Levin and colleagues reported findings from a longitudinal study that investigated the relationship of cognitive measures assessing executive functions with focal brain lesions resulting from TBI. Using a battery of frontal lobe measures, Levin et al. (1993) found significant relationships between performance on each of the cognitive measures, severity of injury, and age. In general, younger (6- to 10-year-olds) severely injured children demonstrated more consistent impairment than a group of older (11- to 16-year-olds) TBI children on measures evaluating concept formation–problem solving, semantic clustering on verbal memory responses, planning, verbal fluency, design fluency, and response inhibitory control. Severely injured older children and adolescents showed impairment relative to normal control children only on measures of concept formation–problem solving, verbal fluency, and design fluency. In addition, frontal lobe lesion size as measured by MRI improved prediction of cognitive test performance over and above that obtained through use of the GCS score alone. Left frontal lesion size significantly improved prediction of performance on measures of response efficiency (percentage of conceptual responses on the Wisconsin Card Sorting Test; Heaton, Chelune, Talley, Kay, & Curtiss, 1993) and response inhibition, and approached significance on verbal fluency. Volume of right frontal lesions significantly improved prediction of scores involving verbal fluency and percentage of semantically clustered responses on a measure of verbal learning and memory, and approached significance on a measure of response inhibition.

Levin et al. (1994) also studied the contribution of frontal lobe lesions to performance on the Tower of London task (TOL; Shallice, 1982). This task involves developing an overall problem-solving schema, generating and organizing subgoals into a sequence of moves, and monitoring performance by keeping the overall plan for sequencing moves in working memory to attain the goal of rearranging three colored beads on pegs using a specific number of moves (Levin et al., 1994). The relationship of injury severity to specific TOL variables was found more consistently in younger (age 6–10) than older (age 11–16) patients. Left and right frontal lobe lesion volume added to the prediction of number of rules broken in performing the TOL task beyond that of the interaction of injury severity and age. Size of orbital and white matter lesions also were determined to be related to the number of broken rules. Volume of dorsolateral lesions increased the ability to predict the number of problems solved on the first trial. In a subsequent cross-sectional study evaluating the utility of three measures of concept formation and problem solving, Levin et. al. (1997) confirmed the sensitivity of the TOL to level of injury severity, with greater impairment in younger than older children. Left frontal lesion volume improved prediction of TOL percentage of problems solved on the first trial and planning time prior to first response. Size of left nonfrontal lesions was sensitive to the number of broken rules.

In addition, the Wisconsin Card Sorting Test (Heaton et al., 1993) performance of TBI children was found to be sensitive to level of injury severity and age, and size of left and right prefrontal lesions and left nonfrontal lesions added to the prediction of card sorting variables beyond that obtained through use of GCS score and age. The Twenty Questions Test (TQT; Mosher & Hornsby, 1966) is a problem-solving task where feedback to questions can help to constrain alternatives and be used to generate hypotheses that help determine which picture the examiner has selected. TQT variables were found to be sensitive to injury severity and age. The prediction of TQT performance was not enhanced by the addition of lesion volume into regression equations beyond the level obtained using the GCS score, age, and their interaction.

Finally, Levin et al. (1996) investigated the factor structure of executive functions in TBI and typically developing children using a battery of tests of purported executive functions. A principal components analysis yielded a 5-factor solution accounting for 79% of the variance as follows: Conceptual-Productivity (Factor 1), Planning (Factor 2), Schema (Factor 3), Cluster (Factor 4), and Inhibition (Factor 5). The size of frontal lobe lesions significantly predicted factor scores for Planning, Schema, and Cluster. Left extrafrontal lesions size also predicted Planning and Schema factor scores. In general, the study by Dennis and the series of studies reported by Levin provide support for relationships between impaired performance on cognitive tasks assessing executive functions and the size and/or location of focal brain lesions. Additional research investigating the relationship of real-world activities such as academic performance and other aspects of adaptive functioning following TBI, with performance on tasks evaluating executive functions and neuroimaging findings, would be particularly useful in facilitating rehabilitation and remedial educational interventions for children who have sustained TBI.

Academic Performance

Academic success is clearly jeopardized when a child sustains a significant TBI. However, research involving academic outcomes following TBI and the nature and associations between postinjury academic performance and neuroanatomical, cognitive, developmental, and environmental variables has been quite limited. Several studies have demonstrated that moderate to severe TBI is associated with reduced academic performance and increased need for special education support services. Klonoff, Low, and Clark (1977) found that over one-fourth of children injured prior to the age of 9 had failed a grade or had received some type of remedial educational services within 5 years of injury. In addition, 21% of the children in the older group were enrolled in special classes in the same 5-year time frame. In a similar vein, Donders (1994) found that 48% of a sample of 6- to 16-year-old mild to severely injured children admitted to a rehabilitation hospital were receiving special education within 1 year of injury. Nearly one-quarter of these children received special education services for more than 50% of the school day. Kinsella and colleagues (1995) reported that 44% of their small sample of moderately and severely injured children and none of the mildly injured children were receiving some type of special educational services 1 year following injury. By 2 years postinjury, Kinsella et al. (1997) found that special educational assistance was required for 31% of their sample, including 7 of the 10 severely injured children. Even more striking were findings reported by Ewing-Cobbs, Iovino, Fletcher, Miner, and Levin (1991), who found that 80% of a sample of moderate to severe TBI children were receiving some type of modified educational program 2 years following injury. Over half of the children had failed a grade within the first year of injury, yet the majority of the children were not identified as eligible for special educational services until after the first postinjury year. In general, these findings clearly suggest that moderate to severe TBI often disrupts academic performance, and increases the probability of receiving special education services. Unfortunately, these services too often may be provided only after significant academic failure has occurred (Ewing-Cobbs et al., 1991).

Several researchers have investigated the effect of TBI on basic academic skills. Shaffer, Chadwick, and Rutter (1980) found that 33% of their sample of school-age TBI children were reading at least 2 years below expectations for age when evaluated approximately 2 years after sustaining a unilateral depressed compound fracture with dural tear and confirmed underlying brain injury. Over the course of a 3-year longitudinal study, Jaffe and associates (1992, 1993, 1995) demonstrated persistent academic deficits in reading recognition, spelling, and computational arithmetic skills in a sample of moderately and severely injured school-age children and adolescents relative to matched controls. In contrast, the achievement test performance of children with mild TBI showed only minor differences relative to their matched controls. Similarly, Asarnow et al. (1995) found no significant differences in performance between groups of mild TBI and non-TBI control children in school grades and school achievement test scores obtained in the immediate preinjury period and at 1 year following injury.

Ewing-Cobbs, Fletcher, and Levin (1995) found evidence of significant deficits in basic academic skills in over one-third of a sample of school-age youth who sustained TBI when evaluated 1 year following injury. These students showed deficits involving either computational arithmetic skills only or broader skill deficiencies involving reading recognition, spelling, and computational arithmetic. In contrast, Kinsella et al. (1995) failed to find significant differences between groups of children with TBI differing in injury severity level on an academic achievement test of basic skills within the first year following injury. However, educational difficulties were reflected in the fact that nearly half of the moderately and severely injured children were receiving special educational assistance at 1 year postinjury, despite no group differences on achievement testing, and 70% of the severely injured children were provided special education at 2 years postinjury. Kinsella et al. (1997) also identified neuropsychological variables assessed at 3 months postinjury that contributed to prediction of change from regular to special educational placement in addition to level of injury severity at 2 years following the injury. Significant predictors included verbal learning, memory, and verbal fluency performance, though only the verbal learning and memory performance significantly enhanced prediction of change in school placement above and beyond that of injury severity.

Recently, Barnes, Dennis, and Wilkinson (1999) demonstrated a significant relationship between age at which TBI was sustained and subsequent reading difficulties. Children injured in the preschool years prior to the onset of formal educational instruction in word decoding skills and children with bilateral or left hemisphere contusions were at greatest risk for later deficiencies in acquiring adequate basic word decoding and reading comprehension skills. Children injured in the primary grades, when decoding skills were being learned, were at particular risk for difficulties in reading comprehension compared with children whose injuries occurred later. Barnes et al. (1999) also found that children with TBI matched with control subjects on word decoding accuracy were significantly slower in word decoding speed (fluency) than matched controls, and that reduced decoding speed was associated with reduced reading comprehension.

The preceding research serves to illustrate several important points related to the impact of TBI on academic functioning. One involves the relatively common finding that academic achievement as assessed by means of standardized achievement tests may not adequately reflect difficulties that children with significant TBI may experience when returning to school (Ewing-Cobbs, Fletcher, & Levin, 1986; Kinsella et al., 1995). Because academic achievement tests tend to assess overlearned, relatively stable academic skills that are often less susceptible to the disruptive effects of TBI, academic test scores often do not adequately identify deficiencies found in actual classroom performance following moderate to severe TBI. Therefore, assessment should not rely solely on traditional tests of academic achievement or on models of special educational need that employ discrepancy models for determination of services, as are commonly employed for determination of developmental learning disorders. Rather, assessment should include careful observation of classroom performance, novel approaches to academic assessment that measure the application of previously or newly learned skills to educational problem solving, and evaluation of neuropsychological skills such as new learning and memory, linguistic variables, attention, and speed of mental processing and motor performance, which are frequently related to academic performance following injury. Additional research is needed to identify the correlates of academic failure following TBI, particularly those involving cognitive regulatory processes that are basic to academic learning and that are disrupted following TBI. Finally, it is hoped that the addition of traumatic brain injury as an educational disability category for special education in the Individuals with Disabilities Education Act (1990) will provide initiation of needed educational services for children with TBI as early as possible in the course of recovery from injury.

Behavioral, Psychosocial, Adaptive, and Family Functioning

There has been limited research investigating behavioral, psychosocial (Fletcher et al., 1996), and family–environmental factors on outcome (Taylor et al., 1995) following pediatric TBI. However, recent research has contributed substantially to increasing the knowledge base in these important areas.

In an important early prospective study, Brown et al. (Brown, Chadwick, Shaffer, Rutter, & Traub, 1981; Rutter, Chadwick, & Shaffer, 1983) found that children with mild TBI showed an increased incidence of behavioral disorder prior to injury, but no increased risk for new psychiatric disorder following injury over the approximate 2-year duration of the study. In contrast, there was a significant increase in new psychiatric disorder in severely injured children and adolescents by 4 months following injury that was at a rate two to three times that of the orthopedic control group and that remained stable throughout the period of study. Brown and colleagues noted the contribution of level of injury severity to prediction of new psychiatric disturbance following TBI children. Of perhaps greater importance, Brown and colleagues (1981) found that psychosocial adversity such as parental marital conflict or psychiatric disorder, and the child's preinjury behavioral characteristics were important factors in predicting new psychiatric disturbance. No specific pattern of behavioral disturbance was consistently noted following severe TBI, with the exception that social disinhibition was common in the first months following injury.

Max and colleagues (Max, Lindgren, et al., 1997; Max, Robin, et al., 1997; Max, Smith, et al., 1997) also investigated risk factors related to the emergence of novel psychiatric disturbances following pediatric TBI in a series of four psychiatric evaluations over a 2-year follow-up period. Consistent with the findings of Brown et al. (1981), Max reported that preinjury family dysfunction was a significant predictor of new psychiatric disturbances throughout the entire 2-year interval. A child's history of a preinjury psychiatric disorder also was predictive of psychiatric disturbance in the first 3 months postinjury, when the child might be particularly vulnerable to the disruptive effects of TBI on behavioral functioning. However, Max hypothesized that the child may be able to overcome the problem, at least in cases of less severe TBI, until such time that prior psychiatric history reemerges as a risk factor, perhaps reflecting the appearance of comorbid conditions related to the original disorder The history of family psychiatric disorder was a significant predictor through the first postinjury year, whereas injury severity was a significant predictor through the first 6 months and from 1 to 2 years postinjury. Consistent with findings from other research (Asarnow et al, 1995; Brown et al., 1981), Max found little evidence for a direct causal link between mild TBI and new behavioral disturbance.

Fletcher and colleagues (Fletcher, Ewing-Cobbs, Miner, Levin, & Eisenberg, 1990) reported a significant decline, persisting throughout the 12-month follow-up, in adaptive behavioral functioning among severely injured TBI children and adolescents carefully screened for premorbid neuropsychiatric disorder. In contrast, there were no significant differences among groups of children with mild, moderate, and severe TBI on scales assessing internalizing or externalizing behavioral adjustment difficulties as reported by parents on the Child Behavior Checklist (CBCL; Achenbach, 1991) through 1 year postinjury. Fletcher et al. (1996) replicated these findings with a larger sample of TBI children, substituting the Personality Inventory for Children—Revised (PIC-R; Wirt, Lachar, Klinedinst, & Seat,

1990), a parent-completed personality inventory, for the CBCL. Parent ratings on the PIC-R did not distinguish severity groups on any of the clinical scales reflecting different aspects of behavioral, emotional, and social adjustment. However, children with severe injuries obtained higher scores than children with mild or moderate injuries on PIC-R scales reflecting cognitive functioning and development. Fletcher et al. (1996) again found significant impairment in adaptive behavior among severely injured children relative to a group of mild and moderate TBI children. Rating scales may be useful in identifying adjustment difficulties before or after injury, but they may not be sufficiently sensitive to document preinjury to postinjury changes in behavior (Fletcher et al., 1996).

A recent retrospective study by Butler, Rourke, Fuerst, and Fisk (1997) identified a typology of psychosocial functioning derived through the use of cluster analytic techniques on PIC-R profiles obtained on average over 2 years following TBI. Subtypes included Normal, Cognitive Deficit, Somatic Concern, Mild Anxiety, Internalized Psychopathology, Antisocial, and Social Isolation. Over half of the children with severe TBI had few or no psychosocial difficulties. However, children with severe injuries were disproportionately represented in the Social Isolation subtype, characterized by younger age at injury, a longer interval between injury and testing, the highest elevations of any subtype on cognitive, academic, and developmental problem scales, and elevations on a scale assessing social isolation, emotional lability, and withdrawal. Based on these findings, the authors noted that children with a pattern of severe, persistent deficits on a wide array of intelligence, neuropsychological, and academic instruments may be at increased risk for problems related to social isolation, withdrawal, and emotional lability.

Few studies have specifically addressed the impact of pediatric TBI on family functioning. Perrott, Taylor, and Montes (1991) assessed a small sample of moderately to severely injured children in the chronic stage of recovery in a variety of areas of cognitive, behavioral, academic, and family functioning. Whereas few intellectual and cognitive difficulties were observed in this sample, problems were reported by parents and teachers that related to poor academic performance, behavior problems, trouble adapting to demands of everyday living, and stressful parent–child relationships compared with siblings who served as the control group. Stressful family relationships, which parents attributed to tensions associated with the TBI child, were reported by about one-half of the parents. No preinjury data was collected for this sample, although the authors hypothesized that the identified problems stemmed from preinjury variables or were acquired following the cognitive recovery.

Yeates and his colleagues (1997) investigated environmental variables as predictors of recovery in groups of TBI and orthopedic control children in the first year following injury. Preinjury family environmental factors were found to significantly predict cognitive and behavioral outcome at 12 months following injury above and beyond that explained by level of injury severity. In addition, preinjury family environment was found to buffer the impact of deficits such as poor memory in severe TBI children from high-functioning families, and to exacerbate the effect of injury in low-functioning families. Severely injured children from poorly functioning families tended to have a less rapid recovery and greater deficits at 12 months postinjury than children from more functional families. In general, Yeates et al. (1997) noted that preinjury family environment was more closely related to behavioral than cognitive outcomes, whereas injury severity was more closely related to cognitive than behavioral outcomes.

Rivara and coworkers (1994) prospectively evaluated a carefully screened sample of 94 children and their families for changes in family functioning and predictors of family outcome from preinjury through the first year following pediatric TBI. Preinjury global functioning and coping resources were regarded as moderate to good in two-thirds of the families, though over half demonstrated at least moderate risk prior to injury from high stress levels and difficult family relationships. Family functioning was generally stable in the first postinjury year in the mild and moderate groups, but showed deterioration in families with severely injured children, based on interviewer ratings. Preinjury family global functioning and coping skills and teacher ratings of the child's preinjury behavior were the best predictors (better than injury severity) of 1-year family functioning in adjusting to the stresses associated with childhood TBI. Rivara and colleagues (1994) also reported that poor academic and cognitive outcomes at one year following injury were related to level of injury severity; preinjury family functioning and child variables were more strongly related to behavioral variables than to academic and cognitive functioning. Conversely, prediction of behavioral outcome at 1 year postinjury was primarily associated with preinjury functioning of the family and child factors, rather than injury severity.

Recent research findings have helped to elucidate the nature and causes of behavioral and psychosocial difficulties that have been noted following TBI in children. In addition, they clearly indicate the importance of preinjury variables involving both the child and the family environment in facilitating understanding and more accurate prediction of both cognitive and behavioral outcome following injury. This type of information promises not only to enhance rehabilitative interventions on behalf of the child with TBI, but also provide needed assistance and support services for the family.

Influence of Age at Injury

Studies of neurobehavioral outcome after pediatric TBI frequently report higher rates of mortality and morbidity in infants and preschool-age children than in school-aged children and adolescents. However, it is unclear to what extent the less favorable outcome in young children is related to TBI secondary to physical child abuse. Although assault caused 5% of all TBIs in children ages 0–4, assault produced 90% of the serious TBIs (Kraus, Rock, & Hemyari, 1990). Moreover, Duhaime and colleagues (1992) identified that 24 % of consecutively injured hospitalized children ages 0–24 months had inflicted TBI. In children ages 0–6 with similar GCS scores and duration of impaired consciousness, cognitive and motor scores obtained at 1 month after the injury were significantly lower in children with inflicted TBI from physical child abuse than in children sustaining noninflicted TBI (Ewing-Cobbs, Kramer, et al., 1998). Therefore, at least a portion of the variability in outcome in young children may be accounted for by the mechanism of TBI, with inflicted TBI producing greater cognitive and motor deficit than noninflicted TBI.

Recovery from TBI may also vary depending on the child's age at injury and the specific function evaluated. Greater intellectual impairment has been documented in children less than 8 years of age than in older children (Brink, Garrett, Hale, Woo-Sam, & Nickel, 1970; Lange-Cosack, Wider, Schlesner, Grumme, & Kubicki, 1979). However, these samples contained infants and young children with brain injuries caused by physical abuse. Longitudinal studies of neuropsychological deficit and recovery in infants and young children have identified persistent widespread reduction in Verbal IQ, Performance IQ, motor, expressive language, receptive language, verbal memory, and visual memory in children with severe TBI in comparison to mild or moderate TBI (Anderson & Moore, 1995; Anderson et al., 1997; Ewing-Cobbs, Miner, Fletcher, & Levin, 1989; Ewing-Cobbs et al., 1997; Ewing-Cobbs, Thompson, Miner, & Fletcher, 1994).

The association between age at the time of TBI and subsequent cognitive development is unclear. Direct comparison of neuropsychological outcome has not been completed in young children, school-age children, and adolescents. Available studies indicate that outcome in most domains is similar in the first 7–8 years of life (Anderson et al., 1997; Ewing-Cobbs et al., 1997). Studies using global outcome ratings for academic, cognitive, social, and vocational domains vary; some found no differences in outcome according to age at injury (Costeff, Groswasser, & Goldstein, 1990), while others identified poorer outcomes in children ages 0–6 than in older children (Filley, Cranberg, Alexander, & Hart, 1987; Kriel, Krach, & Panser, 1989). Several psychometric studies did not identify associations between age at injury and either severity of cognitive sequelae or the rate of recovery of neuropsychological skills (Chadwick, Rutter, Shaffer, & Shrout, 1981; Klonoff et al., 1977) In contrast, other studies have identified greater deficits in younger than older children in reading acquisition, language, attention, memory, visual–motor integration, fine motor speed, and tactile recognition areas (Anderson & Moore, 1995; Anderson et al., 1997;

Barnes et al., 1999; Chapman, 1995; Dennis et al., 1995, 1996; Ewing-Cobbs, Levin, Eisenberg, & Fletcher, 1987; Ewing-Cobbs et al., 1989, 1994; Kaufmann et al., 1993; Levin et al., 1988, 1993; Levin, Ewing-Cobbs, & Eisenberg, 1995; Shaffer et al., 1980; Thompson et al., 1994; Wrightson, McGinn, & Gronwall, 1995). Recovery curves in most areas show initial deficit, some recovery in the first 6–12 months, and then no significant change from 1 to 3 years after TBI. Although long-term outcome measures of children with severe TBI remain stable, they show a persistent deficit in comparison to children with lesser injuries or other comparison groups. It is unclear whether longer term follow-up studies would show a stable, persistent deficit or whether children might evidence delayed deficits characterized by a failure to develop new skills at age-appropriate rates.

The finding of greater impairment following early TBI than TBI sustained in school-aged children and adolescents is consistent with the literature on recovery from early brain insults from other etiologies. Although the immature brain does show developmental sparing in some areas following injury, the majority of outcome studies support the position that brain insults may have more adverse consequences in infants and young children than in school-age children and adolescents. Children may recover well from early focal injury to specific regions of the brain, such as lateralized perinatal lesions with no continuing seizure activity (e.g., Vargha-Khadem, Isaacs, van der Werf, Robb, & Wilson, 1992). However, early diffuse or multifocal brain injury produced by cranial irradiation, infection, endocrinological disturbance, or trauma is associated with greater deficit in young than in older children (Anderson, Smibert, Ekert, & Godber, 1994; Anderson et al., 1997; Ewing-Cobbs et al., 1994, 1997; Radcliffe, Bunin, Sutton, Goldwein, & Phillips, 1994; Rovet, Ehrlich, & Sorbara, 1992; Taylor, Barry, & Schatschneider, 1993). As noted by Taylor and Alden (1997), several mechanisms have been hypothesized to account for the greater disruption in cognitive development in children with early brain injury: greater vulnerability of the immature brain to injury, greater effect on subsequent neuronal development, neural degeneration, or damage to neural systems responsible for skill acquisition. Future studies integrating longitudinal neuropsychological and functional neuroimaging findings may clarify the mechanisms involved in recovery and deficit following early brain injury.

CONCLUSIONS

Late outcome after TBI in children and adolescents is characterized by significant residual cognitive and psychosocial difficulties. The most salient neuropsychological areas of difficulty include Performance IQ, speeded motor skills, verbal learning and memory, focused and sustained attention, discourse, and academic achievement. The severity of cognitive deficit is related to the overall severity of the brain injury as indexed by traditional neurosurgical rating scales. In addition, the presence of focal brain injury contributes to the severity of cognitive deficit. For example, discourse deficits were noted largely in patients with focal left hemisphere involvement compared to those with diffuse or right hemisphere involvement (Ewing-Cobbs, Brookshire, et al., 1998), while executive function deficits were predicted by the volume of prefrontal lesions (Levin et al., 1994, 1997). Age at injury also is related to the quality of outcome; younger children seem disproportionately affected by TBI on indices of reading acquisition, language, attention, memory, visual–motor integration, fine motor speed, and tactile recognition. These cognitive deficits yield major disadvantages in academic, adaptive behavioral, and psychosocial arenas. The child's preinjury cognitive and psychosocial characteristics, coupled with the quality of family functioning, significantly buffer or potentiate posttraumatic difficulties. Although there is a substantial literature on cognitive outcome, the future challenge will be to translate these research findings into academic and cognitive interventions that will assist in reducing morbidity and optimizing outcome after severe TBI.

ACKNOWLEDGMENTS

Preparation of this chapter was supported in part by National Institute of Neurological Disorders and Stroke Grant No. 29462, Accidental and Nonaccidental Pediatric Brain Injury; Grant No. 21889, Outcome of Pediatric Head Injury; and Department of Education Grant No. H133B40002-97. We acknowledge the assistance provided by the University Clinical Research Center at Hermann Hospital and the support of National Institutes of Health Grant No. M01-RR-02558.

REFERENCES

Achenbach, T. (1991). *Manual for the Child Behavior Checklist*. Burlington, VT: University Associates in Psychiatry.

Adams, J. H., Mitchell, D. E., Graham, D. I., & Doyle, D. (1977). Diffuse brain damage of the immediate impact type. *Brain, 100*, 489–502.

Anderson, V., & Moore, C. (1995). Age at injury as a predictor of outcome following pediatric head injury: A longitudinal perspective. *Child Neuropsychology, 1*, 187–202.

Anderson, V., Morse, S. A., Klug, G., Catroppa, C., Haritou, F., Rosenfeld, J., & Pentland, L. (1997). Predicting recovery from head injury in young children: A prospective analysis. *Journal of the International Neuropsychological Society, 3*, 568–580.

Anderson, V., Smibert, E., Ekert, H., & Godber, T. (1994). Intellectual, educational, and behavioral sequelae after cranial irradiation and chemotherapy. *Archives of Diseases in Childhood, 70*, 476–483.

Annegers, J. F., Grabow, J. D., Kurland, L. T., & Laws, E. R. (1980). The incidence, causes, and secular trends of head trauma in Olmstead County, Minnesota, 1935–1974. *Neurology, 30,* 912–919.

Asarnow, R. F., Satz, P., Light, R., Zaucha, K., Lewis, R., & McCleary, C. (1995). The UCLA study of mild closed head injury in children and adolescents. In S. H. Broman & M. E. Michel (Eds.), *Traumatic head injury in children* (pp. 117–146). New York: Oxford University Press.

Barnes, M. A., Dennis, M., & Wilkinson, M. (1999). Reading after closed head injury in childhood: Effects on accuracy, fluency, and comprehension. *Developmental Neuropsychology, 15,* 1–24.

Bawden, H. N., Knights, R. M., & Winogron, H. W. (1985). Speeded performance following head injury in children. *Journal of Clinical and Experimental Neuropsychology, 7,* 39–54.

Brink, J. D., Garrett, A. L., Hale, W. R., Woo-Sam, J., & Nickel, V. L. (1970). Recovery of motor and intellectual function in children sustaining severe head injuries. *Developmental Medicine and Child Neurology, 12,* 565–571.

Brown, G., Chadwick, O., Shaffer, D., Rutter, M., & Traub, M. (1981). A prospective study of children with head injuries: III. Psychiatric sequelae. *Psychological Medicine, 11,* 63–78.

Butler, K., Rourke, B. P., Fuerst, D. R., & Fisk, J. L. (1997). A typology of psychosocial functioning in pediatric closed-head injury. *Child Neuropsychology, 3,* 98–133.

Chadwick, O., Rutter, M., Brown, G., Shaffer, D., & Traub, M. (1981). A prospective study of children with head injuries: II. Cognitive sequelae. *Psychological Medicine, 11,* 49–61.

Chadwick, O., Rutter, M., Shaffer, D., & Shrout, P. E. (1981). A prospective study of children with head injuries: IV. Specific cognitive deficits. *Journal of Clinical Neuropsychology, 3,* 101–120.

Chapman, S. B. (1995). Discourse as an outcome measure. In S. H. Broman & M. E. Michel (Eds.), *Traumatic head injury in children* (pp. 95–116). New York: Oxford University Press.

Chapman, S. B., Culhane, K. A., Levin, H. S., Harward, H., Mendelsohn, D., Ewing-Cobbs, L., Fletcher, J. M., & Bruce, D. (1992). Narrative discourse after closed head injury in children and adolescents. *Brain and Language, 43,* 42–65.

Chapman, S. B., Levin, H. S., Wanek, A., Weyrauch, J., & Kufera, J. (1998). Discourse after closed head injury in young children. *Brain and Language, 61,* 420–449.

Costeff, H., Groswasser, Z., & Goldstein, R. (1990). Long term follow-up review of 31 children with severe closed head trauma. *Journal of Neurosurgery, 73,* 684–687.

Dennis, M., & Barnes, M. A. (1990). Knowing the meaning, getting the point, bridging the gap, and carrying the message: Aspects of discourse following closed head injury in childhood and adolescence. *Brain and Language, 39,* 428–446.

Dennis, M., Barnes, M. A., Donnelly, R. E., Wilkinson, M., & Humphreys, R. P. (1996). Appraising and managing knowledge: Metacognitive skills after childhood head injury. *Developmental Neuropsychology, 12,* 77–103.

Dennis, M., & Lovett, M. W. (1990). Discourse ability in children after brain damage. In Y. Joanette & H. H. Brownell (Eds.), *Discourse ability and brain damage:*

Theoretical and empirical perspectives (pp. 199–223). New York: Springer-Verlag.

Dennis, M., Wilkinson, M., Koski, L., & Humphries, R. P. (1995). Attention deficits in the long term after childhood head injury. In S. H. Broman & M. E. Michel (Eds.), *Traumatic head injury in children* (pp. 165–187). New York: Oxford University Press.

Donders, J. (1993). WISC-R subtest patterns in children with traumatic brain injury. *Clinical Neuropsychologist, 7,* 430–442.

Donders, J. (1994). Academic placement after traumatic brain injury. *Journal of School Psychology, 32,* 53–65.

Duhaime, A. C., Alario, A. J., Lewander, W. J., Schut, L., Sutton, L., Seidl, T., Nudelman, S., Budenz, D., Hertk, R., Tsiaras, W., & Loporchio, S. (1992). Head injury in very young children: Mechanisms, injury types, and ophthalmolgic findings in 100 hospitalized patients younger than two years of age. *Pediatrics, 90,* 179–185.

Ewing-Cobbs, L., Brookshire, B. L., Scott, M. A., & Fletcher, J. M. (1998). Children's narratives following traumatic brain injury: Linguistic structure, cohesion, and thematic recall. *Brain and Language, 61,* 395–419.

Ewing-Cobbs, L., Fletcher, J. M., & Levin, H. S. (1986). Neurobehavioral sequelae following head injury in children: Educational implications. *Journal of Head Trauma Rehabilitation, 1,* 57–65.

Ewing-Cobbs, L., Fletcher, J. M., & Levin, H. S. (1995). Traumatic brain injury. In B. P. Rourke (Ed.), *Syndrome of nonverbal learning disabilities: Neurodevelopmental manifestations* (pp. 433–459). New York: Guilford Press.

Ewing-Cobbs, L., Fletcher, J. M., Levin, H. S., Francis, D. J., Davidson, K., & Miner, M. E. (1997). Longitudinal neuropsychological outcome in infants and preschoolers with traumatic brain injury. *Journal of the International Neuropsychological Society, 3,* 581–591.

Ewing-Cobbs, L., Iovino, I., Fletcher, J. M., Miner, M. E., & Levin, H. S. (1991). Academic achievement following traumatic brain injury in children and adolescents. *Journal of Clinical and Experimental Neuropsychology, 13,* 93.

Ewing-Cobbs, L., Kramer, L., Prasad, M. P., Canales, D. N., Louis, P. T., Fletcher, J. M., Vollero, H., Landry, S. H., & Cheung, K. (1998). Neuroimaging, physical, and developmental findings following inflicted and noninflicted traumatic brain injury in young children. *Pediatrics, 102,* 300–307.

Ewing-Cobbs, L., Levin, H. S., Eisenberg, H. M., & Fletcher, J. M. (1987). Language functions following closed head injury in children and adolescents. *Journal of Clinical and Experimental Neuropsychology, 9,* 575–592.

Ewing-Cobbs, L., Miner, M. E., Fletcher, J. M., & Levin, H. S. (1989). Intellectual, motor, and language sequelae following closed head injury in infants and preschoolers. *Journal of Pediatric Psychology, 14,* 531–547.

Ewing-Cobbs, L., Prasad, M. P., Fletcher, J. M., Levin, H. S., Miner, M. E., & Eisenberg, H. M. (1998). Attention after pediatric traumatic brain injury: A multidimensional assessment. *Child Neuropsychology, 4,* 35–48.

Ewing-Cobbs, L., Thompson, N. M., Miner, M. E., & Fletcher, J. M. (1994). Gunshot wounds to the brain in children and adolescents: Age and neurobehavioral development. *Neurosurgery, 35,* 225–233.

Filley, C. M., Cranberg, L. D., Alexander, M. P., & Hart, E. J. (1987). Neurobehavioral outcome after closed head injury in childhood and adolescence. *Archives of Neurology, 44,* 194–198.

Fletcher, J. M., Ewing-Cobbs, L., Miner, M. E., Levin, H. S., & Eisenberg, H. M. (1990). Behavioral changes after closed head injury in children. *Journal of Consulting and Clinical Psychology, 57,* 1–13.

Fletcher, J. M., Levin, H. S., Lachar, D., Kusnerik, L., Harward, H., Mendelsohn, D., & Lilly, M. (1996). Behavioral adjustment after pediatric head injury: Relationships with age, severity, and lesion size. *Journal of Child Neurology, 11,* 283–290.

Hayes, R. L., & Dixon, C. E. (1994). Neurochemical changes in mild head injury. *Seminars in Neurology, 14,* 25–31.

Heaton, R. K., Chelune, G. J., Talley, J. L., Kay, G. G., & Curtiss, G. (1993). *Wisconsin Card Sorting Test manual—Revised and expanded.* Odessa, FL: Psychological Assessment Resources.

Individuals with Disabilities Education Act. (1990). Public Law 101–456. Reauthorization of Public Law 94-142. Washington, DC: U.S. Government Printing Office.

Jaffe, K. M., Fay, G. C., Polissar, N. L., Martin, K. M., Shurtleff, H., Rivara, J. B., & Winn, H. R. (1992). Severity of pediatric traumatic brain injury and early neurobehavioral outcome: A cohort study. *Archives of Physical Medicine and Rehabilitation, 73,* 540–547.

Jaffe, K. M., Fay, G. C., Polissar, N. L., Martin, K. M., Shurtleff, H., Rivara, J. B., & Winn, H. R. (1993). Severity of pediatric traumatic brain injury and neurobehavioral recovery at one year: A cohort study. *Archives of Physical Medicine and Rehabilitation, 74,* 587–595.

Jaffe, K. M., Polissar, N. L., Fay, G. C., & Liao, S. (1995). Recovery trends over three years following pediatric traumatic brain injury. *Archives of Physical Medicine and Rehabilitation, 76,* 17–26.

Jordan, F. M., & Murdoch, B. E. (1990). Linguistic status following closed-head injury in children: A follow-up study. *Brain Injury, 4,* 147–154.

Jordan, F. M., Murdoch, B. E., & Buttsworth, D. L. (1991). Closed head injured children's performance on narrative tasks. *Journal of Speech and Hearing Research, 34,* 572–582.

Jordan, F. M., Ozanne, A. O., & Murdoch, B. E. (1988). Long-term speech and language disorders subsequent to closed head injury in children. *Brain Injury, 2,* 175–185.

Kaufmann, P. M., Fletcher, J. M., Levin, H. S., Miner, M. E., & Ewing-Cobbs, L. (1993). Attentional disturbance after pediatric closed head injury. *Journal of Child Neurology, 8,* 348–353.

Kinsella, G., Prior, M., Sawyer, M., Murtagh, D., Eisenmajer, R., Anderson, V., Bryan, D., & Klug, G. (1995). Neuropsychological deficit and academic performance in children and adolescents following traumatic brain injury. *Journal of Pediatric Psychology, 20,* 753–767.

Kinsella, G. J., Prior, M., Sawyer, M., Ong, B., Murtagh, D., Eisenmajer, R., Bryan, D., Anderson, V., & Klug, G. (1997). Predictors and indicators of academic outcome in children two years following traumatic brain injury. *Journal of the International Neuropsychological Society, 3,* 608–616.

Kintsch, W., & van Dijk, T. A. (1978). Toward a model of text comprehension and production. *Psychological Review, 85,* 363–394.

Klauber, M. R., Barrett-Connor, E., Marshall, L. F., & Bowers, S. A. (1981). The epidemiology of head injury: A prospective study of an entire community—San Diego County, California, 1978. *American Journal of Epidemiology, 113,* 500–509.

Klonoff, H., Low, M. D., & Clark, C. (1977). Head injuries in children: A prospective five year follow-up. *Journal of Neurology, Neurosurgery, and Psychiatry, 40,* 1211–1219.

Knights, R. M., Iran, L. P., Ventureyra, E. C., Bentirogrio, C., Stoddart, C., Winogron, W., & Bawden, H. (1991). The effects of head injury in children on neuropsychological and behavioral functioning. *Brain Injury, 5,* 339–351.

Kraus, J. F. (1995). Epidemiological features of brain injury in children: Occurrence, children at risk, causes and manner of injury, severity, and outcomes. In S. H. Broman & M. E. Michel (Eds.), *Traumatic head injury in children* (pp. 22–39). New York: Oxford University Press.

Kraus, J. F., Fife, D., Cox, P., Ramstein, K., & Conroy, C. (1986). Incidence, severity, and external causes of pediatric brain injury. *American Journal of Diseases of Children, 140,* 687–693.

Kraus, J. F., Rock, A., & Hemyari, P. (1990). Brain injuries among infants, children, adolescents, and young adults. *American Journal of Diseases of Children, 144,* 684–691.

Kriel, R. L., Krach, L. E., & Panser, L. A. (1989). Closed head injury: Comparison of children younger and older than six years of age. *Pediatric Neurology, 5,* 296–300.

Lange-Cosack, H., Wider, B., Schlesner, H. J., Grumme, T., & Kubicki, S. (1979). Prognosis of brain injuries in young children (one until five years of age). *Neuropaediatrie,10,* 105–127.

Levin, H. S., Benton, A. L., & Grossman, R. G. (1982). *Neurobehavioral consequences of closed head injury.* New York: Oxford University Press.

Levin, H. S., Culhane, K. A., Mendelsohn, D., Lilly, M. A., Bruce, D., Fletcher, J. M., Chapman, S. B., Harward, H., & Eisenberg, H. M. (1993). Cognition in relation to magnetic resonance imaging in head-injured children and adolescents. *Archives of Neurology, 50,* 897–905.

Levin, H. S. & Eisenberg, H. M. (1979). Neuropsychological impairment after closed head injury in children and adolescents. *Journal of Pediatric Psychology, 4,* 389–402.

Levin, H. S., Ewing-Cobbs, L., & Eisenberg, H. M. (1995). Neurobehavioral outcome of pediatric closed head injury. In S. H. Broman & M. E. Michel (Eds.), *Traumatic head injury in children* (pp. 70–94). New York: Oxford University Press.

Levin, H. S., Fletcher, J. M., Kufera, J. A., Harward, H., Lilly, M. A., Mendelsohn, D., Bruce, D., & Eisenberg, H. M. (1996). Dimensions of cognition measured by the Tower of London and other cognitive tasks in head-injured children and adolescents. *Developmental Neuropsychology, 12,* 17–34.

Levin, H. S., High, W. M., Ewing-Cobbs, L., Fletcher, J. M., Eisenberg, H. M., Miner, M. E., & Goldstein, F. C. (1988). Memory functioning during the first year after closed head injury in children and adolescents. *Neurosurgery, 22,* 1043–1052.

Levin, H. S., Mendelsohn, D., Lilly, M. A., Fletcher, J. M., Culhane, K. A., Chapman, S. B., Harward, H., Kusnerik, L., Bruce, D., & Eisenberg, H. M. (1994). Tower of London performance in relation to magnetic resonance imaging following closed head injury in children. *Neuropsychology, 8,* 171–179.

Levin, H. S., Song, J., Scheibel, R. S., Fletcher, J. M., Harward, H., Lilly, M., & Goldstein, F. (1997). Concept formation and problem-solving following closed head injury in children. *Journal of the International Neuropsychological Society, 3,* 598–607.

Massagli, T. I., Jaffe, K. M., Fay, G. C., Polissar, N. I., Liao, S., & Rivara, J. M. B. (1996). Neurobehavioral sequelae of severe pediatric traumatic brain injury: A cohort study. *Archives of Physical Medicine and Rehabilitation, 77,* 223–231.

Max, J. E., Lindgren, S. D., Robin, D. A., Smith, W. L., Jr., Sato, Y., Mattheis, P. J., Castillo, C. S., & Stierwalt, J. A. G. (1997). Traumatic brain injury in children and adolescents: Psychiatric disorders in the second three months. *Journal of Nervous and Mental Disease, 185,* 394–401.

Max, J. E., Robin, D. A., Lindgren, S. D., Smith, W. L., Jr., Sato, Y., Mattheis, P. J., Stierwalt, J. A. G., & Castillo, C. S. (1997). Traumatic brain injury in children and adolescents: Psychiatric disorders at two years. *Journal of the American Academy of Child and Adolescent Psychiatry, 36,* 1278–1285.

Max, J. E., Smith, W. L., Jr., Sato, Y., Mattheis, P. J., Castillo, C. S., Lindgren, S. D., Robin, D. A., & Stierwalt, J. A. G. (1997). Traumatic brain injury in children and adolescents: Psychiatric disorders in the first three months. *Journal of the American Academy of Child and Adolescent Psychiatry, 36,* 94–102.

Mendelsohn, D., Levin, H. S., Bruce, D., Lilly, M., Harward, H., Culhane, K. A., & Eisenberg, H. M. (1992). Late MRI findings after head injury in children: Relationship to clinical features and outcome. *Child's Nervous System, 8,* 445–452.

Mosher, F. A., & Hornsby, J. R. (1966). On asking questions. In J. S. Bruner, R. R. Olver, P. M. Greenfield, J. R. Hornsby, H. J. Kenney, M. Maccoby, N. Modiano, F. A. Mosher, D. R. Olson, M. C. Potter, L. C. Reich, & A. M. Sonstroem (Eds.), *Studies in cognitive growth* (pp. 86–102). New York: Wiley.

Murray, R., Shum, D., & McFarland, K. (1992). Attentional deficits in head-injured children: An information processing analysis. *Brain and Cognition, 18,* 99–115.

Pennington, B. F. (1994). The working memory function of the prefrontal cortices: Implications for developmental and individual differences in cognition. In M. M. Haith, J. Benson, R. Roberts, & B. F. Pennington (Eds.), *Future oriented processes in development* (pp. 243–289). Chicago: University of Chicago Press.

Perrott, S. B., Taylor, H. G., & Montes, J. L. (1991). Neuropsychological sequelae, family stress, and environmental adaptation following pediatric head injury. *Developmental Neuropsychology, 7,* 69–86.

Radcliffe, J., Bunin, G. R., Sutton, L. N., Goldwein, J. W., & Phillips, P. C. (1994). Cognitive deficits in long-term survivors of childhood medulloblastoma and other noncortical tumors: Age dependent effects of whole brain radiation. *International Journal of Developmental Neuroscience, 12,* 327–334.

Rivara, J., Jaffe, K., Polissar, N., Fay, G., Martin, K., Shurtleff, H., & Liao, S. (1994). Family functioning and children's academic performance and behavior problems in the year following traumatic brain injury. *Archives of Physical Medicine and Rehabilitation, 75,* 369–379.

Roberts, R. J., & Pennington, B. F. (1996). An interactive framework for examining prefrontal cognitive processes. *Developmental Neuropsychology, 12,* 105–126.

Rovet, J. F., Ehrlich, R. M., & Sorbara, D. L. (1992). Neurodevelopment in infants and preschool children with congenital hypothyroidism. Etiological and treatment factors affecting outcome. *Journal of Pediatric Psychology, 17,* 187–213.

Rutter, M., Chadwick, O., & Shaffer, D. (1983). Head injury. In M. Rutter (Ed.), *Developmental neuropsychiatry* (pp. 83–111). New York: Guilford Press.

Shaffer, D., Bijur, P., Chadwick, O. F. D., & Rutter, M. (1980). Head injury and later reading disability. *Journal of the American Academy of Child Psychiatry, 19,* 592–610.

Shallice, T. (1982). Specific impairments of planning. *Philosophical Transactions of the Royal Society of London, Part B, 298,* 199–209.

Strich, S. J. (1956). Diffuse degeneration of the cerebral white matter in severe dementia following head injury. *Journal of Neurology, Neurosurgery, and Psychiatry, 19,* 163–185.

Strich, S. J. (1970). Lesions in the cerebral hemispheres after blunt head injury. In S. Sevitt & H. B. Stoner (Eds.), *The pathology of trauma* (pp. 166–171). London, BMA House.

Taylor, H. G., & Alden, J. (1997). Age-related differences in outcomes following childhood brain insults: An introduction and overview. *Journal of the International Neuropsychological Society, 3,* 555–567.

Taylor, H. G., Barry, C. T., & Schatschneider, C. W. (1993). School-aged consequences of Haemophilus influenzae Type b meningitis. *Journal of Clinical Child Psychology, 22,* 196–206.

Taylor, H. G., Drotar, D., Wade, S., Yeates, K., Stancin, T., & Klein, S. (1995). Recovery from traumatic brain injury in children: The importance of the family. In S. H. Broman & M. E. Michel (Eds.), *Traumatic head injury in children* (pp. 188–216). New York: Oxford University Press.

Teasdale, G., & Jennett, B. (1974). Assessment of coma and impaired consciousness: A practical scale. *Lancet, 2,* 81–84.

Thompson, N. M., Francis, D. F., Steubing, K. K., Fletcher, J. M., Ewing-Cobbs, L., Miner, M. E., Levin, H. S., & Eisenberg, H. M. (1994). Motor, visual–spatial, and somatosensory skills after closed head injury in children and adolescents: A study of change. *Neuropsychology, 8,* 333–342.

Vargha-Khadem, F., Isaacs, E., van der Werf, S., Robb, S., & Wilson, J. (1992). Development of intelligence and memory in children with hemiplegic cerebral palsy: The deleterious consequence of early seizures. *Brain, 115,* 315–329.

Warschausky, S., Keuman, D., & Selim, A. (1996). Attentional performance of children with traumatic brain injury: A quantitative and qualitative analysis of digit span. *Archives of Clinical Neuropsychology, 11,* 147–153.

Wechsler, D. (1974). *Wechsler Intelligence Scale for Children: Revised.* New York: Psychological Corporation.

Winogron, H. W., Knights, R. M., & Bawden, H. N. (1984). Neuropsychological deficits following head injury in children. *Journal of Clinical Neuropsychology, 6,* 269–286.

Wirt, R. D., Lachar, D., Klinedinst, J. K., & Seat, P. D. (1990). *Multidimensional description of child personality: A manual for the Personality Inventory for Children.* Los Angeles: Western Psychological Services.

Wrightson, P., McGinn, V., & Gronwall, D. (1995). Mild head injury in preschool children: Evidence that it can be associated with a persisting cognitive defect. *Journal of Neurology, Neurosurgery, and Psychiatry, 59,* 375–380.

Yeates, K. O., Blumenstein, E., Patterson, C. M., & Delis, D. C. (1995). Verbal learning and memory following pediatric closed-head injury. *Journal of the International Neuropsychological Society, 1,* 78–87.

Yeates, K. O., Taylor, H. G., Drotar, D., Wade, S. L., Klein, S., Stancin, T., & Schatschneider, C. (1997). Preinjury family environment as a determinant of recovery from traumatic brain injuries in school-age children. *Journal of the International Neuropsychological Society, 3,* 617–630.

PART THREE

SPECIAL ISSUES

CHAPTER THIRTEEN

Social Correlates of Chronic Illness

WENDY B. SCHUMAN
ANNETTE M. LA GRECA

Coping with the challenges of a chronic disease can be very stressful for children, adolescents, and their families. Consequently, for many years, psychologists and health care professionals have been concerned about the impact of chronic physical conditions on children's and adolescents' social and emotional development. Does chronic disease in children and adolescents lead to impaired psychosocial functioning? That is, does this type of stressor represent a risk factor for problems in development?

Early research on the psychosocial characteristics of children with pediatric conditions focused predominantly on comparisons of physically ill and healthy children. A variety of personality and psychological adaptation parameters were studied, including behavior problems, self-esteem, anxiety, depression, and symptoms of psychiatric dysfunction (see reviews by La Greca & Stone, 1985; Varni & Wallander, 1988). Asthma, hemophilia, sickle cell disease, cystic fibrosis, insulin-dependent diabetes mellitus, and childhood cancer were among the chronic conditions considered in this research.

Perhaps the most striking conclusion that can be drawn from these considerable data is that children and adolescents with chronic illness, and their families, do not differ substantially from healthy youngsters in terms of disease-specific personality patterns or prevalence of severe emotional disorders (e.g., Jacobson et al., 1986; Tavormina, Kastner, Slater, & Watt, 1976). In fact, the psychosocial problems that have been observed among some youth with chronic disease may, in fact, be interpreted as normal reactions to real-life stressors (Drotar, 1981; Kellerman, Zelter, Ellenberg, Dash, & Rigler, 1980; Varni, 1983).

At the same time, however, it is also clear that youngsters and families' coping resources are challenged by the onset and course of many pediatric problems. Childhood illness functions as a stressor that, in combination with other variables, "may contribute to increased risk, but is not the sole cause of adjustment problems" (Drotar, 1981, p. 218).

In fact, this perspective of "heightened risk" fits well with more recent reviews. In a meta-analysis of the literature on the psychosocial adjustment of children with chronic conditions, Lavigne and Faier-Routman (1992) found a range of effect sizes. Compared to healthy comparison youth and normative samples, children with certain physical disorders (e.g., cancer, asthma, juvenile rheumatoid arthritis) showed mild to moderate differences in adjustment (effect sizes between .25 and .49); children with other problems (e.g., cerebral palsy, diabetes mellitus, cleft lip/palate) had moderate to large effect sizes (.50 to .74). For several disorders, including seizure disorders, inflammatory bowel disease, deafness, cardiac disorders, and burns, the analyses revealed very large effect sizes of .75 or more, indicating significant adjustment problems in children with these disorders as compared to healthy controls. Based on this review, it appears that youth with chronic conditions are at greater risk for psychosocial problems than healthy youth, and that this risk increases with more serious or life-threatening conditions.

Furthermore, although many studies of pediatric populations have focused on general psychological adaptation, some reviews have suggested that *social adjustment* might be an area of special vulnerability for children with chronic life-disease (e.g., Drotar, 1981; Fisher, Delamater, Bertelson, & Kirkley, 1982; Johnson, 1980; O'Malley, Koocher, Foster, & Slavin, 1979). In fact, these early impressions have been supported by recent studies that have observed peer adjustment difficulties in some children with chronic pediatric conditions (see La Greca, 1990; Nassau & Drotar, 1997; Pless & Nolan, 1991; Spirito, DeLawyer, & Stark, 1991).

Despite these indications, relatively little attention has been devoted to the study of peer relations among children and adolescents with chronic disease (La Greca, 1990, 1992), in comparison to studies of youngsters' emotional functioning and of family issues. At the same time, youngsters' peer relations, and the interplay between peers and chronic disease, is an area of tremendous importance.

For example, we know from the child development literature that the quality of children's peer relationships is a critical component of current and later emotional adjustment (Dunn & McGuire, 1992; Hartup, 1996). In fact, peer ratings of dislike among third graders have been found to be better predictors of emotional problems 10 years later than other traditional child adjustment indices (Cowen, Pederson, Babian, Izzo, & Trost,

1973; see Parker & Asher, 1987, and Kupersmidt, Coie, & Dodge, 1990, for reviews).

We also know that when peer relations are problematic, they represent a stressor for most children. For example, Brown and colleagues (Brown, O'Keefe, Sanders, & Baker, 1986) found that "fear of negative evaluations from others," and "fights with or rejection by a friend" were the most common stressors reported by youngsters 10–18 years of age. Not surprisingly, worry about peer relationships is one of the factors found to have the greatest impact on the emotional well-being of youngsters with chronic health conditions (Wolman, Resnick, Harris, & Blum, 1994).

On the positive side, social support has been shown to be a critical factor in disease adjustment and adaptation (see Cohen & Wills, 1985). Youngsters' friends provide a key source of emotional support (e.g., Cohen & Wills, 1985; Wasserstein & La Greca, 1996) and may, therefore, be important for helping children and adolescents cope with the stress of a chronic disease.

For these reasons, the study of peer relations among children with chronic disease is of considerable importance. In the present chapter, we review available literature on the social aspects of chronic pediatric conditions, giving special attention to the characteristics of certain chronic diseases and their treatments that may interfere with a child's peer relations, as well as to the impact of peer relations on the youngster's ability to manage chronic pediatric conditions. We frame our review around four key questions:

1. Are youngsters with chronic disease at risk for peer relationship problems?
2. Is this risk heightened for those with cognitive aspects to their condition?
3. How do peers help or hinder the process of disease adaptation?
4. How do peers help or hinder day-to-day disease management and treatment?

ARE YOUNGSTERS WITH CHRONIC DISEASE AT RISK FOR PEER RELATIONSHIP PROBLEMS?

Several recent investigations have found limited support for the notion that children with chronic disease may experience social difficulties. These findings are based on child, parent, teacher, and peer reports of such aspects of social adjustment as popularity, friendships, social reputation, and loneliness.

For example, in a series of investigations, Noll and colleagues compared children with cancer with matched classroom control children on several measures such as popularity, friendship, and social reputation. In the first of these studies, Noll, Bukowski, Rogosch, LeRoy, and Kulkarni (1990) found that, based on peers' ratings, children with cancer were less sociable, less prone toward leadership, and more socially isolated and withdrawn than controls. Subsequently, Noll, LeRoy, Bukowski, Rogosch, and Kulkarni (1991) found no differences between the two groups of children in terms of their general acceptance, self-concept, and loneliness; however, the children with cancer were perceived to have greater levels of illness and to be more socially isolated. When teacher report was included as a measure of social reputation, children with cancer were nominated more often for sociability–leadership roles and less often for aggressive-disruptive roles.

Other work similarly suggests limited differences in the peer relations of children affected by chronic disease compared with their classmates. For instance, Graetz and Shute (1995) compared the peer relations of children with asthma with matched classroom controls. They found that, overall, children with asthma had peer relationships that were equivalent to those of their classmates, but the children with asthma were seen by peers as being sicker and missing more school. However, children with more severe asthma, as indicated by a greater frequency of hospitalizations, were less preferred as playmates, perceived as more sensitive–isolated, and endorsed greater feelings of loneliness than did children with less severe forms of asthma.

In a study of children with sickle cell disease, gender appeared to be an important determinant of peers' perceptions of the affected child's social competence (Noll et al., 1996). Girls with sickle cell disease were perceived by peers as being less sociable and less well accepted relative to comparison girls, whereas boys with the disease were perceived as being less aggressive than comparison boys.

Taken together, these recent investigations suggest considerable variability in the peer relations of children with chronic illness, and provide limited support for the idea that chronic disease has a negative impact on peer relations. These studies also underscore the importance of considering various qualitative aspects of social adjustment. Rather than classifying children as having good or poor peer relationships, these recent studies attempt to evaluate such factors as the child's role in the peer group, social reputation, and satisfaction with his or her social status.

It also may be important to go beyond diagnosis to a consideration of the specific characteristics of disease that may put youngsters at risk for peer relationship difficulties. Specifically, diseases that interfere with normal daily activities, impede physical activity, alter appearance, or impair cognitive functioning may affect youngsters' peer relations. While the impact of cognitive impairment is addressed at length in the next section, we review the effect of restrictions and appearance here.

A number of pediatric diseases can impose *restrictions on a child's physical activity*. Examples include asthma, cystic fibrosis, hemophilia, sickle cell disease, and spina bifida, among others. Such diseases may have social consequences, as they limit the youngster's ability to participate fully in peer activities. Not surprisingly, children with chronic illness accompanied by physical limitations seem to encounter more peer social difficulties than healthy controls or those with chronic illness alone (Cadman, Boyle, Sazatmari, & Offord, 1987; Dorner, 1976; Donnelly, Donnelly, & Thong, 1987; Drotar et al., 1981; Hurtig & White, 1986; Kumar, Powers, Allen, & Haywood, 1976; Morgan & Jackson, 1986; Nocon, 1991; Padur et al., 1995). In addition, children who are more physically impaired tend to have more adjustment difficulties than those with less impairment (Cadman et al., 1987; Stein & Jessop, 1984).

For example, about 50% of adolescents with spina bifida, a chronic disorder that often results in physical handicaps and impaired mobility, report feeling socially isolated, and the percentages are even higher for those with severe activity limitations (Dorner, 1976; McAndrew, 1978; see Varni & Wallander, 1988, for a review). Morgan and Jackson (1986) compared healthy controls to adolescents with sickle cell disease, a condition that is associated with small body size and easy fatigability that can limit social sports participation. Adolescents with sickle cell disease reported less satisfaction with their bodies and spent less time in social activities with peers. Other investigators (Hurtig & White, 1986; Kumar et al., 1976) have observed more social withdrawal and social skill difficulties among children and adolescents with sickle cell disease, compared to healthy controls.

It might be expected that pediatric conditions that restrict physical activities produce greater social consequences for boys. The more athletic, extensive, and activity-oriented nature of boys' peer interactions during the school years (Lever, 1978; Waldrop & Halverson, 1975) could present greater obstacles for boys with activity limitations than for girls. In contrast, patterns of interactions among girls reveal preferences for intensive individual or dyadic social activities of a more sedentary nature. Some evidence on gender differences among adolescents with sickle cell disease is consistent with this notion (Hurtig & White, 1986; Noll et al., 1996).

Chronic diseases also may result in *interruption or suspension of normal daily activities*, including unexpected or lengthy absences from school. For example, asthma is the leading cause of school absence in the elementary school years (Nocon, 1991; Padur et al., 1995). One study found that, since starting school, one in three 7-year-old children with asthma had missed more than 50 days of school due to asthmatic symptoms (Speight, Lee, & Hey, 1983). Children with hemophilia or HIV infection may also experience periods in which they are unable to attend school (Lineberger, 1981; Wolters, Brouwers, Moss, & Pizzo, 1994).

Alterations in physical appearance also may put children with chronic disease at risk for social difficulties. Pediatric conditions that affect appearance include chronic obesity, growth hormone deficiency, craniofacial anomalies, burns, and acquired limb deficiency. Children affected by these conditions may experience problems with social acceptance (e.g., Baum & Forehand, 1984; Bull & Rumsey, 1988; Gordon, Crouthamel, Post, & Richman, 1982; Israel & Shapiro, 1985; Kapp-Simon, Simon, & Kristovich, 1992; Lee & Rosenfeld, 1987; Strauss, Smith, Frame, & Forehand, 1985). For example, two recent investigations found that for children with craniofacial anomalies, dissatisfaction with facial appearance is associated with lower self-worth and social acceptance, and with more loneliness and social anxiety (Pope & Ward, 1997a, 1997b). Observations of adolescents with craniofacial conditions suggest that they tend to initiate fewer contacts with peers, receive less frequent positive responses, and engage in fewer conversations than peers without craniofacial anomalies (Kapp-Simon & McGuire, 1997).

Thus, returning to the question of whether youngsters with chronic disease are at risk for peer relationship problems, there appears to be some recent support for the notion that chronic disease has a negative impact on peer relations. However, there also appears to be considerable variability in the peer relations of children with chronic illness. This indicates the importance of considering various qualitative aspects of peer functioning, as well as examining the specific characteristics of disease that may put youngsters at risk.

ARE YOUNGSTERS WITH CHRONIC DISEASE ASSOCIATED WITH COGNITIVE IMPAIRMENTS AT ELEVATED RISK FOR PEER RELATIONSHIP PROBLEMS?

Chronic diseases that are associated with cognitive impairments present a special challenge to social relations. As evident from much of the literature cited throughout this volume, cognitive impairments can be seen with a variety of chronic conditions and treatments, and may range from mild learning disabilities to significant cognitive impairment (e.g., mental retardation). A wide variety of chronic health conditions are associated with cognitive difficulties and impairments, including cerebral palsy, spina bifida, and epilepsy (Nassau & Drotar, 1997; Shepherd & Hosking, 1989). Children with HIV disease are also at substantial risk for developing central nervous system (CNS) impairments, which can range from mild neuropsychological impairments to progressive encephalopathy (Armstrong,

Seidel, & Swales, 1993; Brouwers, Belman, & Epstein, 1991). In addition, cancers that involve brain tissue and some of the treatments for childhood cancer are likely to have CNS complications and impairments (Nassau & Drotar, 1997). Other conditions associated with CNS impairments include congenital heart disease (DeMaso, Beardslee, Silbert, & Fyler, 1990), as well as sickle cell disease, where imaging studies have found subtle cerebral changes related to ischemia, such as abnormalities of cerebral perfusion, brain morphology, and cerebral metabolism (Fabian & Peters, 1984; Gammal et al., 1988; Huttenlocker, Mohr, & Johns, 1984; Wiznitzer et al., 1990). Children and adolescents with these types of chronic conditions may display subtle yet significant neuropsychological deficits that are sometimes associated with learning difficulties (Brown et al., 1993; Wasserman, Wilimas, Fairclough, Mulhern, & Wang, 1991).

Although the specific cognitive correlates of these and other chronic pediatric conditions are discussed in greater depth in other chapters of this volume, here we note the potential linkages between chronic conditions that are associated with cognitive impairments and problems with children's social adjustment. In a recent, comprehensive review, Nassau and Drotar (1997) posit several specific reasons why children with CNS-related chronic health conditions would have trouble developing age-appropriate peer relations. *First*, cognitive impairments, such as below-average intelligence or specific cognitive deficits (e.g., memory or attention problems) associated with CNS-related conditions may interfere with social understanding and subsequently affect peer relations (Dodge & Price, 1994). *Second*, varying degrees of physical handicap (e.g, braces or wheelchairs that are often required for cerebral palsy or spina bifida) could limit children's ability to participate in age-appropriate peer activities (La Greca, 1990) and lead to social isolation or peer rejection. *Finally*, opportunities for peer involvement may be limited for those who must attend special education classes or participate in rehabilitation settings (see Nassau & Drotar, 1997).

Although a variety of instruments have been used to assess youngsters' social competence, available evidence points to problems in peer relations among children and adolescents with CNS-related chronic conditions (Nassau & Drotar, 1997). For example, six studies that used the Social Competence subscale of the Child Behavior Checklist (Achenbach, 1991) to evaluate the social functioning of youth with spina bifida, cerebral palsy, and other chronic physical disorders found that youth with CNS-related conditions were less socially competent than controls or normative samples (Ammerman, Van Hasselt, Hersen, & Moore, 1989; Apter et al., 1991; Wallander, Feldman, & Varni, 1989; Wallander, Varni, et al., 1989; Wallander, Hubert, & Varni, 1988; Wallander, Varni, Babani, Banis, & Wilcox, 1988). In the one study that used sociometric procedures to evaluate peer relations (Center & Ward, 1984), children with spina bifida were found to be less socially accepted than their "normal" classmates.

In addition to the above studies, Radcliffe and colleagues (Radcliffe, Bennett, Kazak, Foley, & Phillips, 1996) found that children who survived brain tumors had high maternal ratings of social problems. Similarly, work by Noll and colleagues (Noll, Ris, Davies, Bukowski, & Koontz, 1992) found that children who survived brain tumors were nominated more often for sensitive–isolated roles by their peers than were their healthy classmates. Furthermore, in an investigation of children with complex congenital heart disease, Casey and colleagues (Casey, Sykes, Craig, Power, & Mulholland, 1996) found that children with congenital heart disease were seen by parents and teachers as more withdrawn than healthy peers, with parents also viewing their children as having more social problems and engaging in fewer social activities.

Of particular interest recently has been the social functioning of children with HIV infection. Neurocognitive deficits such as inattentiveness, overactivity, impulsivity, and difficulty processing information have been related to the neurological effects of HIV (Armstrong et al., 1993; Belman, 1990; Brown & Madan-Swain, 1993). Not surprisingly, HIV-infected children with encephalopathy have been observed to display less adaptive and appropriate behavior than infected children without encephalopathy (Moss, Wolters, Brouwers, Hendricks, & Pizzo, 1996). It is likely that the social stigma associated with HIV infection may also contribute to impaired social functioning for affected children and adolescents.

In summary, available evidence suggests that youngsters with chronic physical conditions that involve cognitive difficulties are at risk for problems in their peer relations. The balance of studies cited by Nassau and Drotar (1997) in their extensive review, and several other recent works (e.g., Casey et al., 1996; Moss et al., 1996; Noll et al., 1992; Radcliffe et al., 1996), support this observation.

WHAT IS THE ROLE OF PEER RELATIONS IN THE PROCESS OF DISEASE ADAPTATION?

It is reasonable to expect that children with good peer relations and a supportive friendship network would have an easier time making positive adaptation to illness and disease than those with problematic social functioning. Indeed, children and adolescents who are isolated or anxious around peers may find the onset and course of disease much more difficult to negotiate in social contexts, and may exhibit greater resistance to disease acceptance.

In support of this position, O'Malley and colleagues (1979) found that adult survivors of childhood cancer who reported a decrease in their social contacts at the time of their cancer diagnosis and treatment were less well adjusted as adults. In a study of children and adolescents newly diagnosed with diabetes mellitus, Jacobson and colleagues (1986) found that young-sters with higher perceived social acceptance had a better adjustment to diabetes. Although youngsters' attitudes toward their disease were predom-inantly favorable, it also was the case that of the children who reported not talking with their friends about diabetes, 27% generally thought they would enjoy school more if they did not have diabetes and 35% reported at least occasionally thinking that their friends would like them better if they did not have diabetes. In a recent qualitative study of cystic fibrosis (Chris-tian & D'Auria, 1997), adolescents reported concern that their cystic fibro-sis would lead to negative reactions from peers and utilized strategies to reduce their sense of difference. These strategies included keeping secrets from peers about their condition and hiding visible differences. These find-ings suggest that children and adolescents have a high degree of concern about the impact of their disease on their peer relations.

Support from peers has emerged as a critical aspect of disease adapta-tion in several studies. For example, Varni and colleagues (Varni, Ruben-feld, Talbot, & Setoguchi, 1989) examined the role of stress and social support as predictors of depressive symptomatology among children with acquired or congenital limb deficiencies. They found that children's per-ceived support from classmates was the variable most strongly associated with low levels of depressive symptomatology even when age, sex, and stress levels were statistically controlled. In subsequent work, Varni and colleagues (Varni, Katz, Colegrove, & Dolgin, 1994) also found classmate support to be the strongest predictor of psychosocial adjustment for chil-dren with cancer.

Similarly, La Greca and colleagues (La Greca et al., 1995; La Greca & Thompson, 1998) have found that adolescents with insulin-dependent diabetes mellitus perceive their friends as providing greater support than families for "feeling good about diabetes" (La Greca, 1992; La Greca, Rap-aport, & Skyler, 1991). Wallander and Varni (1989) found that for chil-dren with various chronic diseases, those with significant social support from both family and peers showed significantly better adjustment than those with social support from only one of these sources. In addition, chronically ill children without significant support from either peers or family displayed more behavioral difficulties. These studies suggest that friends are an important source of social support for youngsters with chronic disease, and are especially important for providing a key source of acceptance and companionship.

Studies such as these have begun to explore the connections between peer functioning and disease adaptation, yet additional efforts in this direc-tion are needed to further our understanding of peer influences in chronic disease. What is especially needed is research that extends beyond cor-relational methodologies and permits a closer examination of bidirectional influences of peers and disease adaptation.

Future investigations should examine the potentially complex inter-play between peer functioning and disease adaptation. Investigations of so-cial competence among chronically ill children (Cadman et al., 1987; Lemanek, Horwitz, & Ohene-Frempong, 1994; Nassau & Drotar, 1995; Wallander et al., 1988) have found rates of social competence problems (20–30%) similar to those seen in school populations of well students (Asher & Dodge, 1986; Coie & Dodge, 1983; Dumas, Neese, Prinz, & Blechman, 1996). Children experiencing social difficulties may find that the life adjustments that accompany chronic disease are an intrusion upon their already precarious social networks, and may encounter difficulty with dis-ease adaptation. On the other hand, high levels of social competence may be a protective and facilitative factor in disease adjustment, although addi-tional research is needed to demonstrate this point.

WHAT IS THE RELATIONSHIP BETWEEN PEER RELATIONS AND DISEASE MANAGEMENT AND TREATMENT?

For many pediatric conditions, daily management will affect the child's day-to-day peer interactions, and may be a source of concern and stress to many, if not all youngsters. Peer interactions, in turn, also have the poten-tial to influence youngsters' treatment adherence. We first review the evi-dence for the role of peers in disease management, and then discuss the ways in which treatment regimens can interfere with normal peer interac-tions.

The Role of Peers in Disease Management

There is reason to believe that peer relations can strongly affect the disease management of chronically ill youngsters. For example, adolescents with cystic fibrosis have reported not adhering to prescribed medication sched-ules because they did not want to be seen as different from others or risk the loss of a romantic relationship (Christian & D'Auria, 1997). When go-ing on dates, for instance, youngsters made conscious decisions to skip medications or take several doses at once upon returning home. However, the youngsters reported that the development of close friendships that pro-vided acceptance, validation, and social support reduced their perceived need to hide visible differences.

Youngsters with diabetes mellitus have also reported that social inter-actions can interfere with their treatment adherence. For example, La Greca and Hanna (1983) interviewed children with diabetes and their mothers regarding the types of barriers they experienced for several aspects of diabetes care. Barriers reported by children and their mothers included forgetting, difficulties with planning, emotional/motivational factors, and social interference. Interestingly, children who reported more barriers were less adherent with their diabetes regimen and had worse metabolic control. Children reported a large percentage of social barriers for several aspects of diabetes care, especially dietary adherence and daily glucose testing (e.g., wanting to eat what friends are eating; not testing glucose because it interferes with peer activities). Surprisingly, mothers generally were unaware of these social barriers to diabetes care.

This type of information underscores the importance of peer influences on treatment adherence. Subsequent work also has supported a positive association between peers and disease management. La Greca and colleagues (La Greca et al., 1995; La Greca & Thompson, 1998) found that adolescents with diabetes reported that their friends provided substantial companionship support for dietary and exercise aspects of diabetes care. The encouragement and companionship of friends regarding exercise and diet increased the youngsters' adherence to these difficult aspects of chronic disease management.

Indeed, more recent findings with ethnic minority youth (Thompson, La Greca, & Shaw, 1997) revealed that African-American adolescents with diabetes who reported high levels of peer support for insulin administration, dietary adherence, and exercise had significantly better levels of metabolic control than those without such peer support. Moreover, family support for diabetes care was unrelated to metabolic control in this group of adolescents.

The preceding studies suggest that peer interactions can both interfere with as well as potentially facilitate treatment adherence. Having close friends who support the treatment regimen may have positive implications for youngsters' disease management. On the other hand, youngsters who are concerned about appearing "different" or who perceive that their regimen may call undue attention to themselves, may be likely to disregard or modify their self-care in the interests of fitting in with peers. It could also be the case that parental concerns about their child's ability to carry out management tasks successfully (e.g., self-inject insulin; take inhalants for asthma) might lead parents to restrict opportunities for overnight stays or extended outings with peers—which could detract from social interactions.

The precise nature of social influences may be determined in large part by individual child characteristics. Youngsters' typical ways of coping with social situations may reveal the manner in which they approach disease-related social situations. For example, children who are shy and easily embarrassed might be inclined to hide their disease status, or avoid daily management tasks that call attention to themselves, whereas those who are outgoing and secure in their peer interactions might even use their illness to serve as good role models of positive health practices for their friends. Further research is needed to document these notions.

Aspects of Disease Management
That Affect Peer Relations

Various aspects of disease management may interfere with the development of peer relationships. Specifically, the management of a number of diseases may require the interruption of daily activities such as school attendance, the restriction of physical activities, alterations in physical appearance, lifestyle modification, or neurocognitive impairments (La Greca, 1990). While treatments that result in CNS complications have already been discussed, the other treatment considerations mentioned are reviewed here.

Several pediatric conditions require treatment plans that result in extended *absences from school*, and consequently from peer contacts. These include hemophilia (Lineberger, 1981), childhood cancer (Lansky, Cairns, & Zwartjes, 1983; Stehbens, Kisker, & Wilson, 1983); renal disease (Fukunishi, Honda, Kamiyama, & Ito, 1993), and HIV infection (Wolters et al., 1994). For instance, children with leukemia and solid tumors typically are absent between 35 and 40 days of school during the first year of cancer treatment (Stehbens et al., 1983). It is not surprising, then, that others have found children with cancer to be less sociable and more isolated than their classmates (Noll, Bukowski, Davies, Koontz, & Kulkarni, 1993; Noll et al., 1990, 1991). Children who must forgo school and other common peer activities due to their treatment may need to develop alternative strategies for initiating and maintaining friendships (La Greca & Stone, 1985).

Treatment regimens imposing *restrictions on physical activity* include those for asthma, hemophilia, and cancer, among others. These restrictions may be due to physical limitations, or may be intended to prevent the development or worsening of symptoms, as when parents restrict children from activities out of fear of asthma attacks (Miller & Wood, 1991). In addition, investigators have suggested that school personnel or peers may actually exclude some chronically ill children from activities in which they could participate, out of erroneous assumptions about the level of physical abilities required (Turner-Henson, Holaday, Corser, Ogletree, & Swan, 1994). However, the avoidance of sports and other physical activities limits the youngster's opportunities for peer interaction and recognition. It appears that physical restrictions produce greater consequence for boys, due to the athletic, activity-oriented nature of boys' peer interactions during the school years (Hurtig & White, 1986; Lever, 1978; Noll et al., 1996; Waldrop & Halverson, 1975).

Treatment regimens that affect *physical appearance* also can put children at risk for peer relations difficulties. For example, chemotherapy treatment for cancer typically results in hair loss, and corticosteroid medications for renal transplant patients can produce puffy, cushingoid facial features. More subtle physical effects can be observed in Type I diabetes mellitus, where multiple daily insulin injections may result in needle marks and tissue atrophy around injection sites. Similarly, children receiving hemo-dialysis may have unsightly prominent veins on their arms or legs.

Available evidence on the social consequences of these types of treatment regimens suggests that youngsters must be prepared to handle teasing, questions, and comments from peers, in addition to allaying their own concerns about feeling different and unattractive. For instance, about 25% of the adult survivors of childhood cancer recalled losing friends due to peers' fears about cancer contagion or apprehension over their loss of hair or a limb (O'Malley et al., 1979). Moreover, Wasserman and colleagues (Wasserman, Thompson, Wilimas, & Fairclough, 1987) found that 40% of the adolescent and young adult survivors of Hodgkin's disease who had returned to the same schools they had attended prior to treatment reported unpleasant experiences with classmates, such as peers teasing them about their baldness or thinness, avoiding them because of possible contagion, or generally treating them as outcasts. Girls were especially likely to recall hair loss and other cancer treatment side effects as the "worst thing" about their disease. More recently, negatively perceived physical appearance has been related to increased depressive symptoms and social anxiety among pediatric cancer patients (Varni, Katz, Colegrove, & Dolgin, 1995).

In general, the social consequences of conditions or treatments that affect physical appearance may be especially acute during adolescence. Adolescents are already sensitized to their personal appearance, in part as a result of rapid changes in their physical growth and development. The picture is further complicated by typical adolescent concerns regarding sexuality. Thus, the social consequences of pediatric treatments that produce physical changes should be especially acute for this age group, although they are evident for younger children as well.

Gender is another factor that may interact with physical appearance to affect peer functioning. Treatments that limit physical growth and strength may have the most obvious effect on adolescent boys, as their social network typically places considerable emphasis on strength, physical maturation, and athletic ability (Hartup, 1970; Hunt & Solomon, 1942; Jones, 1965; Jones & Bayley, 1950; McGraw & Tolbert, 1953). In contrast, adolescent girls report greater concern about thinness, dieting, and general facial appearance than boys (Cohen, Adler, Beck, & Irwin, 1986; Huon & Brown, 1986). It is no wonder that pediatric treatments that produce hair loss, weight gain, or unwelcome facial changes appear to be especially upsetting to girls (Korsch, Fine, & Negrete, 1978; Korsch et al., 1973; Ryan & Morrow, 1986; Wasserman et al., 1987). In fact, adolescent girls' adherence to pediatric regimens that produce such physical changes may be severely compromised (Korsch et al., 1978).

Disease regimens that require *lifestyle modifications* represent another domain in which to consider peer influences. Lifestyles that involve food restrictions, special diets, complicated exercise routines, or management tasks that could disrupt or draw attention to the child or adolescent may be especially problematic. For regimens that involve lifestyle modifications, one should expect that peers will have an influence on youngsters' treatment adherence.

For example, children with insulin-dependent diabetes mellitus must balance food and exercise in a complicated manner. Children and adolescents with insulin-dependent diabetes mellitus who have friends who value good health practices will have a much easier time with their treatment regimen than those whose friends are actively involved in less healthy lifestyles (La Greca et al., 1995; La Greca & Thompson, 1998). Similarly, self-management programs for asthma teach children to escape or avoid irritants and allergens that can precipitate asthma attacks (Creer, 1987; Creer, Harm, & Marion, 1988). Inevitably, children encounter these precipitants in the course of normal peer activities, yet active efforts to avoid or escape the situation would call attention to the individual. Thus, youngsters must feel comfortable being assertive with peers for this self-management strategy to be effective, otherwise their treatment adherence may suffer.

In light of this, we may need to teach youngsters how to be comfortably assertive with peers while complying with the requirements of the medical regimen (see La Greca & Schuman, 1995). Along these lines, several programs have been designed to promote youngsters' appropriate and assertive responding in disease-related social situations (Follansbee, La Greca, & Citrin, 1983; Gross, Johnson, Wildman, & Mullett, 1981; Kaplan, Chadwick, & Schimmel, 1985; Varni, Katz, Colegrove, & Dolgin, 1993). Further research and evaluation of these kinds of social intervention approaches are indicated.

Moreover, health care professionals should examine ways that youngsters' regimens could better "fit" their lifestyle, so that youngsters do not need to make a forced choice between good self-care and peer acceptance. Food and exercise prescriptions, for example, could be adapted to the types of activities that are likely to be a part of youngsters' regular peer and social interactions.

In summary, peer relations may influence and be influenced by disease management. This complex, bidirectional interplay between social functioning and disease management warrants much closer examination. Moreover, to appreciate the interaction between the individual characteristics of the child and the manner in which disease-related social situations are negotiated, additional research is necessary.

SOCIAL INTERVENTIONS

In recent years, psychological interventions have been developed to address the psychological, developmental, and social challenges faced by children with chronic illness. In a review of the literature examining the effectiveness of such interventions, Bauman and colleagues (Bauman, Drotar, Leventhal, Perrin, & Pless, 1997) found the research to be characterized by numerous theoretical, methodological, and logistic difficulties. Nevertheless, they concluded that there have been several reported interventions that can help children and families cope with the psychological and social consequences of chronic health conditions.

Programs found to have significant efficacy have included interventions designed to promote knowledge and self-management in asthma (Evans et al., 1987; Parcel, Nader, & Tiernan, 1980; Perrin, Maclean, Gortmaker, & Asher, 1992), programs facilitating reintegration of children with cancer in the school setting (Katz, Rubinstein, Hubert, & Blew, 1988; Varni et al., 1993), and interventions providing support and coordination of care among parents of children with a range of conditions (Stein & Jessop, 1984, 1991). These programs provide intervention models that may be applicable in other settings. Although these programs most often made an impact on youngsters' psychiatric or behavioral symptoms, some also demonstrated positive effects on measures of self-efficacy and social competence.

One promising program provided social skills training to children newly diagnosed with cancer (Katz & Varni, 1993; Varni et al., 1993). The training included instruction in social cognitive problem solving, assertiveness training, and handling teasing and name calling associated with changes in physical appearance. The program was presented in three individual 60-minute sessions and also incorporated videotaped modeling by peers, modeling by the instructor, behavioral rehearsal by the child, performance feedback, program generalization and maintenance through home practice and parental participation, relaxation techniques, and follow-up booster sessions. Children receiving this social skills training evidenced fewer behavioral problems and greater classmate and teacher social support and school competence at follow-up than children receiving a standard school reintegration intervention.

Unfortunately, few of the programs providing psychosocial interventions for children with chronic illness have been systematically evaluated (Bauman et al., 1997). Clearly, more methodologically sound evaluations of interventions are needed, particularly given the challenges faced by children and their families. Particularly needed are programs guided by theoretical models and which target the multiple dimensions of psychosocial adjustment (see La Greca & Varni, 1993).

CONCLUSIONS

Several conclusions can be drawn from the literature reviewed on the social correlates of pediatric chronic illness. First, chronic disease appears to be a risk factor for adjustment problems, particularly within the domain of peer relations. Second, chronic illness and treatment may impact peer relations through such factors as the interruption of normal daily activities, restrictions on physical activities, altered physical appearance, and lifestyle modification. In addition, neurocognitive impairments associated with chronic disease appear to increase the risk of peer relationship problems. Third, peer relations play an important role in disease adaptation and management. Peers may be a source of support and acceptance, facilitating adaptation and adherence. Conversely, concern about peer acceptance may lead to poor treatment adherence or interfere with disease adaptation. Finally, intervention programs are being developed to address the psychosocial challenges faced by children with chronic disease, though as yet few have been systematically evaluated.

Future research should continue to consider various dimensions of peer functioning (i.e., social reputation, friendships, loneliness, etc.) and to examine the specific characteristics of disease that may put children at risk for peer relationship difficulties. Investigations should extend beyond correlational methodologies for a closer examination of the bidirectional influences of peers and disease adaptation and management. Future studies also should explore the role of individual child characteristics, including behavioral functioning and personal style, in determining the nature of social influences on disease management. More work also is needed in the development and evaluation of effective interventions to facilitate positive social adjustment in children with chronic disease, particularly regarding appropriate and assertive responding in disease-related social situations.

Investigations in this area will no doubt continue to support the importance of peer relations to the adjustment and well-being of children with chronic disease. Health care professionals have long recognized the importance of the family system to children's disease adaptation. It is now clear that *all* the systems which affect the child, and which are affected by the child's illness, must be considered in order to understand and facilitate the disease adaptation process.

REFERENCES

Achenbach, T. M. (1991). *Manual for the Child Behavior Checklist/4–18 and 1991 Profile*. Burlington: University of Vermont, Department of Psychiatry.

Ammerman, R. T., Van Hasselt, V. B., Hersen, M., & Moore, L. E. (1989). Assessment of social skills in visually impaired adolescents and their parents. *Behavioral Assessment, 11*, 327–351.

Apter, A., Aviv, A., Kamner, Y., Weizman, A., Lehrman, P., & Tyano, S. (1991). Behavioral profile and social competence in temporal lobe epilepsy of adolescence. *Journal of the American Academy of Child and Adolescent Psychiatry, 30*, 887–892.

Armstrong, F. D., Seidel, J. F., & Swales, T. P. (1993). Pediatric HIV infection: A neuropsychological and educational challenge. *Journal of Learning Disabilities, 26*, 92–103.

Asher, S. R., & Dodge, K. A. (1986). Identifying children who are rejected by their peers. *Developmental Psychology, 22*, 444–449.

Baum, F., & Forehand, R. (1984). Social factors associated with adolescent obesity. *Journal of Pediatric Psychology, 9*, 293–302.

Bauman, L. J., Drotar, D., Leventhal, J. M., Perrin, E. C., & Pless, I. B. (1997). A review of psychosocial interventions for children with chronic health conditions. *Pediatrics, 100*, 244–251.

Belman, A. L. (1990). Neurologic syndromes associated with symptomatic human immunodeficiency virus infection in infants and children. In P. B. Kozlowski, D. A. Snider, P. M. Vietze, & H. M. Wisniewski (Eds.), *Brain in pediatric AIDS* (pp. 45–63). Basel, Switzerland: S. Karger.

Brouwers, P., Belman, A. L., & Epstein, L. G. (1991). Central nervous system involvement: Manifestations and evaluation. In P. A. Pizzo & C. M. Wilfert (Eds.), *Pediatric AIDS: The challenge of HIV infection in infants, children and adolescents* (pp. 318–335). Baltimore: Williams & Wilkins.

Brown, J. M., O'Keefe, J., Sanders, S. H., & Baker, B. (1986). Developmental changes in children's cognition to stressful and painful situations. *Journal of Pediatric Psychology, 11*, 343–358.

Brown, R. T., Buchanan, I., Doepke, K., Eckman, J. R., Baldwin, K., Goonan, B., & Schoenherr, S. (1993). Cognitive and academic functioning in children with sickle cell disease. *Journal of Clinical Child Psychology, 22*, 207–218.

Brown, R. T., & Madan-Swain, A. (1993). Cognitive, neuropsychological, and academic sequelae in children with leukemia. *Journal of Learning Disabilities, 26*, 74–90.

Bull, R., & Rumsey, N. (1988). *The social psychology of facial appearance.* New York: Springer-Verlag.

Cadman, D., Boyle, M., Sazatmari, P., & Offord, D. R. (1987). Chronic Illness, disability, and mental and social well-being: Findings of the Ontario Child Health Study. *Pediatrics, 79*, 805–813.

Casey, F. A., Sykes, D. H., Craig, B. G., Power, R., & Mulholland, H. C. (1996). Behavioral adjustment of children with surgically palliated complex congenital heart disease. *Journal of Pediatric Psychology, 21*, 335–352.

Center, Y., & Ward, J. (1984). Integration of mildly handicapped cerebral palsied children into regular schools. *Exceptional Child, 31*, 104–113.

Christian, B. J., & D'Auria, J. P. (1997). The child's eye: Memories of growing up with cystic fibrosis. *Journal of Pediatric Nursing, 12*, 3–12.

Cohen, M., Adler, N., Beck, A., & Irwin, C. E., Jr. (1986). Parental reactions to the onset of adolescence. *Journal of Adolescent Health Care, 7*, 101–106.

Cohen, S., & Wills, T. (1985). Stress, social support, and the buffering hypothesis. *Psychological Bulletin, 98*, 310–357.

Coie, J. D., & Dodge, K. A. (1983). Continuities and changes in children's sociometric status: A five year longitudinal study. *Merrill–Palmer Quarterly, 29*, 261–282.

Cowen, E. L., Pederson, A., Babian, H., Izzo, L. D., & Trost, M. D. (1973). Long-term follow-up of early detected vulnerable children. *Journal of Consulting and Clinical Psychology, 41*, 438–446.

Creer, T. L. (1987). Living with asthma: Replications and extensions. *Health Education Quarterly, 14,* 319–331.

Creer, T. L., Harm, D. L., & Marion, R. J. (1988). Childhood asthma. In D. K. Routh (Ed.), *Handbook of pediatric psychology* (pp. 162–189). New York: Guilford Press.

DeMaso, D. R., Beardslee, W. R., Silbert, A. R., & Fyler, D. C. (1990). Psychological functioning in children with cyanotic heart defects. *Journal of Developmental and Behavioral Pediatrics, 11,* 289–294.

Dodge, K. A., & Price, J. M. (1994). On the relation between social information processing and socially competent behavior in early school age children. *Monographs of the Society for Research in Child Development, 51*(2, Serial No. 213).

Donnelly, J. E., Donnelly, W. J., & Thong, Y. H. (1987). Parental perceptions and attitudes toward asthma and its treatment: A controlled study. *Social Science Medicine, 24,* 431- 437.

Dorner, S. (1976). Adolescents with spinal bifida: How they see their situation. *Archives of Disease in Childhood, 51,* 439–444.

Drotar, D. (1981). Psychological perspective in chronic childhood illness. *Journal of Pediatric Psychology, 6,* 211–228.

Drotar, D., Doershuk, C. F., Stern, R. C., Boat, T. F., Boyer, W., & Matthews, L. (1981). Psychosocial functioning of children with cystic fibrosis. *Pediatrics, 67,* 338–343.

Dumas, J. E., Neese, D. E., Prinz, R. J., & Blechman, E. A. (1996). Short-term stability of aggression, peer rejection, and depressive symptoms in middle childhood. *Journal of Abnormal Child Psychology, 24,* 105–119.

Dunn, J., & McGuire, S. (1992). Sibling and peer relationships in childhood. *Journal of Child Psychology and Psychiatry, 33,* 67–105.

Evans, R. E., Mullally, D. I., Wilson, R. W., Gergen, R. J., Rosenberg, H. M., Grauman, J. S., Edmonds, F. C., & Feinleib, M. (1987). National trends in the morbidity and mortality of asthma in the USA: Prevalence, hospitalization, and death from asthma over two decades: 1965–1984. *Chest, 91,* 655–745.

Fabian, R. H., & Peters, B. H. (1984). Neurological complications of hemoglobin SC disease. *Archives of Neurology, 41,* 289–292.

Fisher, E. B. J., Delamater, A. M., Bertelson, A. D., & Kirkley, B. G. (1982). Psychological factors in diabetes and its treatment. *Journal of Consulting and Clinical Psychology, 50,* 993–1003.

Follansbee, D. J., La Greca, A. M., & Citrin, W. S. (1983). Coping skills training for adolescents with diabetes. *Diabetes, 32*(Suppl. 1), A147.

Fukunishi, I., Honda, M., Kamiyama, Y., & Ito, H. (1993). Influence of mothers on school adjustment of continuous ambulatory peritoneal dialysis children. *Peritoneal Dialysis International, 13,* 232–235.

Gammal, T. E., Adams, R. J., Nichols, F. T., McKie, V., Milner, P., McKie, K., & Brooks, B. S. (1988). Investigation of cerebrovascular disease in sickle cell patients with MRI and CT. *American Journal of Neuroradiology, 7,* 1043–1049.

Gordon, M., Crouthamel, C., Post, E. M., & Richman, R. A. (1982). Psychosocial aspects of constitutional short stature: Social competence, behavior problems, self-esteem, and family functioning. *Journal of Pediatrics, 101*(477), 480.

Graetz, B., & Shute, R. (1995). Assessment of peer relationships in children with asthma. *Journal of Pediatric Psychology, 20,* 205–216.

Gross, A. M., Johnson, W. G., Wildman, H. E., & Mullett, M. (1981). Coping skills training with insulin-dependent preadolescent diabetics. *Child Behavior Therapy, 4,* 141–153.

Hartup, W. W. (1970). Peer interaction and social organization. In P. H. Mussen (Ed.), *Manual of child psychology* (Vol. 2, pp. 361–456). New York: Wiley.

Hartup, W. W. (1996). The company they keep: Friendships and their developmental significance. *Child Development, 67,* 1–13.

Hunt, J., & Solomon, R. L. (1942). The stability and some correlates of group-status in a summer camp group of young boys. *American Journal of Psychology, 55,* 33–45.

Huon, G. F., & Brown, L. B. (1986). Attitude correlates of weight control among secondary school boys and girls. *Journal of Adolescent Health Care, 7,* 178–182.

Hurtig, A. L., & White, L. S. (1986). Psychosocial adjustment in children and adolescents with sickle cell disease. *Journal of Pediatric Psychology, 11,* 411–427.

Huttenlocker, P. R., Mohr, J. W., & Johns, L. (1984). Cerebral blood flow in sickle cell cerebrovascular disease. *Pediatrics, 73,* 615–621.

Israel, A. C., & Shapiro, L. S. (1985). Behavior problems of obese children enrolling in a weight reduction program. *Journal of Pediatric Psychology, 10,* 449–460.

Jacobson, A. M., Hauser, S. T., Wertlieb, D., Wolfsdorf, J. I., Orleans, J., & Vieyra, M. (1986). Psychological adjustment of children with recently diagnosed diabetes mellitus. *Diabetes Care, 9,* 323–329.

Johnson, S. B. (1980). Psychosocial factors in juvenile diabetes: A review. *Journal of Behavioral Medicine, 3,* 95–116.

Jones, M. C. (1965). Psychological correlates of somatic development. *Child Development, 36,* 899–911.

Jones, M. C., & Bayley, N. (1950). Physical maturing among boys as related to behavior. *Journal of Educational Psychology, 41,* 129–148.

Kaplan, R. M., Chadwick, M. W., & Schimmel, L. E. (1985). Social learning intervention to promote metabolic control in Type 1 diabetes mellitus: Pilot experimental results. *Diabetes Care, 8,* 152–155.

Kapp-Simon, K. A., & McGuire, D. E. (1997). Observed social interaction patterns in adolescents with and without craniofacial conditions. *Cleft Palate–Craniofacial Journal, 34,* 380–384.

Kapp-Simon, K. A., Simon, D. J., & Kristovich, S. (1992). Self-perception, social skills, adjustment, and inhibition in young adolescents with craniofacial anomalies. *Cleft Palate–Craniofacial Journal, 29,* 352–356.

Katz, E. R., Rubinstein, C. L., Hubert, N. C., & Blew, A. (1988). School and social reintegration of children with cancer. *Journal of Psychosocial Oncology, 6,* 123–140.

Katz, E. R., & Varni, J. W. (1993). Social support and social cognitive problem-solving in children with newly diagnosed cancer. *Cancer, 71,* 3314–3319.

Kellerman, J., Zelter, L., Ellenberg, L., Dash, J., & Rigler, D. (1980). Psychological effects of illness in adolescents: I. Anxiety, self-esteem, and perception of control. *Journal of Pediatrics, 97,* 126–131.

Korsch, B. M., Fine, R. N., & Negrete, V. F. (1978). Noncompliance in children with renal transplants. *Pediatrics, 61,* 872–876.

Korsch, B. M., Hegrete, V. F., Gardner, J. E., Weinstock, C. L., Mercer, A. S., Grushkin, C. M., & Fine, R. N. (1973). Kidney transplantation in children:

Psychosocial follow- up study on child and family. *Journal of Pediatrics, 83,* 399–408.

Kumar, S., Powers, D., Allen, J., & Haywood, L. J. (1976). Anxiety, self-concept, and personal and social adjustments in children with sickle cell anemia. *Journal of Pediatrics, 88,* 859- 863.

Kupersmidt, J. B., Coie, J. D., & Dodge, K. A. (1990). The role of poor peer relationships in the development of disorder. In S. R. Asher & J. D. Coie (Eds.), *Peer rejection in childhood* (pp. 274–305). Cambridge: Cambridge University Press.

La Greca, A. M. (1990). Social consequences of pediatric conditions: Fertile area for future investigation and intervention. *Journal of Pediatric Psychology, 15,* 285–307.

La Greca, A. M. (1992). Peer influences in pediatric chronic illness: An update. *Journal of Pediatric Psychology, 17,* 775–784.

La Greca, A. M., Auslander, W. F., Greco, P., Spetter, D., Fisher, E. B., & Santiago, J. V. (1995). I get by with a little help from my family and friends: Adolescents' support for diabetes care. *Journal of Pediatric Psychology, 20,* 449–476.

La Greca, A. M., & Hanna, N. (1983). Diabetes related health beliefs in children and their mothers: Implications for treatment. *Diabetes, 32*(Suppl. 1), 66.

La Greca, A. M., Rapaport, W. S., & Skyler, J. S. (1991). Emotions: A critical factor in diabetic control. In M. B. Davidson (Ed.), *Diabetes mellitus* (3rd ed., pp. 327–354). New York: Churchill Livingstone.

La Greca, A. M., & Schuman, W. B. (1995). Adherence to prescribed medical regimens. In M. C. Roberts (Ed.), *Handbook of pediatric psychology* (2nd ed., pp. 55–83). New York: Guilford Press.

La Greca, A. M., & Stone, W. L. (1985). Behavioral pediatrics. In N. Schneiderman & J. T. Tapp (Eds.), *Behavioral medicine: The biopsychosocial approach* (pp. 255–291). Hillsdale, NJ: Erlbaum.

La Greca, A. M., & Thompson, K. (1998). Family and friend support for adolescents with diabetes. *Analise Psicologica, 16,* 101–113.

La Greca, A. M., & Varni, J. W. (1993). Interventions in pediatric psychology: A look toward the future [editorial]. *Journal of Pediatric Psychology, 18,* 667–679.

Lansky, S. B., Cairns, N. U., & Zwartjes, W. (1983). School attendance among children with cancer: A report from two centers. *Journal of Psychosocial Oncology, 1,* 75–82.

Lavigne, J. V., & Faier-Routman, J. (1992). Psychological adjustment to pediatric physical disorders: A meta-analytic review. *Journal of Pediatric Psychology, 17,* 133–157.

Lee, P. D., & Rosenfeld, R. G. (1987). Psychosocial correlates of short stature and delayed puberty. *Pediatric Clinics of North America, 34,* 851–863.

Lemanek, K. L., Horwitz, W., & Ohene-Frempong, K. (1994). A multiperspective investigation of social competence in children with sickle cell disease. *Journal of Pediatric Psychology, 19,* 443–456.

Lever, J. (1978). Sex differences in the complexity of children's play and games. *American Sociological Review, 43,* 471–483.

Lineberger, H. P. (1981). Social characteristics of hemophilia clinic population. *General Hospital Psychiatry, 3,* 157–163.

McAndrew, I. (1978). Adolescents and young people with spina bifida. *Developmental Medicine and Child Neurology, 21,* 619–629.

McGraw, L. W., & Tolbert, J. W. (1953). Sociometric status and athletic ability of junior high school boys. *Research Quarterly, 24*, 72–80.

Miller, B. D., & Wood, B. I. (1991). Childhood asthma in interaction with family, school and peer systems. A developmental model for primary care. *Journal of Asthma, 28*, 405–414.

Morgan, S. A., & Jackson, J. (1986). Psychological and social concomitants of sickle cell anemia in adolescents. *Journal of Pediatric Psychology, 11*, 429–440.

Moss, H. A., Wolters, P. L., Brouwers, P., Hendricks, M. L., & Pizzo, P. A. (1996). Impairment of expressive behavior in pediatric HIV-infected patients with evidence of CNS disease. *Journal of Pediatric Psychology, 21*, 379–400.

Nassau, J. H., & Drotar, D. (1995). Social competence in children with IDDM and asthma: Child, teacher, and parent reports of children's social adjustment, social performance, and social skills. *Journal of Pediatric Psychology, 20*, 187–204.

Nassau, J. H., & Drotar, D. (1997). Social competence among children with central nervous system-related chronic health conditions: A review. *Journal of Pediatric Psychology, 22*, 771–793.

Nocon, A. (1991). Social and emotional impact of childhood asthma. *Archives of Disease in Children, 66*, 458–460.

Noll, R. B., Bukowski, W. M., Davies, W. H., Koontz, K., & Kulkarni, R. (1993). Adjustment in the peer system of adolescents with cancer: A two year study. *Journal of Pediatric Psychology, 18*, 351–364.

Noll, R. B., Bukowski, W. M., Rogosch, F. A., LeRoy, S., & Kulkarni, R. (1990). Social interactions between children with cancer and their peers: Teacher ratings. *Journal of Pediatric Psychology, 15*, 43–56.

Noll, R. B., LeRoy, S., Bukowski, W. M., Rogosch, F. A., & Kulkarni, R. (1991). Peer relationships and adjustment of children with cancer. *Journal of Pediatric Psychology, 16*, 307- 326.

Noll, R. B., Ris, M. D., Davies, W. H., Bukowski, W. M., & Koontz, K. (1992). Social interactions between children with cancer or sickle cell disease and their peers: Teacher ratings. *Journal of Developmental and Behavioral Pediatrics, 13*, 187–193.

Noll, R. B., Vannatta, K., Koontz, K., Kalinyak, K., Bukowski, W. M., & Davies, W. H. (1996). Peer relationships and emotional well-being of youngsters with sickle cell disease. *Child Development, 67*, 423–436.

O'Malley, J. E., Koocher, G., Foster, D., & Slavin, L. (1979). Psychological sequelae of surviving childhood cancer. *American Journal of Orthopsychiatry, 49*, 608–616.

Padur, J. S., Rapoff, M. A., Houston, B. K., Barnard, M., Danovsky, M., Olson, N. Y., Moore, W. V., Vats, T. S., & Lieberman, B. (1995). Psychosocial adjustment and the role of functional status for children with asthma. *Journal of Asthma, 32*, 345–353.

Parcel, G. S., Nader, P. R., & Tiernan, K. (1980). A health education program for children with asthma. *Journal of Developmental and Behavioral Pediatrics, 1*, 128–132.

Parker, J. G., & Asher, S. R. (1987). Peer relations and later personal adjustment: Are low-accepted children at risk? *Psychological Bulletin, 102*, 357–389.

Perrin, J. M., Maclean, W. E., Gortmaker, S. L., & Asher, K. A. (1992). Improving the psychological status of children with asthma: A randomized controlled trial. *Journal of Developmental and Behavioral Pediatrics, 1992*, 241–247.

Pless, I. B., & Nolan, T. (1991). Revision, replication and neglect: Research on maladjustment in chronic illness. *Journal of Child Psychology and Psychiatry, 32,* 347–365.

Pope, A. W., & Ward, J. (1997a). Factors associated with peer social competence in preadolescents with craniofacial anomalies. *Journal of Pediatric Psychology, 22,* 455–469.

Pope, A. W., & Ward, J. (1997b). Self-perceived facial appearance and psychosocial adjustment in preadolescents with craniofacial anomalies. *Cleft Palate–Craniofacial Journal, 34,* 396–401.

Radcliffe, J., Bennett, D., Kazak, A. E., Foley, B., & Phillips, P. C. (1996). Adjustment in childhood brain tumor survival: Child, mother, and teacher report. *Journal of Pediatric Psychology, 21,* 529–539.

Ryan, C. M., & Morrow, L. A. (1986). Self-esteem in diabetic adolescents: Relationship between age at onset and gender. *Journal of Consulting and Clinical Psychology, 54,* 730–731.

Shepherd, C., & Hosking, G. (1989). Epilepsy in schoolchildren with intellectual impairment in Sheffield: The size and nature of the problem and the implications for service provision. *Journal of Mental Deficiency Research, 33,* 511–514.

Speight, A. N. P., Lee, D. A., & Hey, E. N. (1983). Underdiagnosis and undertreatment of asthma in childhood. *British Medicine Journal, 286,* 1253–1256.

Spirito, A., DeLawyer, D., & Stark, L. (1991). Peer relations and social adjustment of chronically ill children and adolescents. *Clinical Psychology Review, 11,* 539–564.

Stehbens, J. A., Kisker, C. T., & Wilson, B. K. (1983). School behavior and attendance during the first year of treatment for childhood cancer. *Psychology in the Schools, 20,* 223–228.

Stein, R. E. K., & Jessop, D. J. (1984). Does pediatric home care make a difference for children with chronic illness?: Findings from the pediatric ambulatory care treatment study. *Pediatrics, 73,* 845–853.

Stein, R. E. K., & Jessop, D. J. (1991). Long term effects of a pediatric home care program. *Pediatrics, 88,* 490–496.

Strauss, C. C., Smith, K., Frame, C., & Forehand, R. (1985). Personal and interpersonal characteristics associated with childhood obesity. *Journal of Pediatric Psychology, 10,* 337–343.

Tavormina, J. B., Kastner, L. S., Slater, P. M., & Watt, S. L. (1976). Chronically ill children: A psychologically and emotionally deviant population? *Journal of Abnormal Child Psychology, 4,* 99–110.

Thompson, K. M., La Greca, A. M., & Shaw, K. H. (1997). *Ethnic differences in family and friend support adolescents with diabetes.* Unpublished manuscript, University of Miami, Coral Gables, FL.

Turner-Henson, A., Holaday, B., Corser, N., Ogletree, G., & Swan, J. H. (1994). The experiences of discrimination: Challenges for chronically ill children. *Pediatric Nursing, 20,* 571–577.

Varni, J. W. (1983). *Clinical behavioral pediatrics: An interdisciplinary biobehavioral approach.* New York: Pergamon Press.

Varni, J. W., Katz, E. R., Colegrove, R., & Dolgin, M. (1993). The impact of social skills training on the adjustment of children with newly diagnosed cancer. *Journal of Pediatric Psychology, 18,* 751–768.

Varni, J. W., Katz, E. R., Colegrove, R., & Dolgin, M. (1994). Perceived social support and adjustment of children with newly diagnosed cancer. *Journal of Developmental and Behavioral Pediatrics, 15,* 20–26.

Varni, J. W., Katz, E. R., Colegrove, R., & Dolgin, M. (1995). Perceived physical appearance and adjustment of children with newly diagnosed cancer: a path analytic model. *Journal of Behavioral Medicine, 18,* 261–278.

Varni, J. W., Rubenfeld, L. A., Talbot, D., & Setoguchi, Y. (1989). Determination of self-esteem in children with congenital/acquired limb deficiencies. *Journal of Developmental and Behavioral Pediatrics, 10,* 13–16.

Varni, J. W., & Wallander, J. L. (1988). Pediatric chronic disabilities: Hemophilia and spina bifida as examples. In D. K. Routh (Ed.), *Handbook of pediatric psychology* (pp. 190–221). New York: Guilford Press.

Waldrop, M. F., & Halverson, C. F. (1975). Intensive and extensive peer behavior: Longitudinal and cross-sectional analyses. *Child Development, 46,* 19–26.

Wallander, J. L., Feldman, W. S., & Varni, J. W. (1989). Physical status and psychosocial adjustment in children with spina bifida. *Journal of Pediatric Psychology, 14,* 89–102.

Wallander, J. L., Hubert, N. C., & Varni, J. W. (1988). Child and maternal temperament characteristics, goodness of fit, and adjustment in physically handicapped children. *Journal of Clinical Child Psychology, 17,* 336–344.

Wallander, J. L., & Varni, J. W. (1989). Social support and adjustment in chronically ill and handicapped children. *American Journal of Community Psychology, 17,* 185–201.

Wallander, J. L., Varni, J. W., Babini, L., Banis, H. T., DeHaan, C. B., & Wilcox, K. T. (1989). Disability parameters, chronic strain, and adaptation of physically handicapped children and their mothers. *Journal of Pediatric Psychology, 14,* 23–42.

Wallander, J. L., Varni, J. W., Babani, L., Banis, H. T., & Wilcox, K. T. (1988). Children with chronic physical disorders: Maternal reports of their psychological adjustment. *Journal of Pediatric Psychology, 13,* 197–212.

Wasserman, A. L., Thompson, E. I., Wilimas, J. A., & Fairclough, D. L. (1987). The psychological status of survivors of childhood/adolescent Hodgkin's disease. *American Journal of Diseases of Children, 141,* 626–631.

Wasserman, A. L., Wilimas, J. A., Fairclough, D. L., Mulhern, R. K., & Wang, W. (1991). Subtle neuropsychological deficits in children with sickle cell disease. *American Journal of Pediatric Hematology/Oncology, 13,* 14–20.

Wasserstein, S., & La Greca, A. M. (1996). Can peer support buffer against behavioral consequences of parental discord? *Journal of Clinical Child Psychology, 25,* 177–182.

Wiznitzer, M., Ruggieri, P. M., Masaryk, T. J., Ross, J. S., Modic, M. T., & Berman, B. (1990). Diagnosis of cerebral vascular disease in sickle cell anemia patients by magnetic resonance angiography. *Journal of Pediatrics, 117,* 551–555.

Wolman, C., Resnick, M. D., Harris, L. J., & Blum, R. W. (1994). Emotional well-being among adolescents with and without chronic conditions. *Journal of Adolescent Health, 15,* 199–204.

Wolters, P. L., Brouwers, P., Moss, H. A., & Pizzo, P. A. (1994). Adaptive behavior of children with symptomatic HIV infection before and after zidovudine therapy. *Journal of Pediatric Psychology, 19,* 47–61.

CHAPTER FOURTEEN

Returning to School
after a Serious Illness
or Injury

AVI MADAN-SWAIN
LAURA D. FREDRICK
JAN L. WALLANDER

It has been estimated that one in every five children under 18 years of age (12 million nationwide) has a chronic illness and that 5% are affected by either a severe disorder or multiple disorders (Newacheck & Stoddard, 1994). In recent years dramatic medical advances in the treatment of chronic illness in children and adolescents have increased both the life expectancy and functional capability of these youth. With the medical management gains, unfortunately, have emerged new problems regarding the reintegration of these youth into school settings. Adjustment issues in school can be the result of direct (primary) effects of the illness or its treatment, including central nervous system (CNS) sequelae, or a function of indirect (secondary) consequences of the illness such as fatigue, absenteeism, psychological stress, or distress (Thompson & Gustafson, 1996).

At some time during their school careers many children and adolescents diagnosed with a chronic illness will require some type of special consideration by the school. Although most of these youth will not require specific special education placement, many will need coordinated school interventions (e.g., regular classroom accommodations with frequent breaks because of fatigue, modification of classroom assignments and homework) to maximize attendance and thereby facilitate educational and social growth (Sexson & Madan-Swain, 1993, 1995). The process of reintegrating the child or adolescent into school after a prolonged absence and monitoring adequate attendance and achievement requires intensive cooperative efforts among health care providers, school personnel, the child or adolescent, and the family (Sexson & Madan-Swain, 1993, 1995).

This chapter will review literature regarding the potential impact a chronic illness may have on the child or adolescent's school attendance and performance. Because the course of an illness likely interacts with school reentry, Rolland's (1990) chronic illness typology is selected for this chapter to review specific chronic conditions. According to Rolland (1990), chronic illness follows three courses: progressive (i.e., disease that is generally continually symptomatic or progressive in severity, e.g., cystic fibrosis, spina bifida); constant (i.e., where an initial event occurs and after an initial period of recovery the chronic phase is characterized by some clear-cut deficit or limitation in function, e.g., traumatic brain injury, spinal cord injury, burns); and relapsing (i.e., the illness follows an episodic course, alternating periods of stability and low levels of symptoms with periods of symptom exacerbation, e.g., asthma, colitis, cancers in remission, sickle cell disease, epilepsy). The course of a chronic illness is further complicated by the degree of incapacitation imposed on the child or adolescent and the outcome (i.e., fatal, possibly fatal [contributing to a shortened lifespan], and nonfatal). Based on the available literature, chronic illnesses and injuries that follow a constant, progressive, or relapsing course are selected in order to examine the interaction of the chronic illness and school reentry. Both direct and indirect adjustment correlates are outlined for a variety of chronic illnesses. Phases of school reentry are outlined, along with the tasks to be accomplished. Finally, suggestions for future research directions in the field of school reentry are presented.

IMPACT OF CHRONIC ILLNESS
Epidemiological Studies

Increased risk for school performance difficulties in children with chronic illness has been well documented (Sexson & Madan-Swain, 1995). One of the earliest and most comprehensive studies examining the educational consequences of physical illness in school-age children was the Isle of Wight study (Rutter, Tizard, & Whitmore, 1970), whose purpose was to examine both direct and indirect consequences of chronic illness. The sample included two groups of children: those with brain-related medical conditions and those without documented brain-related medical conditions. Results revealed below-average intellectual functioning for the children with brain-related illnesses and significantly delayed reading achievement, frequently requiring special education services. In contrast, intellectual functioning of the group of children with non-brain-related illnesses was normally distributed and similar to that of children in the general population. While the youth in this second group also evidenced reading problems, they were nonetheless able to function within regular class placement. Findings from this investigation were interpreted to suggest that the intellectual and academic difficulties experienced by children with brain-related illnesses were likely the direct consequence of the medical illness, while the school-related difficulties experienced by children with non-brain-related illnesses are more likely the indirect consequences of the medical condition (e.g., absenteeism).

Similarly, results from the Ontario Child Health Study, another large-scale investigation examining school performance of children with chronic illness, revealed that almost half of the children classified as having both a chronic illness and a disability had repeated a grade or were receiving remedial educational services, relative to 15% of children diagnosed with a chronic illness but without a disability, and 12% of healthy children (Cadman, Boyle, Szatmari, & Offord, 1987). A subsequent epidemiological study (Gortmaker, Walker, Weitzman, & Sobel, 1990) examining the psychological risk in children with physical illness revealed that children with chronic health conditions were at significantly higher risk for grade failure and special education placement relative to their healthy peers. However, children with chronic illness were not at increased risk for suspension or expulsion. Findings from both these investigations are limited because of their reliance on subjective reports from parents regarding school performance, the lack of objective measures to assess academic achievement (e.g., school records, standardized achievement testing), and the lack of specificity pertaining to brain involvement.

There also have been some epidemiological studies of academic and adjustment difficulties experienced by children with specific types of chronic illness. For example, using the 1988 U.S. National Health Interview Survey on Child Health, Fowler and associates (Fowler, Davenport, & Garg, 1992) examined school functioning in children diagnosed with asthma. When compared to their healthy peers, findings indicated that children diagnosed with asthma had slightly higher rates of grade failure but similar rates of suspension or expulsion. Furthermore, children with asthma were rated by their parents as having twice the rate of learning disabilities relative to their healthy counterparts. Additionally, differences in risk for school problems emerged as a function of demographic and illness variables. Among families from low socioeconomic backgrounds, children with asthma had twice the risk for grade failure than did healthy children. Again, consistent with the general study of chronic illness (Gortmaker et al., 1990), objective indexes of school performance were not obtained, and the findings primarily were based on parental report.

Clinical Studies

Interest in studying the school performance of adolescents with chronic illness is reflected in the growing literature in this area. For example, Howe, Feinstein, Reiss, Molock, and Berger (1993) evaluated school performance, employing standard achievement tests among three groups of adolescents: those diagnosed with brain-related chronic physical illness (e.g., cerebral palsy), those diagnosed with non-brain-related chronic illness (e.g., cystic fibrosis), and a healthy comparison group. Results indicated that both groups of chronically ill adolescents scored significantly below the healthy comparison group on school achievement. Further, adolescents with brain-related illnesses scored significantly lower than the healthy group in mathematics, reading, and general knowledge, whereas the adolescents with the non-brain-related illnesses scored significantly lower than the healthy peers only in mathematics.

In a similar investigation, Fowler, Johnson, and Atkinson (1985) examined school functioning through utilization of objective school data for a large sample of children diagnosed with a variety of chronic health conditions. Children with chronic health conditions scored significantly lower than their healthy counterparts, although their scores were well within the average range. In addition, approximately one-quarter of the chronic illness sample had repeated a grade, and nearly one-third were receiving special education services. Children with seizure disorders, sickle cell disease, and spina bifida were especially at risk for repeating a grade, poor scores on standardized achievement tests, and special education placement. Race and socioeconomic background were found to account for a considerable amount of the variance in achievement scores for the chronic illness group.

Summary

Taken together, the results from the epidemiological and clinical investigations clearly indicate that some children and adolescents with chronic illness are at increased risk for school problems. This risk is particularly apparent in children who experience cognitive impairment as a direct consequence of the illness, such as those with sickle cell disease who suffer strokes, or as a consequence of the treatment, such as side effects of radiation or chemotherapy for the treatment of leukemia. On occasion the cognitive impairment results in major performance difficulties, such as those experienced by children with traumatic brain injury.

While some children with chronic illness do not experience cognitive impairment per se, nonetheless they fail to maximize their potential relative to their healthy peers (Sexson & Madan-Swain, 1993). This may be explained best by mediating processes such as absenteeism, emotional difficulties reflected in depression or anxiety, temporary illness or treatment-related effects such as problems with attention, fatigue, and lethargy, and functional limitations on activity. In addition, attitudes of parents and school personnel toward the school reentry process also may contribute to these learning problems.

CORRELATES OF SCHOOL ADJUSTMENT

Given the considerable evidence of increased risk for school problems in children with chronic illness, we now examine the factors that contribute to this increased risk. First, we examine the direct (primary) effects of the illness on school functioning: neurocognitive sequelae of the illness and the iatrogenic CNS effects of the treatment. We specifically examine the learning, academic, and behavioral problems of children diagnosed with chronic illnesses that follow a constant (e.g., spina bifida, traumatic brain injury), progressive (e.g., juvenile insulin-dependent diabetes mellitus), or relapsing (e.g., epilepsy, sickle cell disease, asthma, childhood cancer) course, with emphasis on brain-related chronic illnesses or injuries. Second, we examine the indirect (secondary) consequences of illness on school functioning: absenteeism, psychological factors associated with chronic illness, and peer relations.

Neurocognitive Sequelae of Illness

Within the past several years there has been a growing body of research examining the neurocognitive profile of children diagnosed with insulin-dependent diabetes mellitus. While there is little consensus in the literature regarding specific neurocognitive deficits, an association has been demonstrated between visual–spatial deficits and earlier onset of diabetes mellitus. In addition, there is some evidence to suggest an association between verbal deficits and later disease onset, suggesting that various brain regions may have different critical periods of vulnerability related to the effects of diabetes mellitus (Rovet, Ehrlich, Czuchta, & Akler, 1993). Additionally, it also has been noted that children with disease onset before age five, those who experience severe hypoglycemia or hyperglycemia, or children experiencing frequent episodes of mild-to-moderate hypoglycemia are more likely to be at increased risk for neurocognitive deficits (Rovet et al., 1993). This chronic health condition may be classified as progressive, with gradual onset, and is generally considered to be nonincapacitating. However, a small subset of this population is at risk for learning problems. Additionally, school performance problems and peer difficulties are more likely to emerge during adolescence when teenagers are required to adhere to a strict medical regimen while they struggle with the typical developmental tasks that are characteristic of adolescence.

Spina bifida is a malformation of the CNS and, consequently, there is potential risk for neurocognitive sequelae in children with this condition. Spina bifida follows a constant course and may be physically incapacitating. A recent comprehensive review of the neuropsychological functioning of children with spina bifida and/or hydrocephalus revealed that while verbal abilities are generally intact, these children evidence difficulty with tasks involving visuospatial and tactile perception; rapid, precise, or sequenced movement; and "executive control" functions. In addition, various academic areas are affected, including arithmetic calculation, spelling, and reading comprehension (Wills, 1993).

Following even a severe traumatic brain injury, approximately 75% of the youth will regain ambulatory abilities and self-care skills, but at least two-thirds will continue to evidence long-term cognitive difficulties (Boyer & Edwards, 1991). In fact, a common problem is that many children with traumatic brain injury appear physically "normal," but experience significant cognitive processing difficulties that are not necessarily detectable on routine examinations. With increasing severity of injury, children exhibit corresponding deficits in adaptive problem-solving skills, memory, speed of processing, language, perceptual–motor skills, intelligence, and academic performance relative to peers (Dalby & Obrzut, 1991; Jaffe et al., 1993). Memory impairment is the most frequently observed and persistent cognitive change following traumatic brain injury (Begali, 1992; Jaffe et al., 1993; Levin et al., 1988). These children experience poor memory for learning new information compared to more remote or "old" memories. This difficulty may result in a slow yet steady decline in academic performance over time. Thus, as their peers advance in knowledge, the child or adolescent with a traumatic brain injury may not.

Epilepsy and sickle cell disease are brain-related diseases that follow a relapsing course. Epilepsy is considered by many to be the most prevalent chronic neurological disorder in children (Bolter, 1986) and has been implicated as a cause of impaired cognitive, academic, behavioral, and emotional functioning. It appears that epilepsy may disrupt learning by a number of mechanisms ranging from variations in ability to sustain attention to incoming information to more permanent reduction of information-processing capacity (Binnie, Channon, & Marston, 1990). Available literature suggests that even after controlling for IQ, children diagnosed with epilepsy are at greater risk for experiencing school difficulties relative to their healthy peers. Academic difficulties are greatest in arithmetic, spelling, reading comprehension, and word recognition (Gourley, 1990). Boys with epilepsy may be more likely to underachieve at school and be more impaired with respect to reading skills (Stedman, Van Heyningen, & Lindsey, 1982). This is consistent with the findings noted in the Isle of Wight study (Rutter et al., 1970), which indicated that more than twice as many children diagnosed with epilepsy evidenced serious reading comprehension problems relative to a group of children without seizure disorders.

There is a growing body of literature attesting to the fact that children with sickle cell disease are at risk for school problems secondary to CNS effects of the illness itself (Brown, Armstrong, & Eckman, 1993). Research findings indicate lower intellectual functioning and greater neuropsychological deficits in patients with sickle cell disease compared with sibling controls (e.g., Brown, Buchanan, et al., 1993; Wasserman, Wilimas, Fairclough, Mulhern, & Wang, 1991). Programmatic research conducted by Brown and colleagues (Brown, Buchanan, et al., 1993) has demonstrated associations among neuropsychological functions, socioeconomic background, and hemoglobin, suggesting that deficits in cognitive functioning in part may be attributable to social class and to the possible etiological effects of reduced oxygen delivery.

Iatrogenic Effects of Treatment

Children with chronic illness also may require treatments for their illness that may have iatrogenic effects on cognitive functioning and, hence, on school achievement. Iatrogenic effects may range from mental status changes associated with particular pharmacological agents (e.g., difficulties with attention and concentration secondary to steroids) or prophylactic therapies, including cranial radiation or intrathecal chemotherapy employed to prevent infiltration of neoplasms in the CNS.

There continues to be considerable debate regarding the effects of asthma medications on cognitive functioning and learning. Overall findings regarding the iatrogenic effects of Theophylline, a broncodilator, on learning and attention in children with asthma are variable (for reviews see Creer & Gustafson, 1989). Similarly there has been some concern regarding the use of corticosteroids to treat asthma as they may negatively impact learning, mood, and behavior. For example, there is some evidence for subtle, reversible, dose-dependent effects on memory and recall (Bender, Lerner, & Kollasch, 1988). However, findings from these studies need to be judiciously interpreted because of methodological limitations (Celano & Geller, 1993).

There is considerable evidence documenting the iatrogenic effects of treatment for childhood cancer. Children with leukemia receive CNS prophylactic treatment to prevent the infiltration of leukemic cells into the CNS. Although this protocol has increased the rate of survival, it has had deleterious effects on neurocognitive functioning. Several reviews of existing studies show evidence of iatrogenic effects of CNS prophylaxis, particularly cranial irradiation in patients diagnosed with leukemia (Fletcher & Copeland, 1988; Madan-Swain & Brown, 1991). More recently, evidence suggests intrathecal chemotherapy may have deleterious effects even in the absence of radiation therapy (Brown et al., 1992, 1996, 1998). Documented neurocognitive deficits after completion of medical therapy include impairment on tasks of higher-order functioning and specific learning disabilities in mathematics (Brown et al., 1992); mild fine-motor impairments (Brown et al., in press); poor academic performance in reading, arithmetic calculation, and spelling (Brown et al., 1996); and diagnosable learning disabilities in reading and mathematics (Brown et al., 1992, 1998).

Youth diagnosed with brain tumors also are treated with high-dose cranial radiation and chemotherapy, and similar deleterious CNS effects have been reported (Glauser & Packer, 1991). Moreover, there is some evidence that the extent of the radiation therapy (i.e., focal vs. whole brain) in patients with brain tumors may be associated with the degree of neurocognitive difficulties (Kun, Mulhern, & Crisco, 1983). The most common neurocognitive sequelae is in the area of nonverbal abilities, attention and concentration, (Fletcher & Copeland, 1988), short-term memory, speed of processing, visual–motor coordination, and sequencing ability (Cousens, Ungerer, Crawford, & Stevens, 1991).

In summary, children with diagnosable learning problems, either pre-existing or subsequent to the onset of the chronic illness, may be at greater risk for school reentry problems. In particular, obvious CNS involvement related to the disease or injury itself (e.g., traumatic brain injury) or as a result of toxicities associated with medical treatments (e.g., leukemia treatment) may result in documented learning difficulties that require special education placement. Prolonged or brief absences, such as in the case of children diagnosed with asthma, Crohn's disease, or sickle cell disease, may significantly impact school performance. Children who were only marginally academically successful prior to the onset of the illness may be more vulnerable to educational difficulties associated with intermittent school absences. Additionally, academic deficits are most likely to be manifested in academic skill areas that build upon previous knowledge (Chekryn, Deegan, & Reid, 1987). While the majority of the children with chronic illnesses will be able to return to their regular classrooms with minimal modifications, many will sustain delays and need to "catch up" on missed work, resulting in anxiety and possibly complicating both attendance and functioning in school.

Absenteeism

School attendance is frequently used as a measure of disease-related functional capacities of children and adolescents with chronic illness (Cook, Schaller, & Krischer, 1985; Fowler et al., 1985; Weitzman & Siegel, 1992). Attending school is important to children's academic, social, and emotional development. It is a highly normative experience. Yet children and adolescents with chronic illness can potentially miss large amounts of school due to illness exacerbation, minor illnesses or health problems, adverse treatment side effects, hospitalizations, and outpatient clinic appointments.

Studies of children and adolescents with chronic illness consistently have shown higher rates of school absence for these youth than for children without a chronic illness (Cook et al., 1985; Fowler et al., 1985; Weitzman, Walker, & Gortmaker, 1986). However, there is variability in the literature regarding the rates and patterns of absenteeism across chronic illnesses that likely reflects the variable manifestations and course of these medical conditions. Relative to their healthy peers, children diagnosed with asthma have higher absenteeism rates, characterized by frequent brief absences. This trend, however, seems to diminish with increasing age (Parcel, Gilman, Nader, & Bunce, 1979). Rates of absenteeism that are four times higher than that of the general school-age population have been found for children with cancer (Stehbens, Kisker, & Wilson, 1983). However, in contrast to the children diagnosed with asthma, the pattern of school attendance in children diagnosed with cancer is characterized by one long period of absence at the time of diagnosis and initiation of treatment, followed by regular short absences for follow-up treatment or monitoring of progress (Charlton et al., 1991).

Absenteeism rates for children with cystic fibrosis and sickle cell disease have been among the highest, with children missing the equivalent of nearly 1 month of each school year (Fowler et al., 1985). Even among children with sickle cell disease where disease severity is mild, absence rates are high (Thompson & Gustafson, 1996), presumably related to low-grade pain experiences. Although children with insulin-dependent diabetes mellitus have fewer absences than for other chronic illnesses (Fowler et al., 1985), they have more absences than their healthy peers (Ryan, Longstreet, & Morrow, 1985).

Numerous factors have been associated with absenteeism in children with chronic illness. Medical factors include the course of the illness (i.e., constant, progressive, or relapsing), onset (i.e., acute or chronic), degree of incapacitation and physical restrictions (Fowler et al., 1985), and the type of treatment (CNS chemotherapy) (Cairns, Klopovich, Hearne, & Lansky, 1982). Demographic factors associated with lower rates of school attendance include parental education (Charlton et al., 1991; Cook et al., 1985), gender (i.e., female) (Cairns et al., 1982; Charlton et al., 1991; Fowler et al., 1985), and birth position (Cairns et al., 1982).

Psychological Factors Associated with Chronic Illness

The child's emotional response to an illness also may impact school functioning. Clearly, psychosocial and emotional factors play an important role in school functioning for children with chronic illness by affecting attendance and influencing the child's ability to effectively engage in the academic process or social milieu while at school. Prolonged absences with little peer contact create social discomfort for the child or adolescent with a chronic illness. Illness-related stress, psychological distress, concerns about peer reactions to physical changes, and the lack of confidence in both physical and academic abilities may contribute to the child's willingness to attend school and to perform when in school. Frequently, these issues are developmentally related. Peers in elementary school are concerned that the disease is contagious, while adolescent peers are likely to avoid interaction because of fears of associating with someone who is different (Davis, 1989).

Anxiety over returning to school results when a child or, particularly, an adolescent is confronted with major physical changes such as hair loss secondary to chemotherapy, disfigurement associated with burns, or amputation necessitated by trauma or diseases (Blakeney, 1994). Physical limitations hindering full participation in the regular school curriculum may contribute to difficulties interacting with peers and ultimately hamper return to school. Students' concerns about physical appearance frequently result in mental health services (Henning & Fritz, 1983). Interestingly, while the fear of peer rejection regarding physical changes is paramount prior to the return to school, most youth ultimately find that the fundamental social and emotional support for their return to school comes from classmates who have been educated about their particular disease (Chekryn et al., 1987).

However, one fairly complicated emotional obstacle to school reentry is that of school phobia or separation anxiety. An incidence of school refusal five times that found in the general population has been reported among chronically ill children (Henning & Fritz, 1983). Lansky and colleagues (Lansky, Lowman, Vata, & Gyulay, 1975) also found an increased incidence of school phobia in youth 10 years or older who were diagnosed with cancer. Psychosocial regression was significant in all age groups. Parents endorsed feelings of vulnerability and the children were reported to foster separation anxiety associated with school refusal. The symptom onset was insidious with physical complaints initially leading to parent-sanctioned school absences, and ultimately to school refusal.

Peer Relations

One of the objectives in lessening the psychosocial impact of chronic childhood illness is to avoid disrupting the normal processes of child development. Children with chronic illness are at risk for peer difficulties because of negative reactions to their physical changes and from the disruption of social contact brought about by the illness. Any major physical change threatens the child's body image, and ultimately self-esteem, potentially causing discomfort in peer relations. Adolescents, in particular, express specific concerns about the changes in their appearance, fears of peer ridicule or teasing, and discomfort in discussing the illness with classmates and teachers. This is particularly salient with adolescents diagnosed with gastrointestinal diseases such as Crohn's disease. While the literature generally indicates that the majority of youth who have experienced a severe injury such as burns achieve satisfactory psychological adaptation to their illness (Blakeney, 1994; Blakeney, Herndon, Desai, Beard, & Wales-Sears, 1988), a small segment of this population does not fare as well. In fact, Tarnowski and colleagues (Tarnowski, Rasnake, Linscheid, & Mullick, 1989) found clinically significant behavioral problems for children with chronic illnesses, as measured by parental ratings.

Social support has been found to serve as a protective factor in adaptation to chronic illness (Thompson & Gustafson, 1996). Wallander and Varni (1989) examined the unique contribution of family and peer support with children diagnosed with a variety of chronic illnesses including Type I diabetes mellitus, spina bifida, juvenile rheumatoid arthritis, cerebral palsy, and chronic obesity. Results from this investigation indicated that children with high levels of both family and peer social support evidenced significantly lower levels of internalizing and externalizing behavior problems than children with social support from only one of these sources. These findings were interpreted to suggest that children with chronic conditions can potentially benefit from efforts to improve social support in school by such means as social skills training.

PHASES OF SCHOOL REENTRY

Meeting the educational needs of children with chronic illness requires cooperative and coordinated efforts among the medical treatment team, school personnel including teachers, classmates, administrators, school psychologists, and counselors, and the children and their families. These groups are integral components to "school reentry" particularly following diagnosis, or after a prolonged absence. Successful school reentry is focused on meeting the unique needs of the individual child or adolescent, ensuring continued academic and social skill development by appropriately modifying the school environment, and assisting parents to be effective advocates for their children.

While there is a burgeoning body of clinical literature describing the school reentry process for various populations including cancer, traumatic brain injury, and burns, there is scant empirical data available. The findings from data-driven studies focusing on children or adolescents diagnosed with cancer provide the best information currently available to guide comprehensive integrated school reentry efforts. For example, findings from the school reentry investigation by Katz and colleagues (1992) indicate that, compared to pretest measures, youth diagnosed with cancer who received a structured intervention program exhibited fewer parent-reported internalizing problems, and according to their classroom teachers were socially better adjusted relative to the comparison group.

School reentry programs typically share the common goal of preparing the chronically ill children, the family, and school personnel for transition back into the typical routine of attending school (Davis, 1989; Katz et al., 1992; Lefebvre & Arndt, 1988). Programs vary in terms of the formality and structure of services provided, but the underlying premises are the same (Blakeney, 1994; Katz, Rubenstein, Hubert, & Blew, 1988; Katz et al., 1992). What follows is the identification of three major phases of school reentry, together with the challenges, roles, and responsibilities of the various groups of individuals involved in the process. Phase 1 begins soon after diagnosis and includes hospitalization and the development of a school reentry plan. This phase focuses on assessing the child's school behavior and parents' involvement with the school prior to the illness, arranging interim educational programs prior to school return, and educating peers. Phase 2 includes contact and education of school personnel by the medical team, who focus on educating school personnel by providing information regarding the child's illness and treatment, including scheduling medical treatments and their adverse side effects, planning for absences, anticipating psychosocial adjustment issues, such as the reaction of school personnel and other children to the child, and developing an individualized educational plan. Emphasis during this phase is placed on preparing the teacher and classmates for the child's imminent reentry. The final phase is for follow-up contact with school personnel and parents. This phase occurs after the child returns to school and continues as needed to provide essential ongoing monitoring to ensure that the child or adolescent is indeed attending school.

Phase 1: Initial Hospitalization and Plans for Reentry

During the initial hospitalization the medical team plays a primary role to both the child and the family by stressing the importance of returning to school. The medical team must convey the message that while the illness or accident is a disruption to life which for some youth will require new ways of performing activities (e.g., having to move at a slower pace than prior to their illness), with time and practice, in most instances they will be able to resume premorbid activities. The importance of returning to school is stressed with both the child or adolescent and the family.

With the parents' permission, a member of the treatment team should contact the child's school to notify school personnel of the child's status, obtain premorbid information regarding the child's academic and social functioning, and elicit any concerns from the school's perspective. As soon as the child or adolescent is medically stable, school instruction is incorporated into the child's daily inpatient treatment program. If hospitals do not have school programs, then schoolwork can be forwarded from the school and a parent or staff member can function as a teacher.

Parents may be reluctant to allow the child with a chronic illness or injury back to school for a variety of reasons. Parents may not agree with the medical team when they determine the child or adolescent is physically ready to return to school. They also may want to protect their child from potential hurt, ridicule, and/or rejection by other children. Parents are susceptible to their own emotions and feelings of guilt and may become too protective and overly responsive to their child's physical complaints or expressions of anxiety related to rejection and ridicule. Understanding the importance of the child's reintegration, parents may provide support by also contacting the child's school, keeping the teacher and classmates informed of medical progress, and encouraging mutual communication between the ill or injured child and his or her peers (Davis, 1989; Lefebvre & Arndt, 1988).

With the family's consent, the teacher or counselor should inform the class about their classmate's chronic illness or injury. Communication with the hospitalized child may be encouraged through cards, e-mail, phone calls, weekly newsletters, class meetings conducted with a speakerphone to include the classmate, audiotaped class discussions of a high-interest topic with comments from the teacher to include the classmate, and, when possible, visits from classmates to the hospital. If peers stay in close contact the chronically ill child may find it easier to return to school and as a result be less likely to experience anxiety related to school reentry (Sexson & Madan-Swain, 1995).

School reentry is critical. Even adolescents who have withdrawn from school prematurely prior to the injury should be expected to become involved in some structured educational or vocational program. Most importantly, the adolescent cannot be allowed to withdraw into the safety of isolation, receiving no new information, feedback from others, or social support. If adolescents, particularly those who have sustained physical changes, are allowed to withdraw, they may experience the daily isolation as confirmation that they are, in fact, incompetent and physically unattractive.

Phase 2: Contact and Education of School Personnel

Teachers

The extent to which school personnel can successfully facilitate the reentry process will be partially determined by the attitudes of school personnel

(Sexson & Madan-Swain, 1995). It is likely that many teachers lack the necessary information or experience with chronic illnesses and are susceptible to all the fears, anxieties, and failings of the general public. Having a child with a serious chronic illness or injury returning to their classroom is a new experience for most teachers. Limited knowledge about the disease, preconceived notions about certain disorders, and the vulnerability communicated by the change in the child's appearance or energy level may cause teachers to arrive at the premature or erroneous conclusion that the child is likely to die (Ross, 1984). Teachers may be overwhelmed, unsure of how to approach the child, and uncomfortable in seeking information from parents who are already stressed from the illness experience and unable to deal with their own anxieties about the situation. Lacking this information, teachers may be overly sympathetic and reluctant to challenge the student to his or her potential (Ross, 1984). Conversely, teachers may be unable to recognize true limitations, thus exerting unrealistic expectations, which may lead to frustration and discouragement. Teachers also may worry that they will be unable to handle the medical issues that could arise (Blakeney, 1994). These fears may cause the teacher to be increasingly more protective, overreacting to even minor complaints, isolating the child, decreasing the child's self-confidence, limiting peer acceptance and, as a result, further hampering the child's normalization process (Ross, 1984).

In order to provide a reinforcing classroom where students are successful, teachers need specific information regarding the illness or injury and its possible impact on school performance and general development. This allows the teacher to adapt instruction to ensure that the child is successful. Initially, reinforcement should be provided to the chronically ill child reentering school simply for returning to school and for participating in the classroom activities. This reinforcement should be delivered at a rapid pace at the beginning of each instructional session (Zanily, Dagged, & Pestine, 1995). In addition, teachers need to analyze the function of behaviors in which the child is likely to engage upon returning to the classroom. Many of these behaviors may provide avoidance from participating in school tasks (e.g., Iwata, Dorsey, Slifer, Bauman, & Richman, 1994). Once avoidance is determined to be the function of the behavior, the teacher must determine if this avoidance is reinforcing because the tasks are academically too difficult, either due to missed instruction or the cognitive difficulties associated with the illness, or because of adverse side effects of treatments, such as fatigue.

Educational Assessment and Programming

It is inappropriate to rely on a one-time assessment to determine the academic functioning level and educational needs of children diagnosed with chronic illness. Repeated assessments are needed to determine whether abilities that typically emerge developmentally are negatively impacted by the injury or diseases and/or subsequent treatments delivered at an early age. The assessment should include psychoeducational testing to be completed annually by a clinical or pediatric psychologist, a neuropsychologist, or a school psychologist who is employed by the school system, as well as a criterion-referenced assessment completed by the classroom teacher. The assessment tools selected for the psychoeducational evaluation are critical. Typically, global measures of intellectual and cognitive functioning are not likely to be adequate indicators of the needs of children who have experienced CNS disease and treatment or traumatic brain injury. Instead, the assessment battery should include neurocognitive measures of processing speed, cognitive flexibility, attention and concentration, language, memory, and visual–spatial and visual–motor abilities. This will allow the development of an educational plan that targets weaknesses but also builds upon areas of strength. Teachers need to be aware that the child may have difficulty with the development of skills, and for this reason the educational program should strengthen those skills present at the time of treatment and foster the development of strategies to aid in the acquisition of later skills. Based on the nature of the deficits, educational plans should adequately facilitate the child's learning.

One important consideration for young children is to ensure that they become competent readers. Most children need regular systematic instruction in reading so that they may become competent readers. If children are frequently absent during this instruction they are likely to have difficulty learning to read, which will quickly compound exponentially unless addressed. One specific method is to identify portable, systematic reading instruction that may be easily implemented both with the hospital and homebound instruction.

In addition to instructional program considerations, children should be allowed to use technology as an aid or to adapt procedures as needed. For example, children may use tape recorders to capture lectures and other oral instructions, word processors to produce work that would otherwise be handwritten, and calculators to perform calculations used in the application of mathematical concepts. Equally important is the consideration of the removal of time constraints and writing requirements in test taking.

Educational programs need to accommodate children's frequent absences due to hospitalizations, dual homebound/school-based schooling during treatment, and, when necessary, environmental adaptations for children requiring wheelchairs or walking devices. Adjustment in school rules may need to be made regarding the wearing of particular garments (e.g., allowing hats for those students who have lost their hair secondary to the medical treatment) and the provision of access to a quiet area for rest when children become fatigued during periods of low blood counts, or pain crises (Armstrong & Horn, 1995).

Although some children with chronic illness may have prolonged absences from school, for most, the pattern of school absences is multiple brief absences that accumulate over the school year. This pattern often leaves the child behind in schoolwork with few available educational resources. While homebound instruction is available, it frequently is limited to only a few hours per week of actual instruction. For the well-motivated student this limited individual instruction may allow successful academic progress. However, the social isolation concomitant with homebound instruction places the chronically ill child at risk for difficulties with ongoing psychosocial development.

Classroom Presentation

To ease the transition back into the classroom, members from the medical team may visit the school and present information regarding the chronic illness. The child is generally given the opportunity to provide information during the presentation, but may elect not to do so if this poses a discomfort. Anecdotal literature on reentry presentations for children who have sustained burns illustrates content areas that may typically be addressed in the presentation (Blakeney, 1994), including injury etiology, hospital care, physical implications, and use of special procedures or equipment (e.g., splints, masks, pressure garments). While the words and methods selected to communicate vary with the target audience, the content remains the same. The format may be adapted for classroom presentations on other chronic illnesses and injury.

Parental Support

If the school provides a reinforcing environment for the child's return and if the parents' behavior of encouraging the child to return to school is reinforced by school personnel, the transition will proceed more smoothly. One way to reinforce the parents' efforts is to provide frequent positive communication about the school reentry process. For the first few days it may be necessary to phone the parents several times during the day to assure them that the reentry is progressing well and to reassure them that the child is experiencing no adjustment difficulties. Over time, the frequency of the contacts may be faded as the parents view the success of their child's return to the classroom.

Phase 3: Follow-Up Contact

Central to this phase is continued communication among the family, school personnel, and medical team. Even after the child returns to school, it is important that school personnel remain in close contact with an identified medical team member so that school-related concerns can be easily discussed. Such communication allows the school to inform the medical team of increasing absences and to seek information regarding how to address the issue. The medical team can assist with the development of decision rules that are acceptable to the school and family. These rules can be used to determine when a child may stay home from school and when attendance is mandatory. Because the decision rules may change depending on the course of the illness, continual contact must be maintained, particularly for children diagnosed with relapsing illnesses (e.g., asthma, Crohns disease).

CONCLUSIONS AND FUTURE DIRECTIONS

School reentry is a dynamic, ongoing process that requires continuous cooperation and commitment among the medical team, family, and school from initial hospitalization through follow-up contact. Regardless of whether the chronic illness follows a constant, progressive, or relapsing course (Rolland, 1990), the child's return to school poses a significant stressor. Yet, reentry to school is imperative. With the importance of school reentry comes a need to establish a scientific basis for enhancing this process. Several questions must be considered in an effort to facilitate school reentry.

1. To what extent is the reentry process disease specific? Whereas there are a few programs that have been evaluated and published addressing school reentry for children with specific illnesses, such as cancer (Katz et al., 1992) and burns (Blakeney, 1994), further work is needed to extend these efforts to other chronic conditions. On the one hand, school reentry can appear to be a relatively generic challenge. Thus, it is possible that these existing illness-specific programs could be applied to other illnesses with only minor modification. However, this type of generalizability of reentry programs is an empirical question warranting the evaluation of a generic school reentry program across various chronic illnesses. Finding common approaches across illnesses would be helpful. On the other hand, some types of illnesses may require differential attention to reentry issues, which may be evaluated based on Rolland's (1990) conceptualization of illness typology.

2. If the school reentry process is not disease specific, does it vary according to Rolland's (1990) typology? This should be delineated initially through a qualitative analysis, and then empirically validated on a larger scale using objective data from several sources (e.g., medical team, parents, child or adolescent, and teacher). For example, relapsing illnesses such as asthma and sickle cell disease require ongoing adjustments from all parties. As a specific example, the school would need to modify attendance policies

so that the child who must miss large numbers of school days is not retained simply because of the number of absences. Alternatively, a child or adolescent who has sustained a traumatic brain injury may have a long follow-up reentry phase, as recovery may initially be slow, but once a child with this illness is in school, attendance should not be an issue.

3. Regardless of whether the process is disease specific, typology specific, or generic to all diseases, what is the impact of the developmental stage of the child or adolescent? Development would likely interact with reentry phase and type of illness. This three-way interaction has been all but ignored thus far. The needs of children reentering school will vary according to their developmental stage. For example, while peers are important at all stages, they play a critical role during adolescence. At this stage, school becomes an important arena for experimenting with different social roles and exploring one's evolving sexuality. Having a chronic illness can readily interfere with these important socialization processes during adolescence. To achieve truly successful school reentry requires attention to these developmental issues.

In conclusion, the questions are complex and the research designed to answer them will have to consider their interactive nature. In this chapter we delineated a three-phase reentry process that may be applied to Rolland's (1990) disease typology. However, this conceptualization of the problem will have to be validated through empirical research. As these data are gathered, it may be necessary to revise aspects of the proposed three-phase reentry process.

REFERENCES

Armstrong, F. D., & Horn, M. (1995). Educational issues in childhood cancer. *School Psychology Quarterly, 10,* 292–304.

Begali, V. (1992). *Head injury in children and adolescents: A resource and review for school and applied professionals* (2nd ed.). Brandon, VT: Clinical Psychology Publishing.

Bender, B. G., Lerner, J. A., & Kollasch, E. (1988). Mood and memory changes in asthmatic children receiving corticosteroids. *Journal of the American Academy of Child and Adolescent Psychiatry, 27,* 720–725.

Binnie, C. D., Channon, S., & Marston, D. (1990). Learning disabilities in epilepsy: Neurophysiological aspects. *Epilepsia, 31*(Suppl. 4), S2–S8.

Blakeney, P. (1994). School reintegration. In K. J. Tarnowski (Ed.), *Behavioral aspects of pediatric burns* (pp. 217–239). New York: Plenum Press.

Blakeney, P., Herndon, D., Desai, M., Beard, S., & Wales-Sears, P. (1988). Long-term psychological adjustment following burn injury. *Journal of Burn Care and Rehabilitation, 9,* 661–665.

Bolter, J. F. (1986). Epilepsy in children: Neuropsychological effects. In J. B. Obrzut

& G. W. Hynd (Eds.), *Child neuropsychology: Vol. 2. Clinical practice* (pp. 59–81). New York: Academic Press.

Boyer, M. G., & Edwards, P. (1991). Outcome 1 to 3 years after severe traumatic brain injury in children and adolescents. *Injury, 22,* 315–320.

Brown, R. T., Armstrong, F. D., & Eckman, J. R. (1993). Neurocognitive aspects of pediatric sickle-cell disease. *Journal of Learning Disabilities, 26,* 33–45.

Brown, R. T., Buchanan, I., Doepke, K., Eckman, J. R., Baldwin, K., Goonan, B., & Schoenherr, S. (1993). Cognitive and academic functioning in children with sickle-cell disease. *Journal of Clinical Child Psychology, 22,* 207–218.

Brown, R. T., Madan-Swain, A., Pais, R., Lambert, R. G., Sexson, S. B., & Ragab, A. (1992). Chemotherapy for acute lymphocytic leukemia: Cognitive and academic sequelae. *Journal of Pediatrics, 121,* 885–889.

Brown, R. T., Madan-Swain, A., Walco, G. A., Cherrick, I., Ievers, C. E., Conte, P. M., Vega, R., Bell, B., & Lauer, S. J. (1998). Cognitive and academic late effects among children previously treated for acute lymphocytic leukemia receiving chemotherapy as CNS prophylaxis. *Journal of Pediatric Psychology, 23,* 333–340.

Brown, R. T., Sawyer, M. B., Antoniou, G., Toogood, I., Rice, M., Thompson, N., & Madan-Swain, A. (1996). A 3-year follow-up of the intellectual and academic functioning of children receiving central nervous system prophylactic chemotherapy for leukemia. *Journal of Developmental and Behavioral Pediatrics, 17,* 392–398.

Cadman, D., Boyle, M., Szatmari, P., & Offord, D. R. (1987). Chronic illness, disability, and mental and social well-being: Findings of the Ontario Child Health Study. *Pediatrics, 79,* 805–813.

Cairns, N. U., Klopovich, P., Hearne, E., & Lansky, S. B. (1982). School attendance of children with cancer. *Journal of School Health, 52,*152–155.

Celano, M. P., & Geller, R. J. (1993). Learning, school performance, and children with asthma: How much at risk? *Journal of Learning Disabilities, 26,* 23–32.

Charlton, A., Larcombe, I. J., Meller, S. T., Morris-Jones, P.H., Mott, M. G., Potton, M. W., Tranmer, M.D., & Walker, J. J. P. (1991). Absence from school related to cancer and other chronic conditions. *Archives of Diseases in Childhood, 66,* 1217–1222.

Chekryn J., Deegan, M., & Reid, J. (1987). Impact on teachers when a child with cancer returns to school. *Children's Health Care, 15,* 161–165.

Cook, B. A., Schaller, K., & Krischer, J. P. (1985). School absence among children with chronic illness. *Journal of School Health, 55,* 265–267.

Cousens, P., Ungerer, J. A., Crawford, J. A., & Stevens, M. (1991). Cognitive effects of childhood leukemia therapy: A case for four specific deficits. *Journal of Pediatric Psychology, 16,* 475–488.

Creer, T. L., & Gustafson, K. E. (1989). Psychological problems associated with drug therapy in childhood asthma. *Journal of Pediatrics, 115,* 850–855.

Dalby, P. R., & Obrzut, J. E. (1991). Epidemiological characteristics and sequelae of closed head injured children and adolescents: A review. *Developmental Neuropsychology, 7,* 35–68.

Davis, K. G. (1989). Educational needs of the terminally ill student. *Issues in Comprehensive Pediatric Nursing, 12,* 235–245.

Fletcher, J. M., & Copeland, D. R. (1988). Neurobehavioral effects of central nervous system prophylactic treatment of cancer in children. *Journal of Clinical and Experimental Neuropsychology, 10,* 495–538.

Fowler, M. G., Davenport, M. G., & Garg, R. (1992). School functioning of U.S. children with asthma. *Pediatrics, 90,* 939–944.

Fowler, M. G., Johnson, M. P., & Atkinson, S. S. (1985). School achievement and absence in children with chronic health conditions. *Journal of Pediatrics, 106,* 683–687.

Glauser, T. A., & Packer, R. J. (1991). Cognitive deficits in long-term survivors of childhood brain tumors. *Child's Nervous System, 7,* 2–12.

Gortmaker, S. L., Walker, D. K., Weitzman, M., & Sobel, A. M. (1990). Chronic conditions, socioeconomic risks and behavioral problems in children and adolescents. *Pediatrics, 85,* 267–276.

Gourley, R. (1990). Educational policies. *Epilepsia, 31* (Suppl. 4), S59–S60.

Henning, J., & Fritz, G. K. (1983). School reentry in childhood cancer. *Psychosomatics, 24,* 261–269.

Howe, G. W., Feinstein, C., Reiss, D., Molock, S., & Berger, K. (1993). Adolescent adjustment to chronic physical disorders: I. Comparing neurological and nonneurological conditions. *Journal of Child Psychology and Psychiatry, 14,* 1153–1171.

Iwata, B. A., Dorsey, M. F., Slifer, K. J., Bauman, K. E., & Richman, G. S. (1994). Towards a functional analysis of self-injury. *Journal of Applied Behavior Analysis, 27,* 197–209.

Jaffe, K. M., Fay, G. C., Polissar, N. L., Martin, K. M., Shurtleff, H., Rivara, J. B., & Winn, H. R. (1993). Severity of pediatric traumatic brain injury and neurobehavioral recovery at one year—A cohort study. *Archives of Physical Medicine and Rehabilitation, 74,* 587–595.

Katz, E. R., Rubenstein, C. L., Hubert, N. C., & Blew, A. (1988). School and social reintegration of children with cancer. *Journal of Psychosocial Oncology, 6,* 123–140.

Katz, E. R., Varni, J. W., Rubenstein, C. L., Blew, A., & Hubert, N. (1992). Teacher, parent, and child evaluative ratings of school reintegration intervention for children with newly diagnosed cancer. *Children's Health Care, 21,* 69–75.

Kun, L. E., Mulhern, R. K., & Crisco, J. J. (1983). Quality of life in children treated for brain tumors: Intellectual, emotional, and academic function. *Journal of Neurosurgery, 58,* 1–6.

Lansky, S. B., Lowman, J. T., Vata, T., & Gyulay, J. (1975). School phobia in children with malignant neoplasms. *American Journal of Diseases of Children, 129,* 42–46.

Lefebvre, A. M., & Arndt, E. M. (1988). Working with facially disfigured children: A challenge in prevention. *Canadian Journal of Psychiatry, 33,* 453–458.

Levin, H. S., High, W. M., Ewing-Cobbs, L., Fletcher, J. M., Eisenberg, H. M., Miner, M. E., & Goldstein, F. C. (1988). Memory functioning during the first year after closed head injury in children and adolescents. *Neurosurgery, 22,* 1043–1052.

Madan-Swain, A., & Brown, R. T. (1991). Cognitive and psychosocial sequelae for children with acute lymphocytic leukemia and their families. *Clinical Psychology Review, 11,* 267–294.

Newacheck, P. W., & Stoddard, J. J. (1994). Prevalence and impact of multiple childhood chronic illnesses. *Journal of Pediatrics, 124,* 40–48.

Parcel, G. S., Gilman, S. C., Nader, P. R., & Bunce, H. (1979). A comparison of absenteeism rates of elementary school children with asthma and nonasthmatic schoolmates. *Pediatrics, 64,* 878–881.

Rolland, J. S. (1990). The impact of illness on the family. In R. E. Rakel (Ed.), *Textbook of family practice* (4th ed., pp. 80–100). Philadelphia: Saunders.

Ross, J. W. (1984). Resolving nonmedical obstacles to successful school reentry for children with cancer. *Journal of School Health, 54,* 84–86.

Rovet, J. F., Ehrlich, R. M., Czuchta, D., & Akler, M. (1993). Psychoeducational characteristics of children and adolescents with insulin-dependent diabetes mellitus. *Journal of Learning Disabilities, 26,* 7–22.

Rutter, M., Tizard, J., & Whitmore, K. (1970). *Education, health, and behavior.* London: Longmans, Green.

Ryan, C. M., Longstreet, C., & Morrow, L. A. (1985). The effects of diabetes mellitus on the school attendance and school achievement of adolescents. *Child: Care, Health, and Development, 11,* 229–240.

Sexson, S. B., & Madan-Swain, A. (1993). School reentry for the child with chronic illness. *Journal of Learning Disabilities, 26,* 115–125.

Sexson, S. B., & Madan-Swain, A. (1995). The chronically ill child in the school. *School Psychology Quarterly, 10,* 359–368.

Stedman, J., Van Heyningen, R., & Lindsey, J. (1982). Educational underachievement and epilepsy: A study of children from normal schools admitted to a special hospital for epilepsy. *Early Childhood Development Care, 9,* 65–82.

Stehbens, J. A., Kisker, C. T., & Wilson, B. K. (1983). School behavior and attendance during the first year of treatment for childhood cancer. *Psychology in the Schools, 20,* 223–228.

Tarnowski, K. J., Rasnake, L. K., Linscheid, T. R., & Mullick, J. A. (1989). Behavioral adjustment of pediatric burn victims. *Journal of Pediatric Psychology, 14,* 607–615.

Thompson, R. J., Jr., & Gustafson, K. F. (1996). *Adaptation to chronic childhood illness.* Washington, DC: American Psychological Association.

Wallander, J. L., & Varni, J. W. (1989). Social support and adjustment in chronically ill and handicapped children. *American Journal of Community Psychology, 17,* 185–201.

Wasserman, A. L., Wilimas, J. A., Fairclough, D. L., Mulhern, R. K., & Wang, W. (1991). Subtle neuropsychological deficits in children with sickle-cell disease. *American Journal of Pediatric Hematology/Oncology, 13,* 14–20.

Weitzman, M., & Siegel, D. M. (1992). What we have not learned from what we know about excessive school absence and school dropout. *Developmental and Behavioral Pediatrics, 13,* 55–58.

Weitzman, M., Walker, D. K., & Gortmaker, S. (1986). Chronic illness, psychosocial problems, and school absences. *Clinical Pediatrics, 25,* 137–141.

Wills, K. E. (1993). Neuropsychological functioning in children with spina bifida and/or hydrocephalus. *Journal of Clinical Child Psychiatry, 22,* 247–265.

Zanily, L., Dagged, J., & Pestine, H. (1995). The influence of the pace of teacher attention on preschool children's engagement. *Behavior Modification, 19,* 339–356.

CHAPTER FIFTEEN

Family Issues

LAMIA P. BARAKAT
ANNE E. KAZAK

The ecological perspective on understanding chronic illness in children focuses attention on the contextual factors that influence adjustment (Kazak, 1992). The effects of chronic illness in children are viewed as extending beyond the expected physical manifestations to complex, reciprocal influences among the illness and its treatment, the affected child, the child's family and its subsystems, the medical setting, the school system, and the wider community. The family context as it interplays with aspects of chronic illness is the focus of this chapter.

The strains of childhood chronic illness on the family are unlimited. No list of potential stressors can do justice to its pervasive impact. Among stressors described by families are juggling the demands of the illness and medical treatment, facing uncertainties about the future well-being and mortality of the child as well as dealing with emotional, academic, and occupational limitations of the child, financial strains, changes in roles and routines, communication breakdowns with family, friends, and neighbors, and lack of leisure time (Holroyd & Guthrie, 1986; Sokol et al., 1996). Additional stressors unrelated to the chronic illness may tax existing family resources. Low socioeconomic status, prior deaths in the family, and low levels of social support or integration in the community are stressors that make the burden of chronic illness difficult to carry.

Despite the significantly high levels of stress experienced by families of children with chronic illness, families have been found to be remarkably competent in adapting. Current research approaches families within a framework of resilience that leads to identification of competencies, resources, and risks in order to delineate aspects of the illness and of family functioning that differentiate those families who adapt well from those who do not. Family patterns and interactions that may serve to improve children and their families' adaptation to chronic illness are identified.

A general overview of theoretical approaches to understanding children with chronic illness and their families is followed by a discussion of findings regarding family functioning and its role in child, parent, and sibling adjustment. Next, a review of findings on the influences of cognitive aspects and illness severity on the family is presented. Finally, we present our own research with childhood cancer survivors and their families to explore further the complex relationships among medical late effects of illness, illness severity, parent and child perceptions of the child's functioning, and family adaptation.

THEORETICAL APPROACHES TO UNDERSTANDING FAMILY FUNCTIONING

Risk, resource, and resilience factors, which change over time, mediate the relationship between the demands of chronic illness and adjustment by improving one's ability to cope (Kazak, 1989). Cognitive aspects of illness and family functioning are among the risk and resilience factors associated with adaptation. Family functioning is conceptualized also as an adjustment outcome. A number of models based on the stress and coping framework of adaptation to the diagnosis and treatment of chronic illness in children have been posited and tested. A sample of the most frequently cited models in theory, research, and practice are described herein.

Disability–Stress–Coping Model

Wallander and Varni (1992), through their work with families of children with spina bifida, proposed a disability–stress–coping model in which risk and resistance factors play a role in the adaptation of children with chronic illness and their families. Among the risk factors are disease parameters, functional limitations, and psychosocial stressors. Resistance factors include personal resources (competence, problem-solving ability), appraisal and coping, and family and social support resources.

There is ample support for various aspects of this model, with the exception of the role of illness type or severity (Wallander, Varni, Babani, Banis, et al., 1989; Wallander, Varni, Babani, DeHaan, et al., 1989). Greater financial resources, use of adaptive coping strategies, and satisfaction with social support as well as child temperament and maternal competence have been linked to better adjustment outcomes for children and their families. Additionally, the number of illness-related and non-illness-related stressors, mothers' level of optimism, and social support network size have been related to children and their families' adjustment as hypothesized in the disability–stress–coping model (Barakat & Linney, 1992; Drotar, Agle, Eckl, & Thompson, 1997).

Thompson, Gustafson, George, and Spock (1994) provide a similar model, identified as the transactional stress and coping model, but include discussion of cognitive processes in adaptation. They suggest that the relationship between illness and adjustment outcomes is based on the transaction between biomedical, developmental, and psychosocial processes. Mother and child adaptational processes, including appraisal of the illness, self-efficacy, locus of control, coping strategies, family functioning and social support are proposed mediators of the illness and adjustment relationship. In the work of Thompson and colleagues, illness and demographic variables account for a small percentage of the variance in mother and child outcome, with the psychosocial mediators accounting for a much larger portion.

Patterson (1988) has expanded the stress and coping models in the Family Adjustment and Adaptation Response (FAAR) model to discuss the role of family and community systems and subsystems. The FAAR model differentiates adjustment of families to the illness based on demands and resistance capabilities and adaptation of families to repeated crises over time. Importantly, Patterson emphasizes the reciprocal impact of illness on the family and the family on illness.

Family Systems–Illness Model

Rolland (1990) has developed the family systems-illness model to guide understanding and exploration of the adaptation of individuals with chronic illness and their families. Rolland proposes that chronic illness results in threatened and perceived loss for the ill individual as well as the family members (e.g., loss of function, change in roles).

Three dimensions of illness and families must be taken into account in assessing the process of family adaptation. The first dimension involves psychosocial illness-related factors such as illness onset (acute, gradual), course (progressive, constant, relapsing), outcome (fatal, shortened lifespan, sudden death, no effect), and level of incapacitation. Certainly an acute, life-threatening illness will have different implications than a gradual, progressive illness resulting in a shortened lifespan. Phases of the natural history of the illness make up the second dimension, with differential effects on the family depending on whether one is in the initial crisis/diagnosis phase, an acute flare-up of the chronic illness, or the terminal stage. Family systems variables are the third dimension. These variables include the role of the illness in the family's developmental life cycle (e.g., is the child with chronic illness entering school, or is the adolescent with chronic illness leaving for college?), belief systems about illness that are influenced by the family's prior experiences with illness (e.g., illness in the grandparent generation), ethnicity, culture, family cohesion, adaptability, and communication. Developmental events for the family are often delayed until there is some resolution of the illness; however, "when the patient recovers, often the family does not" (Penn, 1983, p. 23).

Based on these illness and family dimensions, Rolland (1990) suggests that families must not give up on major family goals (such as sending an adolescent to college) in order to adapt but must readjust their goals (e.g., the adolescent attends a college close to home). Also, families must develop a meaning for the illness that reestablishes the families' sense of competence and control. Similarly, Fiese (1997) discusses the transactional model of mutual influence of the environment, that is, the family, on the child and the child on the environment, with proximal variables (parent–child interaction) and distal variables (family of origin experiences) influencing this transaction. Through this model, Fiese stresses the importance of assessing the meaning assigned to illness and the perception of illness events as experienced by families in order to understand the transaction between the child with chronic illness and the parents.

FAMILY FUNCTIONING

In many reviews (Ievers & Drotar, 1996; Kazak, 1991) and studies (Foley, Barakat, Herman-Liu, Radcliffe, & Molloy, in press; Gowers, Jones, Kiana, North, & Price, 1995; Hamlett, Pellegrini, & Katz, 1992), no differences in family functioning between families of children with chronic illness and comparison groups or norms for scales are reported. The lack of findings regarding general family functioning does not necessarily translate into no risk for families of children with chronic illness (Kazak, 1989). It may be essential to look beyond measures of general family functioning and instead to examine patterns of family interaction within a systems perspective, that is, to understand the interactions of subsystems within the family on a daily basis (Kazak, 1997) and variations in patterns over time. Many studies addressing patterns of interaction use measures of family cohesion (emotional closeness), family adaptability/flexibility (in order to meet varying demands), and family expressiveness or communication. In particular, the circumplex model of family functioning (Olson, Sprenkle, & Russell, 1979) has been cited frequently. Originally, it described family functioning on two dimensions, an enmeshed to disengaged continuum and a rigid to flexible continuum. Cohesion and adaptability are each, respectively, at the midpoints on these continua.

Families of children with chronic illness may be more cohesive and less flexible than families of healthy children. Meijer and Oppenheimer (1995), in a study of children with controlled and uncontrolled asthma, found that both groups had more cohesive, rigid, and overprotective families, with the controlled asthma group showing more cohesion, rigidity, and over-protection than the uncontrolled asthma group.

As suggested in the family systems–illness model, family functioning may vary by age of the child with chronic illness and by stage of the illness or treatment. It has been found that family cohesion is higher in families of infants and preschoolers with chronic illness and lower for school-age children (Northam, Anderson, Adler, Werther, & Warne, 1996). Similarly, in a sample of children with insulin-dependent diabetes mellitus (IDDM) and children with asthma, older children had less cohesive and adaptable families than younger children and girls had more cohesive families than boys (Holden, Chmielewski, Nelson, & Kager, 1997). It may be that families adjust to the demands of illness by becoming closer emotionally to younger children (and girls) while being more distant and controlling with school-age children (and boys) given their differing, developmentally influenced demands and needs. Both age groups and genders in these studies had adequate levels of adjustment, which indicates that various family structures and interactions may lead to adjustment, depending on the unique situation of the family.

A stronger association between family cohesion, adaptability, and adjustment has been found for adolescent cancer survivors recently off treatment and survivors off treatment over 5 years compared with survivors off treatment for intermediate periods of time (Rait et al., 1992). In addition, family cohesion was significantly lower than norms in these survivors. In fact, 40% of families were classified as disengaged. Coupled with findings of increased cohesion during the treatment phase, it is suggested that survivor families may disengage after treatment is complete in an extreme attempt to regain a sense of normality and allow their adolescents to gain independence. This reaction has been referred to as "family retreat" (Rait et al., 1992).

In an examination of family functioning that went beyond general family functioning or measures of cohesion and adaptability, Silver, Stein, and Dadds (1996) examined the role of family structure on the relationship of illness severity to child adjustment. They found that family structure may impact the child's adjustment to chronic illness. Two-parent families and families with the mother and another adult relative in the home showed better adjustment than single-parent families and mothers living with a stepfather or other partner. Additionally, the link between illness severity and child adjustment was strongest for the mother plus unrelated partner structure and weakest for the two-parent family structure. The risk that these family structures pose may be due to stressors associated with the structure. Single-parent families and mothers living with unrelated partners may face low socioeconomic status, isolation from extended families and the community, or other stressors unrelated to the chronic illness while two-parent families may have a larger pool of resources on which to draw to face the challenges of the illness.

The finding of differences in patterns of interaction for families of children with chronic illness should not be interpreted as an indication of dysfunction. These family patterns may represent attempts to adapt to the demands of the illness that may lead to better adjustment. It is speculated that increased closeness and greater rigidity enable families to organize to meet the challenges of demanding treatment regimens and the threat of harm to their children. This interpretation is supported in findings of positive adjustment in children with chronic illness and their parents and in studies showing these parents to have a greater sense of competence in parenting than normative samples (Hoffmann, Rodrigue, Andres, & Novak, 1995). As an example, treatment for brain tumors often requires the child and family to be at the hospital daily for cranial irradiation treatment which is preceded or followed by surgery and/or chemotherapy; treatment for IDDM involves a complex regimen of daily blood glucose testing, insulin shots, and maintaining a proper diet. For successful adherence, families have to muster immense resources to organize, set strict rules and structure with their children, and support family members' emotional needs.

Child Adaptation and Family Functioning

Research on children with chronic illness shows a wide range of adjustment outcomes, from resilience (Gowers et al., 1995) to problematic adaptation (Daniels, Moos, Billings, & Miller, 1987; Hamlett et al., 1992; Hoffmann et al., 1995). For example, Janus and Goldberg (1995) found that children with congenital heart disease have higher levels of behavior problems as reported by their mothers compared with their siblings and with age-matched norms.

The link between parent and child adjustment in pediatric conditions is established, as is the role of family functioning (Drotar, 1997; Kazak, 1997). Although Daniels and colleagues (1987) found that parent dysfunction and family stressors but not family functioning were related to adjustment of children with rheumatic disease, others generally report a link between family functioning, parent–child interaction, and child adjustment. Davis, Tucker, and Fennell (1996) reported that family cohesion and expressiveness were related to adaptive functioning and behavioral adjustment among children with renal disease, in which one group had transplants and one group was in renal failure. Similarly, Hamlett et al. (1992) reported that family functioning, including family cohesion and family conflict, were related to the increased internalizing behavior problems seen in children with asthma, with greater cohesion, less conflict, and more support linked to better adjustment. Further work has supported the link between family cohesion, expressiveness, control and conflict with the adjustment of children with liver disease (Hoffmann et al., 1995) and spina bifida (Murch & Cohen, 1989). Once more, greater cohesion, greater expressiveness, greater control, and less conflict are related to better child adjustment.

Regarding parent–child interaction, child persistence and self-reliance and effective use of maternal resources in problem-solving tasks with the mother have been related to better adjustment outcomes for children with epilepsy (Pianta & Lothman, 1994). These results were robust even when controlling for the effects of disease (intelligence, severity) and demographic factors.

Lavigne and Faier-Routman (1993), in a review of studies of children with physical disorders, reported that disease/disability, parent/family, and child characteristics are related to child adjustment. Parent/family factors (parent adjustment, family functioning, family stress) are stronger predictors than disease/disability parameters (severity, prognosis, functional status). Child factors (self-concept, temperament, coping) were the strongest predictors of child adjustment, perhaps because of shared variance in the measures. Furthermore, in a recent review, Drotar (1997) reported that generally parent or family functioning measures are related to child adjustment. However, these family measures account for only a small portion of the variance in outcome. He suggests that future research on children with chronic illness and their families include more than one informant or family-level data, develop and use illness-specific measures, take into account the illness course in understanding adjustment, and use a prospective design.

Parent Adaptation and Family Functioning

The literature reflects varying adjustment outcomes for parents of children with chronic illness. Parenting stress, parenting sense of competence, coping strategies, and social support seem to differentiate those parents who adapt successfully from those who do not.

Generally, parents of children with chronic illness use adaptive coping strategies, including problem-focused strategies such as at-risk strategies (complying with treatment) and information seeking, and emotion-focused strategies such as encapsulation (normalizing family life, attempting to find meaning in the illness) (Barakat & Linney, 1995; Birenbaum, 1990). Baine, Rosenbaum, and King (1995) asked parents of children with IDDM and with cystic fibrosis to rank aspects of caregiving for a child with chronic illness that reduced stress and prevented worries. Rankings were similar across the two groups of parents and included parental involvement to enhance a sense of control, provision of emotional support, consistency and continuity in the medical care of their child, and education and information. Some researchers have suggested that parents of chronically ill children rely on these coping strategies more than do parents of healthy children or community samples (Birenbaum, 1990; Boyer & Barakat, 1996). The relationship between coping and parent adjustment has been supported repeatedly (Barakat & Linney, 1995; Ievers & Drotar, 1996).

Social support is a powerful mediating factor in the adjustment of parents of children with chronic illness (Kazak, 1997). It appears that families of children with chronic illness are not more isolated than families of healthy children (Kazak, 1991). Some differences in their networks have been identified, such as greater density (members of the network who know each other) and a larger role for professionals (Kazak, 1992), although others report no differences in network size and satisfaction (Barakat & Linney, 1992). Less isolated families with more available support, greater satisfaction with support, and less dense networks show the best adjustment (Barakat & Linney, 1992; Ievers & Drotar, 1996; Kazak, 1992).

Traditional gender roles in approaching caregiving tasks in families of children with chronic illness have been found (Brown & Barbarin, 1996). Mothers seem to be the most at risk for adjustment problems as they take more responsibility for, devote more time to, and feel more stress related to medical tasks, spending time with other family members, completing household chores, and keeping family and friends informed than do fathers (Brown & Barbarin, 1996; Kazak, 1992). Fathers have been found to spend more time addressing household and medical expenses but experience just as much responsibility and worry for this caregiving task as do mothers. In related findings, mothers of children with congenital heart disease and cystic fibrosis reported higher levels of parenting stress related to personal variables (such as depression, role restriction, sense of competence) than fathers, whereas fathers reported more child-related parenting stress (distractibility, lack of reinforcement to the parent) (Goldberg, Morris, Simmons, Fowler, & Levison, 1990).

These gender differences in stressful aspects of chronic illness may translate into use of different coping strategies and may influence family adjustment outcomes. For children with spina bifida, Holmbeck and colleagues (1997) found that mothers experienced increased social isolation and denial and decreased active coping, adaptability to change, parenting satisfaction, and perceived parental competence compared with mothers of healthy children. Fathers of children with spina bifida experienced less restricted roles, increased venting of emotions in coping and psychological symptoms, and decreased parenting satisfaction. Coping was related to adjustment both in the spina bifida and the comparison group, with less behavioral disengagement (or giving up), more adaptability to change in self and family, and less venting of emotions related to better adjustment outcomes. Regarding family outcomes, McCubbin and colleagues (1983) identified three patterns of coping used by parents of children with chronic illness that were differentially related to family functioning: (1) maintaining family integration, cooperation, and optimism; (2) maintaining social support and psychological stability; and, finally, (3) communication with medical staff and other families. For mothers, maintaining family integration and communication with medical staff were related to family cohesion and maintaining social support was related to family expressiveness. For fathers, maintaining family integration was related to family cohesion and communication with medical staff was related to family organization and control.

Sibling Adaptation and Family Functioning

Siblings of children with cancer report a number of changes in themselves and their families as a result of the diagnosis and treatment of chronic illness. They report that their parents focus more of their attention on the ill sibling and less attention on them and that their parents are more worried and tired (Menke, 1987). Siblings also report that they themselves worry about the physical and emotional well-being of their ill siblings, and they find difficulty in their sibling's limitations. Routines and plans are disrupted, and family separations are frequent (Barbarin et al., 1995; Menke, 1987; Sargent et al., 1995).

The impact of these changes on the siblings' adjustment is not clear. Although some studies have shown detrimental effects on siblings, such as difficulties accepting the illness and internalizing and externalizing behavior problems (Barbarin et al., 1995), others have demonstrated siblings to be resilient (Janus & Goldberg, 1995). Adjustment problems prior to the diagnosis of the sibling are not a reliable predictor of problems postdiagnosis (Barbarin et al., 1995). It seems that siblings may exhibit an initial psychological reaction to the illness, with increased academic difficulties or internalizing and externalizing behavior problems followed by a gradual return to their previous level of functioning (Menke, 1987). Older siblings, in particular, report some positive effects of the illness, such as increased supportiveness, patience, and understanding of the ill sibling, increased maturity and independence, and more attention from family members other than parents and from family friends (Menke, 1987; Sargent et al., 1995). In summary, it seems that some aspects of sibling adjustment may suffer from the strains of chronic illness, such as the emergence of behavior problems, while other aspects, such as social competence, academic adjustment, conflict with the ill sibling, and physical health, may improve or stay the same (Barbarin et al., 1995).

Prospective Studies of Chronic Illness in Children and Family Functioning

Few longitudinal studies have been conducted to examine how the functioning of families and children may change over time and what factors may prospectively influence adjustment. The exceptions address the adjustment of children with cancer and their families. Family functioning changes over the course of the illness and treatment, and it concurrently and prospectively influences child and parent adjustment. Kupst and her colleagues (Kupst & Schulman, 1988; Kupst et al., 1995) examined the functioning of children and their families over a 10-year period spanning the diagnosis of leukemia to the survivor phase, and supported the importance of coping, parent, and family factors. In Kupst et al.'s work, survivors and their families showed adequate adjustment over the study period with parent and child adjustment related to each other and improving over time. A positive association of mother coping with child coping and a negative association of child-perceived psychological adjustment and child academic adjustment were found. Previous coping, level of family support, open family communication, and lack of non-illness-related stressors were related to current coping.

Current family cohesion and expressiveness were associated with child psychological and social adjustment at three time points: at diagnosis with childhood cancer and six and nine months postdiagnosis (Varni, Katz, Colgrove, & Dolgin, 1996). Also, family conflict was associated with child adjustment at diagnosis but not at 6 and 9 months postdiagnosis. In our own work (Kazak & Barakat, 1997) with a small sample of families assessed while their children were on treatment for cancer and then after treatment ended, we found that parenting stress and problematic parent–child interaction reported while a child was on treatment were related to reports of mother and father anxiety and posttraumatic stress symptoms after treatment was completed.

The role of family functioning in influencing the adaptation of children to bone marrow transplantation (BMT) was examined by Phipps and Mulhern (1995). They reported that children's social competence and total self-concept scores declined from pre- to post-BMT assessment. Family expressiveness increased from pre- to post-BMT. Family functioning was unrelated to pre-BMT child adjustment. However, post-BMT family cohesion and expressiveness were related to fewer child behavior problems and more social competence. Family conflict presented as a risk factor for poor adjustment. These families and their children, having arrived at BMT as a treatment option, had likely experienced a history of illness-related stressors prior to the BMT. The results of this study indicate that BMT posed a discrete stressor for these children and their families and that family functioning played a role in the children's successful adaptation to BMT.

These prospective studies generally indicate that family functioning changes over the course of a chronic illness and does influence adjustment concurrently and prospectively. Family influence lies more in patterns of interaction than in gross measures of family functioning and may be specific to the demands of the particular stage of illness or its treatment.

THE ROLE OF COGNITIVE ASPECTS AND
ILLNESS SEVERITY IN FAMILY FUNCTIONING

Breslau (1985) has noted that damage to the central nervous system is the key to predicting the adjustment of children with disabilities. It seems evident that illness severity and cognitive aspects that may limit the functioning of children with chronic illness and increase the stress of caring for them will influence the adaptation of the family. The stress and coping and family systems–illness models cited earlier include the disease parameters of cognitive limitations and illness severity among risk factors. However, these factors have shown inconsistent or weak relationships to adjustment. In contrast, psychosocial variables, including appraisal of the illness and its severity (also included in these models), have been more strongly associated with adaptation.

The literature is scant on the impact of cognitive aspects on family functioning. We now discuss the impact of disease parameters, differentiating cognitive aspects and illness severity, on family functioning and the impact of family functioning on these disease parameters.

Cognitive Aspects

Special education placement, used to represent possible cognitive sequelae of cancer treatment, was linked to lower social and academic competence and more behavior problems but not to general family functioning in a group of children treated for hypothalamic brain tumors (Foley et al., in press). Special education placement also has been identified as a risk factor for poor adjustment outcomes in young adolescent cancer survivors (Kazak, Christakis, Alderfer, & Coiro, 1994). Specifically, those survivors in special education placements demonstrated lower self-concept, social competence, and social support and higher trait anxiety than survivors without learning disabilities.

Cranial irradiation (XRT) appears to result in long-term cognitive deficits (Stehbens et al., 1991). In a comparison of childhood leukemia survivors, those treated with chemotherapy plus XRT and those treated with chemotherapy only, children with XRT were found to be at greater risk for behavioral problems, lower academic achievement, and lower social competence (Deasy-Spinetta, Spinetta, & Oxman, 1988). Similarly, Mulhern, Wasserman, Friedman, and Fairclough (1989) reported that functional impairments and a history of XRT in survivors of cancer placed survivors at risk for academic and adjustment problems, whereas cosmetic impairments did not.

In a unique study of children treated for brain tumors that examined the impact of disease and family factors measured at diagnosis on intellectual and behavioral functioning about 2 years later, Carlson-Green, Morris, and Krawiecki (1995) reported that intellectual functioning was best explained by disease (fewer treatment modalities, less time off treatment) and family (two-parent families, less use of coping by mothers) factors. Behavioral adjustment for the children was best explained only by family factors, not disease parameters.

Thus, cognitive aspects or sequelae of illness have been associated with long-term adjustment in children with chronic illness but not necessarily to family functioning. An exception to these findings is in a sample of children with liver disease, in which disease severity and cognitive functioning were not associated with social competence (Hoffmann et al., 1995).

Breslau (1990) employed a regression design to address the question of whether cognitive limitations have a direct effect on the adjustment of children and their families or serve to make children and their families more vulnerable to illness demands and other stressors. Findings were that children with physical disabilities with brain dysfunction demonstrated greater risk for depression and inattention than a comparison group of able-bodied children. Family cohesion was associated with child adjustment. Main effects, but not interactions, were found for both brain involvement and family cohesion, indicating that their relation to child adjustment was no stronger than that found for the comparison group. These findings do not support the hypothesis that children with disability with brain dysfunction are more vulnerable to stress than other children, but they do support the association between cognitive aspects and child and family adjustment.

Illness Severity

Illness severity seems to account for only a small portion of the variance in adjustment (up to 10%) (Daniels et al., 1987) or is one among a number of factors (family cohesion, family conflict, maternal social support) that influence outcome for children (Hamlett et al., 1992) and their parents (Van Dongen-Melman et al., 1995). In children with asthma, uncontrolled asthma status has been related to less family cohesion, poorer parental interaction in problem solving, and more family flexibility (Meijer & Oppenheimer, 1995).

In contrast to the aforementioned findings, in a sample of boys with hemophilia with and without HIV infection, generally low rates of family stress were reported and severity of the illness was not associated with family functioning (Bussing & Burket, 1993). Also, in samples of children with moderate to severe head injuries as measured by the Glasgow Coma Scale and days to orientation, severity of the injury has not been related to family functioning (Perrott, Taylor, & Montes, 1991). Similarly, Holroyd and Guthrie (1986) reported that parental stress and adjustment were associated more with the demands of the illness than with the severity of illness. Higher parental stress was associated with children with neuromuscular disease (Duchenne's dystrophy), who required more management than comparison children with cystic fibrosis and renal disease.

There has been some support for the "marginality hypothesis" first put forward by Pless and Pinkerton (1975). This hypothesis proposes that less severely ill children in comparison with those who are severely impaired are more at risk for problems in psychological and social adjustment because they are not accepted by or do not fit in with both their healthy peers and their severely ill counterparts. Holmbeck and Faier-Routman (1995) examined the relationship between spinal level lesion, shunt status, family relationships, and psychological adjustment in children with spina bifida. They found that mothers of children with higher level lesions (or greater severity) reported greater attachment to their children, less family conflict, and greater willingness to encourage independence in their children. Children with shunts showed poorer school performance and decreased cognitive competence, although shunt status was not related to family functioning.

Overall, then, objective factors such as cognitive aspects and illness severity seem to relate to functioning in a complex manner (see also Kupst & Schulman, 1988). In line with Thompson et al.'s (1994) and Fiese's (1997) writings on the importance of appraisal of the illness, our work suggests that it may be most productive and relevant for interventions to examine the influence of child and parent perceptions of the impact of the illness on the child and family's functioning. With a large sample of childhood cancer survivors and their parents, we discovered that parent and child appraisals of life threat associated with cancer and its treatment in the past and present ("My child could still die") and appraisals of the intensity of the treatment ("My child's cancer treatments were hard/scary") were consistently related to child, parent, and family adjustment. However, intensity of the treatment and severity of medical late effects as rated by a pediatric oncologist and history of XRT were not associated with adjustment (Barakat et al., 1997; Kazak et al., 1997; Stuber et al., 1997).

We found similar results in our work with children treated for hypothalamic brain tumors, in which perceived change in the child's academic, social, and behavioral functioning as rated by parents was strongly correlated with general family functioning whereas special education placement, intensity of treatment and severity of medical late effects as rated by a pediatric oncologist were not related family functioning (Foley et al., 1999). We believe that these findings provide strong evidence for the importance of child and parent subjective appraisals or perceptions of changes in child and family functioning due to chronic illness over the influence of the more objective cognitive aspects and illness severity factors.

FAMILY ISSUES RELATED TO
LONG-TERM CANCER SURVIVAL

The overall rate of survival from childhood cancer is now in the range of 60–70% due to advances in treatment (Granowetter, 1994). With these advances, treatments have become more toxic and are associated with high morbidity and, in some cases, mortality, as, for example, with bone marrow transplantation (Meister & Meadows, 1993). Specific chemotherapy regimens have been linked to sterility or delayed puberty; heart, growth, hearing, and vision problems; and an increased risk (20 times) of developing a second cancer. Cranial irradiation treatment and intrathecal chemotherapy may lead to progressive cognitive deficits, although modified and reduced dosages in recent years and consideration of child age at treatment have decreased the morbidity. A great deal of attention has focused on identifying these physical sequelae or medical late effects of treatment. Less attention has been placed on understanding the link between this aggressive approach to cancer treatment, the presence of medical late effects, and the adjustment of children, parents, and families.

Prior researchers have reported some difficulties among childhood cancer survivors compared to healthy children. Survivors with learning problems seem to be at increased risk in particular in the area of social relationships. In general, survivors of brain tumors have shown the most risk for poor academic and social adjustment. Overall, however, survivors are functioning within the normal range on standardized measures of psychological adjustment. Although parents may report some distress, family functioning and general adaptation are not problematic. Taken as a whole, these findings seem to indicate that children and their families survive the stresses of childhood cancer treatment showing remarkable resilience.

Some have explained the findings of resilience by positing that survivors and their parents use denial as a coping mechanism to minimize the effects of childhood cancer treatment on their long-term functioning (Kupst et al., 1995). This denial, if it is in fact at work, may be adaptive and part of children's and their families' attempts to resume "normal" routines, interactions, and developmental goals following the disruption of the diagnosis and treatment.

In an alternative approach to understanding the findings of adequate adjustment in survivors, a growing body of research in the area of pediatric cancer survivorship likens cancer to a traumatic event and draws on the trauma literature to shed light on the reactions of children and their parents. The guiding principle is that the diagnosis of cancer and its subsequent treatment present a life-threatening situation to the child and family to which they may respond on an individual level with symptoms resembling posttraumatic stress disorder (PTSD). These symptoms include reexperiencing of the diagnosis or aspects of the treatment, avoidance of situations that serve as reminders of the cancer and its treatment, physiological arousal when reminded of the cancer, sleep disturbance, difficulty concentrating, and hypervigilance to physical symptoms (in oneself or one's child).

The trauma framework to chronic illness is implicit in subject matter of some studies. Cohen (1995) described the uncertainty faced by parents of children with chronic illness. These parents must learn to manage uncertainty regarding illness course, recurrence, and potentially reduced lifespan. Cohen found, in interviews with parents of children with cancer, hemophilia, cystic fibrosis, and congenital heart disease, that routine medical appointments, regular physical symptoms like a fever, changes in the child's medical regimen, negative outcomes for other children from their treatment center, and the child's achieving developmental milestones all triggered this uncertainty. In another sample, parents (particularly mothers) of cancer survivors were found to experience uncertainty and loneliness, but they denied feelings of distress (Van Dongen-Melman et al., 1995).

With a more explicit use of the trauma framework, Pelcovitz and colleagues (1996), using a structured diagnostic interview, found that 54% of mothers of survivors of childhood cancer in their sample experienced a lifetime diagnosis of PTSD, whereas 25% were currently diagnosed with PTSD. These scores were higher than those found for a comparison group of mothers of healthy children. Illness severity, social support, and general maternal distress were unrelated to PTSD diagnosis. Children with cancer also have shown symptoms of PTSD following bone marrow transplantation (Stuber, Nader, Yasuda, Pynoos, & Cohen, 1991).

In our research, we hypothesized that survivors of childhood cancer and their parents may show a subdiagnostic cluster of symptoms of posttraumatic stress with emphasis on reexperiencing and heightened arousal. These symptoms were thought to be related to memories of the cancer and its treatment, ongoing concerns about medical late effects, and worries about the future due to the real risk of recurrence or the development of a second cancer. This hypothesis explained the findings of some difficulties in behavior problems for survivors and some elements of distress for parents, which typically were outside of the clinical range. That is, we hypothesized that the difficulties experienced by children and their parents would be specific to the cancer and its treatment and not necessarily generalized or global in content. In addition, posttraumatic stress symptoms, if experienced by survivors and parents, might influence family development and functioning.

Next, we report our findings from a multisite study of childhood cancer survivors involving 309 families of survivors of childhood cancer and 219 families of healthy children (Barakat et al., 1997; Kazak et al., 1997, 1998; Stuber et al., 1997). Children with all cancers with the exception of brain tumors were included in the sample. The survivors had been off treatment for a mean of 5.86 years, with an average current age of 13.53 years and an average age at diagnosis of 5.83 years. The comparison group was recruited through the pediatric practices at each site. The project involved an initial phase of paper-and-pencil measures designed to assess the presence of posttraumatic stress symptoms in child survivors and their parents as well as correlates of distress (life events, parental social support, family functioning, intensity of treatment, severity of medical late effects, perceived intensity of treatment, and life threat). The second phase involved in-depth semistructured interviews to examine those aspects of childhood cancer diagnosis and treatment that contribute to posttraumatic stress symptoms and to assess the level of PTSD in the survivors and their parents.

Parents of childhood cancer survivors reported more posttraumatic stress symptoms related to the childhood cancer than parents of healthy children dealing with primarily moderate level child-related stressors (Barakat et al., 1997; Kazak et al., 1997). Although a high percentage of parents fell in the severe range of symptoms, their average score was not in the clinical range. In addition, the childhood cancer survivors themselves did not report increased symptoms compared to their healthy peers. From the interview phase, using a semistructured interview designed specifically to assess aspects of cancer and its treatment related to posttraumatic stress symptoms, mothers continually reexperienced memories centered on worry that their child would become sick again, worry about their child having pain, feeling scared that their child could die, and finding out that their child had cancer (Kazak, Stuber, Barakat, & Meeske, 1996). For survivors, shots, hair loss, staying in the hospital, bone marrow aspirations and spinal taps, and pain were the most frequently reexperienced memories. Mothers experienced significant fear, helplessness, and horror associated with the cancer and its treatment. The survivors experienced significant fear.

We then examined which factors were related to posttraumatic stress symptoms in response to the childhood cancer diagnosis and its treatment. We examined this in two ways, through regression and path analyses. For survivors, we found that their appraisal of life threat at the time of treatment and their perception of treatment as "hard" and "scary," their level of anxiety, non-illness-related stressors, female gender, their social support, and family functioning were related to posttraumatic stress symptoms (Stuber et al., 1997). For parents, symptoms of posttraumatic stress were related to trait anxiety, belief that their child could still die from the cancer, parent perceptions of the intensity of treatment and the size of their social support networks (Kazak et al., 1998). As stated previously, documented intensity of treatment, medical late effects, history of cranial irradiation, time off treatment, and age at diagnosis were not associated with posttraumatic stress symptoms. Time since the end of treatment was related to child symptoms in the path-analytic study (Stuber et al., 1997) but unrelated to child posttraumatic stress symptoms in the regression analyses (Barakat et al., 1997).

CONCLUSION

Family functioning is affected in subtle ways by chronic illness in children, and chronic illness in children is affected by family functioning. The role of cognitive factors in family functioning is complex, with some indication of detrimental effects and other indications of continued family coping with these problems. As part of assessment and intervention with families, the burden of care for the child along with parent and child perceptions of child functioning seem central to child and parent adaptation, in addition to the overall well-being of the family.

Preventive interventions are suggested in which child and parent perceptions of cognitive factors and the impact of the illness may be modified to improve the long-term adaptation of the family. Interventions will be most effective if they are provided before the family's perceptions of children's cognitive functioning produce a pattern of reciprocal interactions that serve to reinforce these perceptions. It is essential to work with families from the point of diagnosis of chronic illness to provide a realistic but optimistic framework for understanding children's capabilities and needs. These interventions also must take into account developmental processes in families. As the children grow older, families must be able to reassess and then reintegrate the meaning of the cognitive factors for their children and their families.

In addition to addressing perceptions, it is necessary to facilitate positive changes in family interactions directly (e.g., interactions around homework, rules and responsibilities in the home, peer relationships). Interactions that promote development of children's competencies, as opposed to those that reinforce cognitive factors or limitations, are likely to improve children's and their families' overall functioning. The role of related systems, such as the school, church, and medical treatment team, in influencing perceptions and interactions must be addressed.

Finally, improvement of parent resources and coping will be beneficial in improving the functioning of families dealing with the strains of treatment for chronic illness and cognitive changes. Family-to-family contact and support through multiple family groups may be an integral and beneficial part of bolstering children's and their parents' resources. As families utilize resources and experience support, they will be able to respond more flexibly and successfully in their family interactions, thus promoting continued family development and long-term adaptation.

REFERENCES

Baine, S., Rosenbaum, P., & King, S. (1995). Chronic childhood illnesses: What aspects of caregiving do parents value? *Child: Care, Health, and Development,* 21(5), 291–304.

Barakat, L. P., Kazak, A. E., Meadows, A. T., Casey, R., Meeske, K., & Stuber, M. L. (1997). Families surviving childhood cancer: A comparison of posttraumatic stress symptoms with families of healthy children. *Journal of Pediatric Psychology,* 22(6), 843–859.

Barakat, L. P., & Linney, J. A. (1992). Children with physical handicaps and their mothers: The interrelation of social support and maternal adjustment, and child adjustment. *Journal of Pediatric Psychology, 17*(6), 725–739.

Barakat, L. P., & Linney, J. A. (1995). Optimism, appraisals, and coping in the adjustment of mothers and their children with spina bifida. *Journal of Child and Family Studies, 4*(3), 303–320.

Barbarin, O. A., Sargent, J. R., Sahler, O. J. Z., Carpenter, P. J., Copeland, D. R., Dolgin, M. J., Mulhern, R. K., Roghmann, K. J., & Zeltzer, L. K. (1995). Sibling adaptation to childhood cancer collaborative study: Parental views of pre- and post diagnosis adjustment of sibling of children with cancer. *Journal of Psychosocial Oncology, 13*(3), 1–20.

Birenbaum, L. K. (1990). Family coping with childhood cancer. *Hospice Journal, 6*(3), 17–33.

Boyer, B. A., & Barakat, L. P. (1996). Self-reported and observed distress and coping by mothers of children with leukemia during painful procedures. *American Journal of Family Therapy, 24*(3), 236–250.

Breslau, N. (1985). Psychiatric disorders in children with physical disabilities. *Journal of the American Academy of Child Psychiatry, 24*, 87–94.

Breslau, N. (1990). Does brain dysfunction increase children's vulnerability to environmental stress? *Archives of General Psychiatry, 47*(1), 15–20.

Brown, K. A. E., & Barbarin, O. A. (1996). Gender differences in parenting a child with cancer. *Social Work in Health Care, 22*(4), 53–71.

Bussing, R., & Burket, R. C. (1993). Anxiety and intrafamilial stress in children with hemophilia after the HIV crisis. *Journal of the American Academy of Child and Adolescent Psychiatry, 32*(3), 562–567.

Carlson-Green, B., Morris, R. D., & Krawiecki, N. (1995). Family and illness predictors of outcome in pediatric brain tumors. *Journal of Pediatric Psychology, 20*(6), 769–784.

Cohen, M. H. (1995). The triggers of heightened parental uncertainty in chronic, life-threatening childhood illness. *Qualitative Health Research, 5*(1), 63–77.

Daniels, D., Moos, R. H., Billings, A. G., & Miller, J. J. (1987). Psychosocial risk and resistance factors among children with chronic illness, healthy siblings, and healthy controls. *Journal of Abnormal Child Psychology, 15*(2), 295–308.

Davis, M. C., Tucker, C. M., & Fennell, R. S. (1996). Family behavior, adaptation, and treatment adherence of pediatric nephrology patients. *Pediatric Nephrology, 10*, 160–166.

Deasy-Spinetta, P., Spinetta, J. J., & Oxman, J. B. (1988). The relationship between learning deficits and social adaptation in children with leukemia. *Journal of Psychosocial Oncology, 6*(3/4), 109–121.

Drotar, D. (1997). Relating parent and family functioning to the psychological adjustment of children with chronic health conditions: What have we learned? What do we need to know? *Journal of Pediatric Psychology, 22*(2), 149–166.

Drotar, D., Agle, D., Eckl, C., & Thompson, P. (1997). Correlates of psychological distress among mothers of children and adolescents with hemophilia and HIV infection. *Journal of Pediatric Psychology, 22*(1), 1–14.

Fiese, B. H. (1997). Family context in pediatric psychology from a transactional perspective: Family rituals and stories as examples. *Journal of Pediatric Psychology, 22*(2), 183–196.

Foley, B., Barakat, L. P., Herman-Liu, A., Radcliffe, J., & Molloy, P. (in press). The impact of childhood hypothalamic/chiasmatic brain tumors on child adjustment and family functioning. *Children's Health Care.*

Goldberg, S., Morris, P., Simmons, R. J., Fowler, R. S., & Levison, H. (1990). Chronic illness in infancy and parenting stress: A comparison of 3 groups of parents. *Journal of Pediatric Psychology, 15*(3), 347–358.

Gowers, S. G., Jones, J. C., Kiana, S., North, C. D., & Price, D. A. (1995). Family functioning: A correlate of diabetic control? *Journal of Child Psychology and Psychiatry, 36*(6), 993–1001.

Granowetter, L. (1994). Pediatric oncology: A medial overview. In D. J. Bearson & R. K. Mulhern (Eds.), *Pediatric psychooncology: Psychological perspectives on children with cancer* (pp. 9–34). New York: Oxford University Press.

Hamlett, K. W., Pellegrini, D. S., & Katz, K. S. (1992). Childhood chronic illness as a family stressor. *Journal of Pediatric Psychology, 17*(1), 33–47.

Hoffmann, R. G., Rodrigue, J. R., Andres, J. M., & Novak, D. A. (1995). Moderating effects of family functioning on the social adjustment of children with liver disease. *Children's Health Care, 24*(2), 107–117.

Holden, E., Chmielewski, D., Nelson, C., & Kager, V. (1997). Controlling for general and disease-effects in child and family adjustment to chronic illness. *Journal of Pediatric Psychology, 22*(1), 15–27.

Holmbeck, G. N., & Faier-Routman, J. (1995). Spinal lesion level, shunt status, family relationships, and psychosocial adjustment in children and adolescents with spina bifida myelomeningocele. *Journal of Pediatric Psychology, 20*(6), 817–832.

Holmbeck, G. N., Gorey-Ferguson, L., Hudson, T., Seefeldt, T., Shapera, W., Turner, T., & Uhler, J. (1997). Maternal, paternal, and marital functioning in families of preadolescents with spina bifida. *Journal of Pediatric Psychology, 22*(2), 167–181.

Holroyd, J., & Guthrie, D. (1986). Family stress with chronic childhood illness: Cystic fibrosis, neuromuscular disease, and renal disease. *Journal of Clinical Psychology, 42*(4), 552–561.

Ievers, C. E., & Drotar, D. (1996). Family and parental functioning in cystic fibrosis. *Developmental and Behavioral Pediatrics, 17*(1), 48–55.

Janus, M., & Goldberg, S. (1995). Sibling empathy and behavioral adjustment of children with chronic illness. *Child: Care, Health, and Development, 21*(5), 321–331.

Kazak, A. E. (1989). Families of chronically ill children: A systems and social-ecological model of adaptation and challenge. *Journal of Consulting and Clinical Psychology, 57*(1), 25–30.

Kazak, A. E. (1992). The social context of coping with childhood chronic illness: Family systems and social support. In A. M. La Greca, L. J. Siegel, J. L. Wallander, & C. E. Walker (Eds.), *Stress and coping in child health* (pp. 262–278). New York: Guilford Press.

Kazak, A. E. (1997). A contextual family/systems approach to pediatric psychology: Introduction to the special issue. *Journal of Pediatric Psychology, 22*(2), 141–148.

Kazak, A. E., & Barakat, L. P. (1997). Parenting stress and quality of life during treatment for childhood leukemia predicts child and parent adjustment after treatment ends. *Journal of Pediatric Psychology, 22*(5), 749–758.

Kazak, A. E., Barakat, L. P. Meeske, K., Christakis, D., Meadows, A. T., Casey, R., Penati, B., & Stuber, M. L. (1997). Posttraumatic stress, family functioning, and social support in survivors of childhood leukemia and their mothers and fathers. *Journal of Consulting and Clinical Psychology, 65*(1), 120–129.

Kazak, A. E., Christakis, D., Alderfer, M., & Coiro, M. J. (1994). Young adolescent cancer survivors and their parents: Adjustment, learning problems, and gender. *Journal of Family Psychology, 8*(1), 74–84.

Kazak, A. E., Stuber, M. L., Barakat, L. P., & Meeske, K. (1996). Assessing posttraumatic stress related to medical illness and treatment: The Impact of Traumatic Stressors Interview Schedule (ITSIS). *Families, Systems, and Health, 14*(3), 365–380.

Kazak, A. E., Stuber, M. L., Barakat, L. P., Meeske, K., Guthrie, D., & Meadows, A. T. (1998). Predicting posttraumatic stress symptoms in mothers and fathers of survivors of childhood cancers. *Journal of the American Academy of Child and Adolescent Psychiatry, 37*(8), 823–831.

Kupst, M. J., Naita, M. B., Richardson, C. C., Schulman, J. L., Lavigne, J. V., & Das, L. (1995). Family coping with pediatric leukemia: Ten years after treatment. *Journal of Pediatric Psychology, 20*(5), 601–617.

Kupst, M. J., & Schulman, J. L. (1988). Long-term coping with pediatric leukemia: A six-year follow-up study. *Journal of Pediatric Psychology, 13*(1), 7–22.

Lavigne, J. V., & Faier-Routman, J. (1993). Correlates of psychological adjustment to pediatric physical disorders: A meta-analytic review and comparison with existing models. *Developmental and Behavioral Pediatrics, 14*(2), 117–123.

McCubbin, H. I., McCubbin, M. A., Patterson, J. M., Cauble, A. E., Wilson, L. R., & Warwick, W. (1983). CHIP—Coping Health Inventory for Parents: An assessment of parental coping patterns in the care of the chronically ill child. *Journal of Marriage and the Family, 45*, 359–370.

Meijer, A., & Oppenheimer, L. (1995). The excitation–adaptation model of pediatric chronic illness. *Family Process, 34*(4), 441–453.

Meister, L., & Meadows, A. T. (1993). Late effects of childhood cancer treatment. *Current Problems in Pediatrics, 23*, 102–131.

Menke, E. M. (1987). The impact of a child's chronic illness on school-aged siblings. *Children's Health Care, 15*(3), 132–140.

Mulhern, R. K., Wasserman, A. L., Friedman, A. G., & Fairclough, D. (1989). Social competence and behavioral adjustment of children who are long-term survivors of cancer. *Pediatrics, 83*(1), 18–25.

Murch, R. L., & Cohen, L. H. (1989). Relationships among life stress, perceived family environment, and the psychological distress of spina bifida adolescents. *Journal of Pediatric Psychology, 14*(2), 193–214.

Northam, E., Anderson, P., Adler, R., Werther, G., & Warne, G. (1996). Psychosocial and family functioning in children with insulin-dependent diabetes at diagnosis and one year later. *Journal of Pediatric Psychology, 21*(5), 699–717.

Olson, D. H., Sprenkle, D., & Russell, C. S. (1979). Circumplex model of marital and family systems: I. Cohesion and adaptability dimensions, family types, and clinical applications. *Family Process, 18*, 3–28.

Patterson, J. M. (1988). Families experiencing stress: I. The family adjustment and adaptation response model. II. Applying the FAAR model to health-related issues for intervention and research. *Family Systems Medicine, 6*(2), 202–237.

Pelcovitz, D., Goldenberg, B., Kaplan, S., Weinblatt, M., Mandel, F., Meyers, B., & Vinciguerra, V. (1996). Post-traumatic stress disorder in mothers of pediatric cancer survivors. *Psychosomatics, 37*, 116–126.

Penn, P. (1983). Coalitions and binding interactions in families with chronic illness. *Family Systems Medicine, 1*(2), 16–25.

Perrott, S. B., Taylor, H. G., & Montes, J. L. (1991). Neuropsychological sequelae, familial stress, and environmental adaptation following pediatric head injury. *Developmental Neuropsychology, 7*(1), 69–86.

Phipps, S., & Mulhern, R. K. (1995). Family cohesion and expressiveness promote resilience to the stress of pediatric bone marrow transplant: A preliminary report. *Developmental and Behavioral Pediatrics, 16*(4), 257–263.

Pianta, R. C., & Lothman, D. J. (1994). Predicting behavior problems in children with epilepsy: Child factors, disease, factors, family stress, and child–mother interaction. *Child Development, 65*, 1415–1428.

Pless, I. B., & Pinkerton, P. (1975). *Chronic childhood disorder: Promoting patterns of adjustment.* London: Kimpton.

Rait, D. S., Ostroff, J. S., Smith, K., Cella, D. F., Tan, C., & Lesko, L. M. (1992). Lives in a balance: Perceived family functioning and the psychosocial adjustment of adolescent cancer survivors. *Family Process, 31*, 383–397.

Rolland, J. S. (1990). Anticipatory loss: A family systems developmental framework. *Family Process, 29*(3), 229–244.

Sargent, J. R., Sahler, O. J. Z., Roghmann, K. J., Barbarin, O. A., Carpenter, P. J., Copeland, D. R., Dolgin, M. J., & Zeltzer, L. K. (1995). Sibling adaptation to childhood cancer collaborative study: Siblings' perceptions of the cancer experience. *Journal of Pediatric Psychology, 20*(2), 151–164.

Silver, E. J., Stein, R. E. K., & Dadds, M. R. (1996). Moderating effects of family structure on the relationship between physical and mental health in urban children with chronic illness. *Journal of Pediatric Psychology, 21*(1), 43–56.

Sokol, D., Ferguson, C., Pitcher, G., Huster, G., Fitzhugh-Bell, K., & Luerssen, T. (1996). Behavioral adjustment and parental stress associated with closed head injury in children. *Brain Injury, 10*(2), 439–451.

Stehbens, J. A., Kaleita, T. A., Noll, R. B., MacLean, W. E., O'Brien, R. T., Waskerwitz, M. J., & Hammond, D. G. (1991). CNS prophylaxis of childhood leukemia: What are the long-term neurological, neuropsychological, and behavioral effects? *Neuropsychology Review, 2*, 147–177.

Stuber, M. L., Kazak, A. E., Meeske, K., Barakat, L. P., Guthrie, D., Garnier, H., Pynoos, R., & Meadows, A. T. (1997). Predictors of posttraumatic stress symptoms in childhood cancer survivors. *Pediatrics, 100*(6), 958–964.

Stuber, M. L., Nader, K., Yasuda, P., Pynoos, R., & Cohen, S. (1991). Stress responses following pediatric bone marrow transplantation: Preliminary results of a prospective longitudinal study. *Journal of the American Academy of Child and Adolescent Psychiatry, 30*, 952–957.

Thompson, R. J., Jr., Gustafson, K. E., George, L. K., & Spock, A. (1994). Change over a 12-month period in the psychological adjustment of children and adolescents with cystic fibrosis. *Journal of Pediatric Psychology, 19*(2), 189–203.

Van Dongen-Melman, J. E. W. H., Pruyn, J. F. A., De Groot, A., Koot, H. M., Hahlen, K., & Verhulst, F. C. (1995). Late psychosocial consequences for parents of children who survived cancer. *Journal of Pediatric Psychology, 20*(5), 567–586.

Varni, J. W., Katz, E. R., Colgrove, R. Jr., & Dolgin, M. (1996). Family functioning predictors of adjustment in children with newly diagnosed cancer: A prospective analysis. *Journal of Child Psychology and Psychiatry, 37*(3), 321–328.

Wallander, J. L., & Varni, J. W. (1992). Adjustment in children with chronic physical disorders: Programmatic research on a disability–stress–coping model. In A. M. La Greca, L. J. Siegel, J. L. Wallander, & C. E. Walker (Eds.), *Stress and coping in child health* (pp. 279–298). New York: Guilford Press.

Wallander, J. L., Varni, J. W., Babani, L., Banis, H. T., DeHaan, C. B., & Wilcox, K. T. (1989). Disability parameters, chronic strain, and adaptation of physically handicapped children and their mothers. *Journal of Pediatric Psychology, 14*(1), 23–42.

Wallander, J. L., Varni, J. W., Babani, L., DeHaan, C. B., Wilcox, K. T., & Banis, H. T. (1989). The social environment and the adaptation of mothers of physically handicapped children. *Journal of Pediatric Psychology, 14*, 371–387.

CHAPTER SIXTEEN

Pharmacological Issues and Iatrogenic Effects on Learning

MARCIE WARTEL HANDLER

GEORGE J. DuPAUL

As a growing number of children and adolescents survive chronic illness and the use of medication as a primary treatment for pediatric disorders increases, many children are returning to school after receiving psychotropic medications or continue to receive pharmacological therapy for their illness following school reentry (DuPaul & Kyle, 1995). Accordingly, psychologists need to understand the impact these agents may have on children's neurocognitive functioning and ability to learn. Furthermore, the impact of pharmacological treatments on academic performance must be examined separately from the illness experience, which may also have some impact on children's learning.

It is beyond the scope of this chapter to address all types of childhood chronic illness. Therefore, we chose to provide information on the cognitive effects of common medications used to treat children with seizure disorders, asthma, cancer, and sickle cell disease because the cognitive sequelae of these diseases have been fairly well researched. In addition, we propose a method for assessing iatrogenic effects of these medications on cognition and suggest measures that may be used in these assessments.

SEIZURE DISORDERS

Although antiepileptic drugs (AEDs) have been fairly effective in the management of many seizure disorders, they have side effects that also must be considered. The impact of AEDs on cognition is particularly important because most children with seizure disorders are in regular school settings (Sachs & Barrett, 1995), although learning problems may occur in up to 50% of children with epilepsy (Thompson, 1987). Some of the AEDs that have been demonstrated to be effective in controlling seizures include carbamazepine, valproic acid, phenytoin, and phenobarbital. The effects of each of these and other AEDs on cognition are briefly discussed in this section and summarized in Table 16.1. The reader is referred to other sources for a more comprehensive review (Carpenter & Vining, 1993; Devinsky, 1995; Vermeulen & Aldenkamp, 1995).

Carbamazepine

Carbamazepine (CBZ; trade name Tegretol) is effective in treating partial and generalized tonic–clonic seizures. Early research suggested that CBZ produced improvements in attention and concentration (Dalby, 1975) as well as problem solving (Schain, Ward, & Guthrie, 1977). Alternatively, some investigators have noted that methodological issues may limit the validity of these findings (Trimble & Cull, 1988). For example, beneficial outcomes may be the result of improved seizure control by CBZ or the discontinuation of more sedating AEDs (e.g., phenobarbital and phenytoin) (Schain et al., 1977). Although nearly all of the AEDs can cause drowsiness (Carpenter & Vining, 1993), some studies have found no significant differences in children's attention prior to and following months of treatment while receiving CBZ (O'Dougherty, Wright, Cox, & Walson, 1987) or after the drug had been discontinued (Aldenkamp et al., 1993). In the short term, however, not long after receiving their daily dose of CBZ, children's attention span (Aman, Werry, Paxton, Turbott, & Stewart, 1990) and reaction time (Mitchell, Zhou, Chavez, & Guzman, 1993) seem to improve.

CBZ in moderate doses may impair learning of new information and memory-scanning rates in children with complex partial epilepsy (O'Dougherty et al., 1987). In one study of children with epilepsy who had been free of various types of seizures, no differences in memory scores were observed 1 month after children were randomly assigned to a CBZ, phenytoin, or sodium valproate group (Forsythe, Butler, Berg, & McGuire, 1991). However, after 6 months of CBZ treatment, recent recall was significantly impaired compared to other AEDs, with this effect being even greater following 1 year of treatment. In addition, the speed of information processing was impaired after 1 month of treatment with both CBZ and phenytoin. CBZ may also adversely affect psychomotor speed, but these ef-

TABLE 16.1. Cognitive Effects of Medications for Pediatric Diseases

Disorder	Class of medications	Specific medications	Cognitive effects of medications
Seizure disorders	AEDs	Carbamazepine (CBZ) (Tegretol)	ST: Increase in attention span and reaction time following daily dose LT: No effect on attention span; decrease in short-term memory, information-processing speed, and psychomotor speed (temporary)
		Valproic acid, valproate (VPA) (Depakote, Depakene)	ST: Decrease in psychomotor speed, auditory–visual integration, and planning following daily dose LT: No effect on attention or memory, FSIQ, VIQ, or PIQ
		Phenytoin (PHT) (Dilantin)	ST: Decrease in attention and information-processing speed; increase in sedation LT: Decrease in visual–motor functioning; lower reading comprehension and accuracy skills than other AEDs; lower VIQ scores at high dose than low dose or control group
	Barbiturates	Phenobarbital (PB)	ST: Decrease in attention and memory LT: Decrease in memory and comprehension; no change in FSIQ scores (1 year); decrease in FSIQ scores (2 years) and after discontinuing medication; lower FSIQ, PIQ than other AEDs (?)
	Benzodiazepines	Diazepam (Valium) Lorazepam (Ativan) Clonazepam (Klonopin)	ST: Increase in sedation; decrease in memory ST: Increase in sedation ST: Increase in sedation
	Nootropics	Piracetam	ST: Increase in attention, memory, orientation, and judgment
Asthma	Bronchodilators Beta-adrenergic agonists	Albuterol	ST: No effect on response speed, visual–motor control, or dexterity
	Methylated xanthine	Theophylline	ST: No effect on cognition, attention, or math and reading achievement test scores; decrease in attention in children with learning or attention problem LT: Increase in attention and verbal memory (6 months)

(continued)

357

TABLE 16.1. *continued*

Disorder	Class of medications	Specific medications	Cognitive effects of medications
	Anticholinergics	Atropine sulfate, ipratropium bromide (Atrovent)	ST: Decrease in reaction time, visual perception, verbal memory, and coordination (in adults)
	Nonbronchodialators		
	Ingested corticosteroids	Prednisone	ST: Decrease in verbal and visual memory (especially at higher doses) LT: No effect on standardized reading and math achievement scores
	Inhaled corticosteroids	Beclomethasone dipropionate (BDP) (Beclovent, Vanceril)	
	Mast cell stabilizer	Cromolyn sodium, disodium cromoglycate (DSG)	ST: Increase in attention, concentration, memory, and visual–spatial planning when compared to theophylline; no studies with control groups
	Antihistamines		
	Traditional	Chlorpheniramine, diphenhydramine	ST: Increase in sedation; decrease in psychomotor reflexes
	Second generation	Loratadine	ST: Improved performance on tests of factual and conceptual knowledge; no sedating effect
Sickle cell disease	Systemic analgesics Opioids	Morphine	ST: Increase in sedation; decrease in concentration
(Pediatric pain)		Meperidine (Demerol) Codeine Fentanyl	ST: Increase in sedation ST: Increase in sedation ST: No effect on alertness

Note. ST, short-term effects; LT, long-term effects; AEDs, antiepileptic drugs; FSIQ, Full Scale IQ score on a Wechsler intelligence test; VIQ, Verbal IQ score on a Wechsler intelligence test; PIQ, Performance IQ score on a Wechsler intelligence test.

fects appear to reverse when medication is discontinued (Aldenkamp et al., 1993).

Valproate or Valproic Acid

Sodium valproate (or valproic acid, VPA; trade names Depakote, Depakene) is a broad-spectrum AED effective in the treatment of absence, myoclonic, tonic–clonic seizures, and partial complex seizures (Carpenter & Vining, 1993), particularly those classified as idiopathic (Legarda, Booth, Fennell, & Maria, 1996). In pediatric populations, it is probably the mostly widely prescribed AED (Legarda et al., 1996) as it is relatively safe in most children except those younger than 2 years old (Sachs & Barrett, 1995). On tests of general cognitive abilities such as the Wechsler Intelligence Scale for Children—Revised (WISC-R; Wechsler, 1974), children who did not suffer any neurological abnormalities or mental retardation treated with VPA did not differ significantly from healthy control children on Full Scale, Verbal, or Performance IQ scores 6 months following treatment (Calandre, Dominguez-Granados, Gomez-Rubio, & Molina-Font, 1990).

In one study, VPA did not appear to have adverse effects on memory or attention when measured in children one year after initialization of treatment (Forsythe et al., 1991). However, despite employing a control group of 31 children, results comparing children receiving VPA to healthy children were not reported. Perhaps VPA has fewer adverse effects than the other AEDs examined in this investigation (CBZ and phenytoin) but still has a negative impact on cognition when compared to healthy control children who do not receive AEDs.

More specific effects on cognition have been found in studies that examined short-term, dose-related changes of AEDs. Children performed significantly worse on tests of psychomotor speed at higher doses (> 20 mg/kg/day) than at lower doses (< 20 mg/kg/day; i.e., before morning medication of VPA was administered) (Aman, Werry, Paxton, & Turbott, 1987). Another study found that children who received higher doses of VPA (> 20 mg/kg/day) performed more poorly on measures of auditory–visual integration and planning than children who received low doses (< 20 mg/kg/day) (Herranz, Arteaga, & Armijo, 1982). Therefore, VPA may impair psychomotor speed and performance on more complex cognitive tasks, but these effects appear to be dose related (Carpenter & Vining, 1993).

Phenytoin

Phenytoin (PHT; trade name Dilantin) is effective in treating generalized tonic–clonic seizures as well as partial simple and partial complex seizures. It can cause problems with sedation (Herranz et al., 1988) and attention

(Carpenter & Vining, 1993) as well as slow information processing speed (Forsythe et al., 1991). In one study, children taking PHT for at least 2 years had significantly lower reading accuracy and comprehension skills than children receiving other AEDs (Stores & Hart, 1976).

PHT also has been noted to effect visual–motor functioning. Children being treated with PHT were found to perform more poorly on visual search tasks both before and after withdrawal of the drug than children receiving CBZ (Aldenkamp et al., 1993; Blennow, Heijbel, Sandstedt, & Tonnby, 1990) or those in a control condition (Blennow et al., 1990). In addition, one study provided data to indicate that children receiving PHT performed more poorly on 10 of 12 tests that measure motor and mental speed than children being treated with CBZ (Aldenkamp et al., 1993).

PHT also appears to have dose-related effects on cognition. In one study of children who had been randomly assigned to either a high-dose, low-dose, or placebo control group, those who had received high doses of PHT had lower mean Verbal IQ scores than children receiving low doses or placebo controls (Nolte, Wetzel, Brugmann, & Brintzinger, 1980).

Phenobarbital

Phenobarbital (PB) is a type of barbiturate used to treat generalized tonic–clonic, partial simple, and partial complex seizures. Although once commonly prescribed, it is used less often today because of its association with behavioral and cognitive effects. Specifically, PB has been associated with deficits in attention and memory (Riva & Devoti, 1996) as well as declines in mental ability (Calandre et al., 1990; Farwell et al., 1990). Children sometimes have been noted as being overactive (Vining et al., 1987), drowsy, and irritable (Camfield et al., 1979; Carpenter & Vining, 1993) when receiving PB as compared to other AEDs or placebos. In addition, in one study of children with epilepsy ranging in age from 6 to 16 years old who had become depressed while receiving PB, those who continued treatment remained depressed at follow-up, 2.5 years later, while those who discontinued PB recovered from their depression (Brent, Crumrine, Varma, Allan, & Allman, 1987). This may be an important issue given that symptoms related to depression can inhibit children's cognitive and school performance (e.g., trouble with concentration) (Kovacs & Goldston, 1991).

Some researchers have measured the iatrogenic effects of PB on general cognitive ability in toddlers with febrile seizures who were randomly assigned to either a placebo group or a PB group using the Stanford–Binet Intelligence Test (Thorndike, Hagan, & Sattler, 1986) and the Bayley Scales of Infant Development (Bayley, 1969). Despite no significant differences between the groups in Full Scale IQ scores following 8–12 months of therapy, memory function was impaired with increasing doses of PB, and comprehension significantly decreased 2 years after being treated with PB for 12 months as compared to 8 months (Camfield et al., 1979). In another double-blind, placebo-controlled randomized study, the mean Full Scale IQ scores were significantly lower (7.03 points) in the active medication group relative to the placebo group (Farwell et al., 1990). Six months after discontinuing the drug, the mean Full Scale IQ was still 5.2 points lower for children who had been taking PB than for those not receiving active medication (Farwell et al., 1990). Other investigators have provided data to indicate that Performance IQ scores actually increase after discontinuation of PB treatment (Riva & Devoti, 1996).

Some studies have compared the cognitive effects of PB with other AEDs. A group of children who ranged in age from 6 to 11 years old who received PB had significantly lower mean Full Scale and Verbal IQ scores than children in a control group, both at baseline and 6 months following initial administration of drug therapy. In contrast, no differences were found between the children in the control group and those receiving VPA (Calandre et al., 1990). In a double-blind, crossover design measuring differences between children receiving either PB or VPA after 6 months of treatment, children who received PB obtained significantly lower scores on the Full Scale and Performance IQ scales, Block Design subtest, and one measure of attention and short-term learning (from a battery of 35 neuropsychological measures administered in the study) (Vining et al., 1987). However, a more recent study found no significant differences in the Full Scale, Verbal, or Performance IQ scores among groups of children before, after 6 months, and after 12 months of treatment with PB, CBZ, or VPA (Chen, Kang, & So, 1996).

Other Antiepileptic Drugs

In contrast to most findings of the iatrogenic effects of AEDs on cognitive processes, beneficial effects on performance tasks have been found in children given piracetam, which is a type of nootropic. When this AED was prescribed either alone or in combination with CBZ, WISC-R subtest scores improved so as to resemble those of children in the control group, whereas those not receiving piracetam demonstrated no improvements (Chaudhry, Najam, De Mahieu, Raza, & Ahmad, 1992). Improvements on the Picture Completion, Picture Arrangement, Block Design, and Object Assembly subtests were interpreted by the investigators as indicating that Piracetam may have beneficial effects on memory, orientation, judgment, and attention.

Benzodiazepines such as diazepam (trade name Valium), lorazepam (trade name Ativan), and clonazepam (trade name Klonopin), often prescribed for anxiety disorders, also have been used as adjunctive medications for seizure disorders. These agents have adverse effects that may include drowsiness, dizziness, irritability, and depressed mood (Carpenter & Vining, 1993). Studies of healthy adolescents indicate that diazepam may also reduce memory performance by inhibiting acquisition of new information (Ghoneim, Hinrichs, & Mewaldt, 1984; Ghoneim, Mewaldt, Berie, & Hinrichs, 1981).

Summary

It appears that various AEDs may impair general mental abilities and specific cognitive functions including attention, memory, processing speed, and reading skills. Because most studies have examined between-group differences, it is not known how large these effects are for specific children, or how such differences over time further affect mental abilities or, more specifically, children's academic achievement in school. However, given that children with epilepsy are more prone to learning problems than children without seizures (Gourley, 1990; Mahapatra, 1990), active attempts should be made to monitor the iatrogenic effects that AEDs may cause.

Methodological problems inherent in most studies examining the iatrogenic effects of AEDs on cognition make it difficult to reach any definitive conclusions. Although some studies have employed randomized control groups of healthy children, and placebo controls, as well as repeated measures, most studies have included small sample sizes of heterogeneous groups of children suffering from various types of seizure disorders or initial cognitive impairments. Given that there are frequently differential medication effects for particular subgroups of children with seizure disorders (Aman et al., 1990; Silverstein, Parrish, & Johnston, 1982), future research should examine the cognitive effects of these agents for specific populations. In addition, research on the iatrogenic effects of AEDs on cognition should include subjects with well-controlled seizures receiving single medications (i.e., monotherapy) to improve experimental control and attempt to control for previous seizure activity that might account for the observed deficits in cognition and learning (Vermeulen & Aldenkamp, 1995). Finally, given that AEDs tend to slow psychomotor speed, measures used to assess cognition should be independent of these skills.

ASTHMA

Asthma is considered to be the most common chronic illness in children and is believed to affect between 6.7% and 12% of children under the age of 18 years old (Burr, Butland, King, & Vaughan-Williams, 1989; Gergen, Mullally, & Evans, 1988). As a result, there is concern that a large number of children may be adversely affected by the medications used to treat asthma. As with any chronic illness, it is important to determine what effects the medication may have on cognition and school performance, aside from the contribution of the illness and school absences on cognition and academic skills. We discuss the cognitive effects of the main types of asthma medication, including bronchodilators (e.g., beta-adrenergic agonists, theophylline, and anticholinergics), nonbronchodilators (e.g., corticosteroids, and cromolyn sodium), and antihistamines (see Table 16.1).

Brochodilator Antiasthma Medication

Beta-Adrenergic Agonists

Beta-adrenergic agonists used with children include albuterol (trade names Proventil, Ventolin), metaproterenol (trade names Alupent, Metaprel), terbutaline (trade names Brethine, Bricanyl), and tolterol (trade name Tornalate) (Hill & Szefler, 1992). They are used to treat mild asthma, exercise-induced breathing problems, and chronic asthma conditions, and are typically administered through metered dose inhalers to hasten their effect directly on the lungs (Hill & Szefler, 1992). When employed to manage chronic asthma, these drugs are often supplemented with theophylline, cromolyn, and/or corticosteroids (DuPaul & Kyle, 1995).

Unfortunately, despite their widespread use in children, virtually no research has been conducted that examines the iatrogenic effects of these drugs on children's cognition and learning. One study of 20 children with chronic asthma who ranged in age from 4 to 14 years old employed a double-blind, crossover placebo design to examine the effects of albuterol. Findings indicated that although albuterol was associated with fine motor tremors, it did not compromise performance on complex perceptual–motor tasks involving response speed, visual–motor control, and dexterity (Mazer, Figueroa-Rosario, & Bender, 1990).

Another study involving 18 adolescents and adults concluded that inhaled albuterol relative to theophylline or the combination of these two drugs did not impair verbal learning and memory, visual memory, mental speed and efficiency, or sustained attention (Joad, Ahrens, Lindgren, & Weinberger, 1986). However, these findings are limited by the fact that the study did not include placebo groups and by the small sample size, with participants who ranged in age from 13 to 70 years old.

Theophylline

Theophylline (or methylated xanthine; trade name Theo-Dur) reduces late asthmatic response and bronchial hyperresponsiveness by increasing beta-adrenergic receptor activity (Celano & Geller, 1993). It is chemically related to caffeine and acts as a central nervous system (CNS) stimulant. Typically, dosage levels increase for children up to the age of 9 years old and decrease at older ages (Milavetz, Vaughn, Weinberger, & Hendeles, 1986). In many cases, theophylline is combined with the corticosteroids in the management of severe, chronic asthma, but is used less extensively than in previous years (Celano & Geller, 1993).

Early research had suggested that theophylline interfered with children's attention and concentration (Furukawa et al., 1988; Rachelefsky et al., 1986; Springer, Goldenberg, Ben Dov, & Godfrey, 1985), memory (Furukawa et al., 1984; Springer et al., 1985), visual–spatial planning, and motor skills (Springer et al., 1985). However, most of these conclusions are relative to groups receiving cromolyn sodium, or have methodological shortcomings such as small sample sizes, lack of placebo control groups, or the failure to include methodologically sound tests of academic achievement (Creer & Bender, 1993; Milgrom & Bender, 1993).

More recent studies have found no changes in cognition as a result of theophylline administration. A recent meta-analysis of 11 studies of children treated with theophylline and 9 studies of children receiving caffeine revealed that neither agent resulted in significant deleterious effects on children's cognition or behavior (Stein, Krasowski, Leventhal, Phillips, & Bender, 1996). Two randomized, double-blind, placebo-controlled crossover designs revealed no treatment-related changes on psychological batteries or on parent and teacher ratings of behavior for children with mild (Rappaport et al., 1989) and moderate asthma (Schlieper, Alcock, Beaudry, Feldman, & Leikin, 1991).

On standardized achievement tests of reading and mathematics, no differences were observed in scores for children with asthma and a sibling control group regardless of whether or not the children with asthma were receiving theophylline (Lindgren et al., 1992). Similarly, no significant differences were found for measures of academic achievement or indices of distractibility and vigilance between severely ill, hospitalized asthmatic children receiving theophylline and a healthy comparison group of chronically ill children (Weldon & McGeady, 1995). Unfortunately, the latter study must be interpreted cautiously because some of the children with asthma continued treatments with beta-agonists, antihistamines, and corticosteroids, and children with other chronic illnesses (e.g., insulin-dependent diabetes mellitus, burns, orthopedic problems) also were receiving various types of medications that have previously been found to affect cognition.

Some researchers have provided support for theophylline-related decrements in verbal memory (Bender & Milgrom, 1992), while others have not found support for these findings (Bender, Lerner, Ikle, Comer, & Szefler, 1991). Similarly, children receiving theophylline have demonstrated nonsignificant positive trends on laboratory measures of attention when compared to asthmatic children not receiving theophylline as well as to a nonasthmatic control group (Rappaport et al., 1989; Schlieper et al., 1991), while other investigations have not provided support for these findings (Bender, Lerner, & Poland, 1991).

There also is evidence for individual variations in children's response to theophylline. Schlieper et al. (1991) found no significant differences on measures of attention between 31 children receiving theophylline and a comparison group; eight children who demonstrated improvements in attention did not differ from the rest of the group on any other variables. Yet the 12 children who exhibited adverse responses to the drug (e.g., more errors and higher distractibility scores) were significantly more likely to have preexisting problems in attention or learning when compared to the other children with asthma. Thus, it appears that children who have attention or academic achievement problems may be at greater risk for additional adverse cognitive effects when treated with theophylline.

Anticholinergics

Anticholinergics such as atropine sulfate and ipratropium bromide (trade name Atrovent) relax smooth muscles in the respiratory tract. They are typically used to manage acute, severe asthma when patients do not respond to more common beta-adrenergic agonist therapy. Despite being less toxic than other antiasthma agents, anticholinergics are used infrequently due to their higher potency (DuPaul & Kyle, 1995).

One anticholinergic, atropine, has been associated with impaired visual perception, reaction time, verbal memory, coordination, and the ability to perform mental calculations in a small sample of healthy adults (Sepp'al'a & Visakorpi, 1983). Despite research on the adverse effects of atropine in adults, no studies could be located that have examined the neuropsychological or cognitive effects of anticholinergics in children.

Nonbronchodilator Antiasthma Medication

Corticosteroids

Corticosteroids are anti-inflammatory agents often used in combination with bronchodilators to manage moderate to severe asthma (Celano & Geller, 1993). They are used to prevent and/or inhibit inflammation of airways and may be administered orally in tablets or inhaled as metered doses of aerosol. Oral corticosteroids such as prednisone, cortisol, and methylprednisolone are usually given in "bursts" consisting of an initial high dose lasting several days followed by a gradual tapering off of the medicine (Bender, 1995). Inhaled corticosteroids such as beclomethasone dipropionate (BDP) (trade names Beclovent, Vanceril) may be more effective than orally administered steroids because the agents deliver medication directly to lung tissue and are associated with less adverse effects than orally administered systematic steroids (Jenkins & Woolcock, 1988).

The most widely studied oral corticosteroid used with children is prednisone. Prednisone has been associated with decreases in verbal and visual memory 8 hours following administration, but these effects seem to dissipate 24 or 48 hours following ingestion (Seuss, Stump, Chai, & Kalisker, 1986). Two other studies also have found that children ranging in age from 8 to 16 years old with severe asthma performed significantly worse on tests of verbal memory on high doses relative to low doses (Bender et al., 1988, 1991). Although no dose-related changes emerged on measures of attention, overactivity, impulsivity, or motor control, children reported significantly more depressive symptoms and anxiety while receiving the high doses of prednisone (Bender et al., 1988, 1991). Furthermore, cognitive and behavioral changes associated with high doses of steroids were more likely to occur among children who had a history of adjustment difficulties or who were from dysfunctional families (Bender et al., 1991). Thus, oral steroids may impair memory, but the effects appear to be mild, transitory, and dose related. They also are likely to be influenced by psychosocial factors.

Despite several reviews on the physiological effects of inhaled (aerosolized) corticosteroids in children, virtually no published research is available regarding the impact of these drugs on children's cognitive or academic functioning. One study reported no differences on reading and mathematics achievement test scores between children with asthma taking inhaled steroids (the specific type was not mentioned) and control children who did not suffer from asthma (Lindgren et al., 1992).

Cromolyn Sodium

Cromolyn sodium (or disodium cromoglycate, DSG) is a mast cell stabilizer administered through a metered dose inhaler which acts as an anti-inflammatory agent by reducing the airway and pulmonary response to irritant stimuli (e.g., specific pollen, food, cold air, exercise) (Celano & Geller, 1993). Given that the beneficial effects of this substance may take up to 4 weeks to appear, it is often preceded with beta-adrenergic and/or corticosteroid treatment.

Cromolyn sodium has gained increasing acceptance partly because of the absence of adverse cognitive and behavioral toxicities relative to theophylline. Three studies have been conducted that have examined the cognitive side effects of these agents in relation to theophylline (Furukawa et al., 1983; Furukawa, Shapiro, Kraemer, Pierson, & Bierman, 1988; Springer et al., 1985). Furukawa et al. (1983) conducted a blind crossover study of six children ages 6–13 years old who first received theophylline and who were subsequently transferred to DSG. Significant improvements were found in attention, concentration, and memory when children were receiving DSG. Similar results were found not only on measures of concentration and memory, but also on assessments of depression and anxiety in a follow-up study of 29 children who ranged in age from 7 to 12 years old (Furukawa et al., 1988).

In another double-blind trial, Springer et al. (1985) evaluated 13 children after they had been receiving each medication (i.e., theophylline and DSG) for 1 month. No differences were found, but when three tests of visual–spatial planning were combined, a significant effect was noted in favor of DSG.

Although this suggests that cromolyn sodium has some advantages over theophylline, the absence of controls in all of these studies limits conclusions regarding the neurocognitive effects of this agent. Furthermore, it is not clear that all children with asthma respond similarly to this drug. For instance, in one study by Springer et al. (1985), four children with average IQ scores performed better on visual–spatial tests when receiving cromolyn sodium than theophylline. However, this improvement was not observed for the nine children with above-average IQ scores.

Antihistamines

Children with asthma are sometimes treated with antihistamines to manage symptoms of chronic coughs and rhinitis. In adults, the most common adverse effects of traditional antihistamines (e.g., chlorpheniramine, diphenhydramine) include drowsiness and impaired psychomotor reflexes (Meltzer, 1990). Second-generation H1 antihistamines (e.g., loratadine, terfenadine, astemizole, and cetirizine) that are now available without prescriptions do not depress the CNS and do not cause subsequent sedation as these medications do not cross the blood–brain barrier (Meltzer, 1990; Norman, 1985). Unfortunately, little research is available regarding the cognitive toxicities of either traditional or nonsedating antihistamines on children.

One study of 52 children with seasonal allergic rhinitis examined the comparison of a traditional antihistamine (diphenhydramine), a nonsedating antihistamine (loratadine), and a placebo condition to matched control children without allergies (Vuurman, van Veggel, Uiterwijk, Leutner, & O'Hanlon, 1993). Baseline assessments and subsequent instruction were conducted when children were asymptomatic and 2 weeks following instruction. During the posttest, children were not receiving medication and were asymptomatic. Although the group receiving the nonsedating antihistamine performed significantly better on tests of factual and conceptual knowledge than the children receiving the sedating antihistamine or placebo, all groups with allergic rhinitis performed more poorly than healthy controls (Vuurman et al., 1993). This finding suggests that children with asthma who are treated with nonsedating antihistamines may experience less cognitive impairment following treatment than their peers who are treated with sedating antihistamines.

In a double-blind crossover study, cognitive performance was measured in 92 children between 8 and 16 years old who were treated for 3 weeks with astemizole (nonsedating) or chlorpheniramine (sedating) antihistamines (Shanon et al., 1993). No adverse effects for either drug or conditions were found on laboratory tests of attention or visual memory. It should be noted that children with asthma were excluded from the investigation, and thus the findings may not generalize to children with asthma who receive antihistamines. Given the widespread use of antihistamines, more controlled studies need to be conducted that compare the cognitive effects of both traditional and nontraditional forms of these agents on children both with and without asthma.

Summary

Antiasthma medications have been found to result in cognitive toxicities. In particular, oral steroids may impair short-term memory and increase depressive symptoms which may result in decreased school performance. Fortunately, these effects are transitory. Recent, well-controlled studies have provided data to suggest that theophylline does not negatively impact cognition for most children, and for those who experience adverse effects from these agents that include problems with behavior and attention, the effects are typically limited to the first few days of treatment (Stein & Lerner, 1993). Preliminary studies of beta-adrenergic agonists, anticholinergics, and cromolyn sodium have not reported adverse effects on neurocognitive functioning. However, the lack of consistency across studies of theophylline and the paucity of research on other antiasthma drugs coupled with some evidence of individual differences in response to antiasthma medications (e.g., theophylline) suggest that further research needs to be conducted prior to drawing definitive conclusions about the effects of these medications on cognition. Given that other factors also have been found to contribute to academic difficulties in children with asthma (including low socioeconomic status and behavioral problems) (Gustadt et al., 1989), studies also need to control for such factors in their clinical trials.

CANCER

The most common form of childhood cancer is leukemia. These include acute lymphocytic leukemia (ALL), acute nonlymphocytic leukemia (ANLL), acute myelocytic leukemia (AML), and chronic myelogenous leukemia (CML). This chapter will focus on ALL because it is the most common of the cancer diagnoses and carries the most favorable prognosis (Brown & Madan-Swain, 1993). Typically, the initial (induction) treatment phase of ALL, which includes a variety of medications, induces remission in approximately 95% of patients (Powers, Vannatta, Noll, Cool, & Stehbens, 1995). CNS-prophylactic (preventative) therapy is provided with either whole-brain cranial radiation therapy (CRT), intrathecal (IT) chemotherapy (injected directly into the spinal cord), or a combination of CRT and IT chemotherapy. These therapies are administered to prevent leukemia cells from entering the CNS. Given the severity of cognitive impairment associated with CRT (e.g., mental retardation, and problems with short-term memory, attention, visual–spatial skills, visual–motor skills, and perception), CRT is at present only employed for children at high risk for CNS involvement. Several reviews of empirical studies examining the neuropsychological effects of CRT in children have been published (Brown & Madan-Swain, 1993; Cousens, Waters, Said, & Stevens, 1988; Fletcher & Copeland, 1988; Mulhern, 1994); however, there has been less attention devoted to the effects of prophylactic chemotherapy for children with ALL (see Table 16.2 for a summary).

In addition, some of the drug therapies that may be used during the induction phase include prednisone, L-asparginase, and donoribicin as well as antineoplastics such as cyclophosphamide, actinomycin-D, vincristine, and doxorubicin. Prophylactic treatment with IT chemotherapy consists of high doses of methotrexate (MTX) administered either alone, or in combination with hydocortisone and cytosine arabinoside (ARA-C). When all three drugs are given, it is called triple intrathecal chemotherapy (TIT). The goal of these chemotherapies is to eliminate cancer cells. They also diminish regular cell growth and as a result they lower blood cell counts, frequently leaving children fatigued. All of these drugs can cause fatigue and lower concentration, which may impede children's school performance (Armstrong & Horn, 1995). In addition, vincristine has been associated with impairment in fine motor coordination, speed, and strength, which also can affect children's school performance (Copeland et al., 1988; Dowell, Copeland, & Judd, 1988).

The few studies examining the iatrogenic effects of IT chemotherapy independently from CRT have examined the neurocognitive sequelae of the various chemotherapies simultaneously. For example, one study compared children with leukemia receiving TIT chemotherapy and combinations of systemic therapy (e.g., vincristine, prednisone, L-asparginase, MTX) to children with solid tumors who had received only systemic chemotherapy. No differences in intelligence, memory, language, or academic achievement were found between the groups following diagnosis and at the 1-year follow-up evaluation (Copeland et al., 1988).

Another investigation compared children with either ALL or AML treated with systemic and IT chemotherapy as a CNS prophylaxis but without radiation to children with various other types of cancers (excluding brain tumors) who did not receive CNS prophylaxis (Brown et al., 1996). Chemotherapy (L-asparginase, 6-mercaptopurine, and MTX) was administered to the children with ALL for 25 months. Although no differences were found between groups immediately after diagnosis, children treated

TABLE 16.2. Cognitive Effects of Chemotherapy for Pediatric Cancer

Chemotherapy agent	Cognitive effects of medication
Triple intrathecal therapy (TIT) Methotrexate (MTX) Hydrocortisone Cytosine arabinoside (ARA-C)	ST: Increase in fatigue and low energy LT: No effect on intelligence, memory, or attention (1 year postdiagnosis); no effect of MTX on FSIQ score (5 years postdiagnosis) but decrease in short- and long-term memory
Systemic chemotherapy drugs Cyclophosphamide Prednisone L-Asparginase Actinomycin-D	ST: Increase in fatigue and low energy
Vincristine	ST: Decrease in fine motor coordination, speed, and strength
Combined systemic and IT Tx TIT, prednisone, vinctistine, L-asparginase, MTX, cyclophosphamide, and 6-mercaptopurine	ST: No effect on overall intelligence, memory, language, or academic achievement immediately after diagnosis LT: No effect on overall intelligence, memory, language, or academic achievement (1 year postdiagnosis)
TIT, prednisone, vinctistine, and 6-mercaptopurine	LT: Lower PIQ scores and fine motor skills but not FSIQ or VIQ; no decrease in reading or math achievement test scores (2–7 years after Tx ended)
MTX, L-asparginase, and 6-mercaptopurine	ST: No effect on overall intelligence or achievement test scores immediately after diagnosis LT: No effect on overall intelligence; reading, spelling, and math achievement test scores were 1 standard deviation lower than a group receiving no IT Tx (3 years postdiagnosis and after Tx ended)
TIT, MTX, L-asparginase, cyclophosphamide, prednisone, and 6-mercaptopurine	LT: No effect (1 year postdiagnosis); decrease in perception, short-term memory, visual–motor performance, receptive and expressive language skills, attention, and concentration (1 year after completing 3 years of Tx); 60% of children exhibited learning disabilities in math (1 year after completing 3 years of Tx)
Specific chemotherapy agents not mentioned	ST: No effect on overall intelligence or achievement test scores LT: Decrease in FSIQ, VIQ, and math achievement scores (6 years after Tx ended)

Note. ST, short-term effects; LT, long-term effects; Tx, treatment; IT Tx, intrathecal treatment; FSIQ, Full Scale IQ score on a Wechsler intelligence test; VIQ, Verbal IQ score on a Wechsler intelligence test; PIQ, Performance IQ score on a Wechsler intelligence test.

with chemotherapy scored approximately 1 standard deviation lower on academic tests of reading, spelling, and arithmetic than did children in the non-CNS prophylactic group 3 years postdiagnosis (i.e., after treatment had ceased). Chemotherapy did not appear to adversely affect mental abilities at any point in time. However, in both of the preceding studies (Brown et al., 1996; Copeland et al., 1988) although the majority of children receiving chemotherapy had ALL, the treatment groups were heterogeneous across types of leukemia, making it difficult to generalize the findings to any specific type of leukemia.

Studies that have included only children with ALL also have found short and long-term declines in intellectual functioning as a function of CNS prophylaxis. In one study, 70% of children under the age of 4 years with ALL receiving systemic and IT chemotherapy demonstrated cognitive deficits in intelligence, language, memory, and visual–motor skills 1 year postdiagnosis, as opposed to 14% of children whose diagnosis was at the age of 5 years or older (Nitschke, Wilson, Bowman, Chaffin, & Sexauer, 1990, cited in Brown & Madan-Swain, 1993). A similar investigation compared young children randomly assigned to either systemic plus IT chemotherapy or systemic chemotherapy and CRT (Ochs et al., 1991). No differences between groups were found and mean scores on intelligence and academic achievement tests did not differ from the normative population. However, both groups demonstrated significant declines in WISC-R Full Scale and Verbal IQ scores as well as arithmetic achievement scores between the first evaluation after induction and the final evaluation, 6 years following termination of treatment. Further, clinically significant decreases in individual test performance (> 15-point decrease from the first to the last evaluation on any of the neuropsychological measures) were found for more than 50% of the children receiving either form of treatment (Ochs et al., 1991). These findings may suggest that children receiving IT chemotherapy as a prophylactic treatment may encounter similar deficits in the areas of academic achievement, albeit milder, as do children receiving CRT.

No differences were found for general intelligence, memory, attention, or concentration for children who were randomly assigned to receive CNS prophylaxis treatment with either IT MTX and high-dose MTX or IT MTX and CRT with sequential therapy 5 years following diagnosis (Mulhern, Wasserman, Fairclough, & Ochs, 1988). Although Full Scale IQ scores did not differ from normative samples, when data were pooled across treatment groups, performance on tests of short- and long-term visual and auditory memory was lower than for normative levels. The authors have interpreted this finding as suggesting that academic deficits experienced by children treated for ALL may be related to memory problems that impair children's acquisition of new skills and information (Mulhern et al., 1988). Unfortunately, no baseline assessment was included to allow for a determination of whether children receiving treatment for

ALL also had cognitive deficits prior to their diagnosis or if impairments in memory occurred in response to prophylactic chemotherapy.

Brown et al. (1992) hypothesized that cognitive and academic abilities in children with ALL receiving only systemic and IT chemotherapy would diminish over time. Participants were 48 children and adolescents ranging in age from 4 to 17 years old who were consecutively referred. None were reported by their parents to have had learning difficulties prior to their cancer diagnosis. Prophylactic treatment consisted of L-asparginase, cyclophosphamide, intravenously administered MTX, and TIT. Subjects received MTX, prednisone, and 6-mercaptopurine during maintenance therapy, which lasted 3 years. The study consisted of children who were assessed at diagnosis, 1 year postdiagnosis when receiving treatment, and 1 year after completing 3 years of therapy (off-therapy group). Consistent with previously reported studies, cognitive impairments were found in the 1-year postdiagnosis group, although children who had the longest duration of treatment and were off-therapy evidenced the most severe cognitive and academic impairments. Specifically, the off-therapy group performed more poorly than the other groups on cognitive tasks tapping perception, short-term memory, attention and concentration, visual–motor performance, and expressive and receptive language skills. Further, 60% of the off-therapy children also exhibited diagnosable learning disabilities in mathematics, even after controlling for school absences. These findings suggest that prophylactic long-term chemotherapy treatment can impair the cognitive functioning of children diagnosed with ALL.

A recent study by Brown et al. (1998) provides additional support for the finding that children with ALL who have received TIT and systemic therapy may experience long-term cognitive deficits. Participants included 47 children and young adults ranging in age at testingfrom 5 to 22 years old. Treatment consisted of TIT as the primary CNS prophylaxis; 6-mercaptopurine, MTX, vincristine, and prednisone for continuation therapy; and intermittent TIT for 2 years as preventative therapy. Subjects' cognitive and academic functioning were assessed when they were off-treatment for 2–7 years. Results indicate that age of diagnosis and length of time off-treatment were not associated with cognitive and academic functioning. Participant' scores on nonverbal tasks (e.g., Performance IQ) were significantly lower than average normative levels, but Full Scale and Verbal IQ levels were not significanty different. Mild deficits in fine motor skills also were found. In contrast to Brown et al. (1992), no significant academic impairments were found in reading or math using standardized achievement tests, yet 43% of the participants were receiving part- or full-fime special education services.

Although the aforementioned investigations suggest that children with ALL who have received prophylactic chemotherapy demonstrate neurocognitive impairment on standardized tests of mental abilities, memory, and academic achievement, these findings do not provide a great deal of information or identify the specific problem that children may actually experience in the classroom setting. One investigation has attempted to bridge the gap between the medical setting and the school setting by asking teachers of children with leukemia (no specific type reported) to complete a questionnaire on an annual basis between 1988 and 1994 (Adamoli et al., 1997). The questionnaire compared the school functioning of children with leukemia (42% of whom were receiving chemotherapy without CRT and 65% of whom were off-therapy) to that of comparison controls identified from the same classrooms as the children with cancer. Significant discrepancies in learning (e.g., staying on-task, memory, signs of reading or mathematics learning disabilities) were found between children with leukemia and their healthy peers for each year that the children were studied.

An item analysis revealed that only a small number of children with leukemia presented serious concerns in learning and as a result inflated the group means (Adamoli et al., 1997). Children who scored in the lowest quartile on a dependent variable received "support to help him or her regain mastery in the affected areas" (p. 129) from the staff psychologist. Unfortunately, the specific nature of this support is unclear, and it is not specified whether any of the participants required special education services (those who were receiving special education prior to the study were excluded). In addition, children who had the highest frequency of learning difficulties were those with leukemia who had received CRT and not chemotherapy. While children with leukemia were reported to attend school less regularly than matched controls, the investigation did not control for the effect of school absences on teacher's ratings of learning performance.

Summary

Studies of the iatrogenic effects of systemic or IT chemotherapy on children with ALL have yielded mixed results. Although chemotherapy may impair mental abilities and academic achievement in children less than 4 years old (Nitschke et al., 1990), chemotherapy has not been found to affect these functions year postdiagnosis in children older than 4 years (Brown et al., 1992, 1996; Copeland et al., 1988). However, the results from longitudinal studies suggest that the effects of chemotherapy on attention, language skills (Brown et al., 1992), memory (Mulhern et al., 1988), and verbal and nonverbal mental abilities, (Brown et al., 1998; Ochs et al., 1991), as well as on arithmetic (Brown et al., 1992; Ochs et al., 1991), reading, and spelling achievement (Brown et al., 1996), may become evident several years after treatment has terminated.

Thus, the effects of chemotherapy in children with ALL must be monitored over the course of several years in order to assess possible learning difficulties and provide appropriate remediation. Investigators have recommended that future studies incorporate longitudinal designs, control groups that control for the cancer experience with larger sample sizes while at the same time attempting to control for the child's age at diagnosis, psychosocial and socioeconomic factors, school absenteeism, degree of illness, and previous educational experiences (Brown & Madan-Swain, 1993; Butler & Copeland, 1993). Although assessing learning by means of teacher ratings is a positive first direction (Adamoli et al., 1997), future studies need to assess classroom achievement and cognitive performance of children with ALL in order to delineate specific deficits that may be associated with chemotherapy.

SICKLE CELL DISEASE

Children and adolescents with sickle cell disease (SCD) frequently experience painful vaso-occlusive episodes in their back, abdomen, chest, and extremities that may require pain management with systemic opioid (narcotic) analgesics. Meperidine (trade name Demerol) and morphine are by far the most common types of opioid analgesic administered to patients with SCD who are hospitalized for painful episodes, although nalbuphine (trade name Nubain), hydromorphone, and acetaminophen with codeine also are used (Pegelow, 1992). In addition, methadone, buprenorphine, alfentanyl, fentanyl, and sufentanyl are used to treat severe pediatric pain (DuPaul & Kyle, 1995). Nonnarcotic analgesics for children commonly include acetaminophen and ibuprofen.

Research exists on the acute physiological side effects of opioid medication (e.g., depressed respiration, urinary retention, constipation, lethargy) for children with SCD (Cole, Sprinkle, Smith, & Buchanan, 1986), and on the neurocognitive and academic sequelae of children with SCD (see Frank, Allison, & Cant, Chapter 8, this volume, or Brown, Armstrong, & Eckman, 1993, for a review). However, an extensive search of medical, psychological, and educational data bases identified no available studies that have examined the iatrogenic effects of analgesics on cognitive functioning in children with SCD.

Furthermore, virtually no information exists on the cognitive effects of these medications that are employed for the management of pediatric pain. Narcotic analgesics such as morphine, meperidine, and codeine have been noted to cause sedation, difficulties in concentration, and "mental clouding" in children (Schecter, 1985; Yaster & Deshpande, 1988). In contrast, fentanyl, which is effective in blocking biochemical and endocrine stress response to painful procedures has not been found to be associated with sedation (Yaster & Deshpande, 1988). Methylprednisolone (MPN) is a corticosteroid also used in the treatment of SCD, but like other medications used in pain management, the cognitive effects of this drug on children are largely unknown.

Thus, research is needed that examines the short- and long-term cognitive effects of pain analgesics not only in children with SCD, but also for children managed for other types of pediatric pain. These studies should control for factors other than medication (e.g., social class, school absenteeism, disease severity, and psychosocial factors such as coping skills, family functioning, and depression) that may also impact the cognitive and academic performance of children with SCD (Brown et al., 1993).

ASSESSING THE IATROGENIC EFFECTS OF PHARMACOLOGICAL AGENTS ON COGNITION

Several authors have described a methodology for assessing the iatrogenic effects of medication on children who may experience physiological or psychological illness (e.g., cancer, asthma, and attention-deficit/hyperactivity disorder) (Armstrong & Horn, 1995; Creer & Bender, 1995; DuPaul & Barkley, 1993). This section builds upon these recommendations and offers suggestions that may be applied by both clinicians and researchers (see Table 16.3).

The first step in assessing the effects of pharmacological agents on cognition is to attempt to control for variables other than medication that are posited to affect children's academic and cognitive functioning. For instance, the child's age, severity of the illness, family functioning, social class, absences from school, presence of comorbid psychological disorders (e.g., depression, anxiety), and classroom factors (e.g., type of task, level of task difficulty, teacher variables) may all impact children's cognition and capacity to learn new material. Given that children with chronic illness often are treated with multiple medications (either for their illness or for comorbid psychological problems), all medications that are administered should be documented and their behavioral effects must be noted (Creer &

TABLE 16.3. Measuring the Cognitive Effects of Medication

1. Control for alternative hypotheses.

2. Determine what effects to measure.

3. Choose appropriate measures that are clinically meaningful, sensitive to repeated administrations, and evaluate a broad range of skills using multiple measures and appropriate methodologies.

4. Determine when to assess.

5. Determine where to assess.

6. Determine who will participate in the assessment.

Bender, 1995). In addition, as only an estimated 50% of children comply with their medication regimens (Litt & Cuskey, 1980), some assurances need to be included to determine that medication is actually being taken at the proper dose and according to the presented schedule.

For investigators using single-subject designs or clinicians working with individual children, controlling for extraneous and confounding factors may be accomplished by including baseline data prior to the administration of medication. For example, one might collect teacher ratings of behavior and observations of classroom performance for a week or two prior to initiating a medication protocol. When it is not possible to obtain baseline data prior to initiating pharmacotherapy, other steps should be taken to document the status of the patient's behavior, academic performance, and/or cognitive functioning through examination of archival records. Typically, information about the child's academic performance is available through perusal of teacher records and/or gradebooks. The degree to which the child has completed work and performed adequately on assignments, tests, and projects can be discerned from these records. If such data continue to be collected following an initiation of a medication treatment, then the clinician may monitor any deleterious effects of these medications on academic performance.

The second step in assessing possible iatrogenic effects of medication is to determine the specific areas to assess. Beyond determining changes in physiological functioning, it is important to assess changes in cognitive skills, academic performance, and behavior control. Specific cognitive skills such as memory, planning, understanding of abstract concepts, verbal abilities, and visual–motor performance might be of greatest interest. It may be even more critical to document pharmacological effects on actual academic performance, as this would be a more direct indicator of possible alterations of the child's functioning in the classroom setting. Along these lines, examination of productivity and accuracy on assigned work, tests, and quizzes should be considered. Finally, medication may lead to changes in behavior control that could have a deleterious impact on a child's ability to succeed in school. Increases in the frequency of both internalizing and/or externalizing symptoms should be monitored on a regular and ongoing basis while the medication is being used.

The third step in monitoring possible iatrogenic effects of medication is to select measures that are clinically meaningful and sensitive to repeated administrations, and that allow for an evaluation of a broad range of skills. Armstrong and Horn (1995) have noted that global measures of intellectual functioning are not likely to help clinicians delineate children's specific needs. They have recommended either the analysis of subtest performance on intelligence tests or inclusion of "standardized, age-normed measures of processing speed, sequential memory, attention and concentration, visual–motor integration, . . . and language functioning" (p. 300) in order to target children's strengths and weaknesses. Although standardized, norm-referenced tests of achievement or specific cognitive skills may be useful in comparing children with same-age peers, they often do not provide information about proper remediation as they are not sensitive to academic changes over short periods of time and they are not associated with learning that frequently takes place in the classroom (Shapiro, 1996).

Measures used to assess the effects of medication need to be ecologically valid to provide psychologists with information that can be utilized by parents and teachers to monitor both short- and long-term cognitive effects. Curriculum-based assessment (CBA) is routed in the assumption that "one should test what one teaches" (Shapiro, 1996, p. 16). Rate- and accuracy-based skill probes provide information that directly relates to interventions because they determine not only children's placement in their local curriculum (e.g., spelling, reading, math, and writing), but identify specific cognitive deficits that require remediation (e.g., multiplication facts, reading comprehension, reading fluency). CBA can be used to compare the academic performance of children with chronic illness not only to their previous level of performance, but also to other children in their school if local norms are developed. Given that test probes are designed to be brief and to allow for frequent and repeated assessments, they may be particularly effective in evaluating short- and long-term cognitive effects of pharmacological agents. Furthermore, because they assess specific academic skills, CBA probes may be especially valid for clinicians who attempt to remediate cognitive deficits in children.

The assessment of various aspects of cognition should also include multiple assessment strategies. In addition to CBA, behavioral assessment techniques (e.g., direct observations of behavior) can be employed to evaluate medication effects. For example, when measuring the effects of medication on attention (either over time or with different doses), one could include parent and teacher ratings of attention, direct observations of attention in the classroom setting or on analogue tasks developed by psychologists or trained observers, and specific measures of productivity and accuracy on actual academic tasks (DuPaul & Barkley, 1993). Ideally, observers (including teachers and parents) are kept blind to the type or dose of medication administered, thus providing the possibility of objective feedback about changes in children's behavior that may be associated with a particular pharmacotherapy.

Direct observations also may provide information about factors in the child's academic environment that may be simultaneously affecting cognitive functioning. For example, if one suspects that a child's attention is negatively affected by medication, it is helpful to know whether the effects are apparent across different types of instructional settings (e.g., independent seatwork and large group instruction) and academic subjects (e.g., reading, math, and science). By combining CBA and behavioral assessment techniques, psychologists may further determine if the teaching environment, the academic tasks, or the particular medication under question may be impairing cognitive and academic performance.

In addition to determining the type of assessment necessary, one also must consider the type of methodology to utilize. Whenever possible, medication effects should be evaluated using placebo controls and double-blind methodology to reduce possible bias by reporters. In group designs, the order of doses should be randomized across subjects to control for possible order effects. When one cannot include children in a control group (either with or without chronic illness) who are not receiving medication, children will need to be compared to themselves while not on medication by using either a baseline or placebo condition. It may be particularly meaningful for clinicians to use test scores from classmates to estimate the average level of performance for same-age classmates not receiving medication from that specific classroom as opposed to generalizing from normative data. Likewise, given the variability in children's responses to medication, single-subject methodologies may be important in understanding individual differences.

The fourth step in evaluating the adverse effects of medication on cognition is to determine when to assess the cognitive effects of pharmacological agents. Given that, in some cases (e.g., cancer), the effects of medication on academic functioning may not be evident for several years following termination of treatment, children will need to be carefully monitored and reevaluated periodically over the course of several years. School records may provide additional information about the child's ability to learn prior to his or her current medical treatment. In addition, during each evaluation, one should assess performance during the time when peak behavioral effects of the medication are believed to occur.

The final steps must be to decide where assessments will be conducted and who will be involved in these evaluations. Despite the importance of evaluating children in their natural environments, this is not always feasible. Many psychologists will conduct evaluations of children's cognitive abilities or performance using standardized tests administered in the clinic setting, or even employ analogue tasks to "simulate" learning experiences. Clinicians need to supplement this type of information with school-based data to ensure that the evaluation is ecologically valid. Therefore, psychologists working outside of the school setting may need to collaborate with school personnel to obtain behavioral and curriculum-based assessment measures. Parents also can provide valuable information about behaviors observed at home related to their child's cognitive and academic functioning. Essentially, accurate and comprehensive evaluations on the effects of pharmacological agents will require communication among professionals across settings (i.e., psychologists, physicians, educators, and parents).

CONCLUSION

Although some studies suggest that medications used to treat children with asthma, seizure disorders, cancer, and pain associated with SCD may place children at greater risk for cognitive and academic problems, too little research has been conducted on the iatrogenic effects of these medications for pediatric populations. Furthermore, most of these studies have methodological difficulties that include small samples that preclude confidence in their results. Furthermore, of the few studies that are available, most have examined short-term effects and have failed to employ assessment measures that are ecologically valid.

We have provided a possible method for assessing the effects of medication on cognition in children with chronic illness that will supply clinicians with valuable information particularly applicable to intervention strategies for these children. However, given that more children with chronic illness are surviving and returning to school, psychologists must be prepared not only to evaluate, but to provide remediation for children whose cognitive processes and academic achievement are compromised by treatment with pharmacological agents. It is anticipated that these types of assessments will provide physicians with information about how to achieve desired therapeutic levels of medication for managing diseases and alleviating symptoms without deleteriously impacting on children's cognition.

REFERENCES

Adamoli, L., Deasy-Spinetta, P., Corbetta, A., Jankovic, M., Lia, R., Locati, A., Fraschini, D., Masera, G., & Spinetta, J. J. (1997). School functioning for the child with leukemia in continuous first remission: Screening high-risk children. *Pediatric Hematology–Oncology, 14,* 121–131.

Aldenkamp, A. P., Alpherts, W. C. J., Blennow, G., Elmqvist, D., Heijbel, J., Nilsson, H. L., Sandstedt, P., Tonnby, B., Wahlander, L., Wosse, E. (1993). Withdrawal of antiepileptic medication in children: Effects on cognitive functioning. The multicenter Holmfrid study. *Neurology, 43,* 41–50.

Aman, M. G., Werry, J. S., Paxton, J. W., Turbott, S. H., & Stewart, A. W. (1990). Effects of carbamazepine on psychomotor performance in children as a function of drug concentration, seizure type, and time on medication. *Epilepsia, 31,* 51–60.

Aman, M. G., Werry, J. S., Paxton, J. W., & Turbott, S. H. (1987). Effects of sodium valproate on psychomotor performance in children as a function of dose, fluctuations in concentration, and diagnosis. *Epilepsia, 28,* 115–124.

Armstrong, F. D., & Horn, M. (1995). Educational issues in childhood cancer. *School Psychology Quarterly, 10,* 292–304.

Bayley, N. (1969). *Bayley Scales of Infant Development.* New York: Psychological Corporation.

Bender, B. G. (1995). Are asthmatic children educationally handicapped? *School Psychology Quarterly, 10,* 274–291.

Bender, B. G., Lerner, J. A., Ikle, D., Comer, C., & Szefler, S. (1991). Psychological change associated with theophylline treatment of asthmatic children: A six-month study. *Pediatric Pulmonology, 11,* 233–242.

Bender, B. G., Lerner, J. A., & Kollasch, E. (1988). Mood and memory changes in asthmatic children receiving corticosteroids. *Journal of the American Academy of Child and Adolescent Psychiatry, 27,* 720–725.

Bender, B. G., Lerner, J. A., & Poland, J. E. (1991). Association between corticosteroids and psychological change in hospitalized asthmatic children. *Annals of Allergy, 66,* 414–419.

Bender, B. G., & Milgrom, H. (1992). Theophylline-induced behavior change in children: An objective evaluation of parents' perceptions. *Journal of the American Medical Association, 267,* 2621–2624.

Blennow, G., Heijbel, J., Sandstedt, P., & Tonnby, B. (1990). Discontinuation of antiepileptic drugs in children who have outgrown epilepsy. Effects on cognitive function, *Epilepsia, 31*(Supp. 4), S50–S53.

Brent, D. A., Crumrine, P. K., Varma, R. R., Allan, M., & Allman, C. (1987). Phenobarbital treatment and major depressive disorder in children with epilepsy. *Pediatrics, 80,* 909–917.

Brown, R. T., Armstrong, F. D., & Eckman, J. R. (1993). Neurocognitive aspects of pediatric sickle cell disease. *Journal of Learning Disabilities, 26,* 33–45.

Brown, R. T., & Madan-Swain, A. (1993). Cognitive, neuropsychological, and academic sequelae in children with leukemia. *Journal of Learning Disabilities, 26,* 74–90.

Brown, R. T., Madan-Swain, A., Pais, R., Lambert, R. G., Sexson, S., & Ragab, A. (1992). Chemotherapy for acute lymphocytic leukemia: Cognitive and academic sequelae. *Journal of Pediatrics, 121,* 885–889.

Brown, R. T., Madan-Swain, A., Walco, G. A., Cherrick, I., Ievers, C. E., Conte, P. M., Vega, R., Bell, B., & Lauer, S. J. (1998). Cognitive and academic late effects among children previously treated for acute lymphocytic leukemia receiving chemotherapy as CNS prophylaxis. *Journal of Pediatric Psychology, 23,* 333–340.

Brown, R. T., Sawyer, M. B., Antoniou, G., Toogood, I., Rice, M., Thompson, N., & Madan-Swain, A. (1996). A three-year follow-up of the intellectual and academic functioning of children receiving central nervous system prophylactic chemotherapy for leukemia. *Developmental and Behavioral Pediatrics, 17,* 392–398.

Burr, M. L., Butland, B. K., King, S., & Vaughan-Williams, E. (1989). Changes in asthma prevalence: Two surveys 15 years apart. *Archives of Disease in Childhood, 64,* 1452–1456.

Butler, R. W., & Copeland, D. R. (1993). Neuropsychological effects of central nervous system prophylactic treatment in childhood leukemia: Methodological considerations. *Journal of Pediatric Psychology, 18,* 319–338.

Calandre, E. P., Dominguez-Granados, R., Gomez-Rubio, M., & Molina-Font, J. A. (1990). Cognitive effects of long-term treatment with phenobarbital and valproic acid in school children. *Acta Neurologica Scandinavica, 81,* 504–506.

Camfield, C. S., Chaplin, S., Doyle, A. B., Shapiro, S. H., Cummings, C., & Camfield, P. R. (1979). Side effects of phenobarbital in toddlers: Behavioral and cognitive aspects. *Journal of Pediatrics, 361–365.*

Carpenter, R. O., & Vining, E. P. G. (1993). Antiepileptics (anticonvulsants). In J. S.

Werry & M. G. Aman (Eds.), *Practitioner's guide to psychoactive drugs for children and adolescents* (pp. 321–346). New York: Plenum Press.

Celano, M. P., & Geller, R. J. (1993). Learning, school performance, and children with asthma: How much at risk? *Journal of Learning Disabilities, 26*, 23–32.

Chaudhry, H. R., Najam, N., De Mahieu, C., Raza, A., & Ahmad, N. (1992). Clinical use of Piracetam in epileptic patients. *Current Therapeutic Research, 52*, 355–360.

Chen, Y. J., Kang, W. M., & So, W. (1996). Comparison of antiepileptic drugs on cognitive function in newly diagnosed epileptic children: A psychometric and neurophysiological study. *Epilepsia, 37*, 81–86.

Cole, T. B., Sprinkle, R. H., Smith, S. J., & Buchanan, G. R. (1986). Intravenous narcotic therapy for children with severe sickle cell pain crisis. *American Journal of Diseases of Children, 140*, 1255–1259.

Copeland, D. R., Dowell, R. E., Fletcher, J. M., Sullivan, M. P., Jaffee, N., Cangir, A., Frankel, L. S., & Judd, B. W. (1988). Neuropsychological test performance of pediatric cancer patients at diagnosis and one year later. *Journal of Pediatric Psychology, 13*, 183–196.

Cousens, P., Waters, J. S., Said, J., & Stevens, M. (1988). Cognitive effects of cranial radiation in leukemia: A survey and meta-analysis. *Journal of Child Psychology and Psychiatry, 29*, 839–852.

Creer, T. L., & Bender, B. G. (1993). Asthma. In R. J. Gatchel & E. B. Blanchard (Eds.), *Psychophysiological Disorders* (pp. 151–203). Washington, DC: American Psychological Association.

Creer, T. L., & Bender, B. G. (1995). Pediatric asthma. In M. C. Roberts (Ed.), *Handbook of pediatric psychology* (2nd ed., pp. 219–240). New York: Guilford Press.

Dalby, M. A. (1975). Behavioral effects of carbamazepine. In J. K. Perry & D. D. Daly (Eds.), *Advances in neurology* (pp. 331–343). New York: Raven Press.

Devinsky, O. (1995). Cognitive and behavioral effects of antiepileptic drugs. *Epilepsia, 36*(Suppl. 2), S46–S65.

Dowell, R. E., Copeland, D. R., & Judd, B. W. (1988). Neuropsychological effects of chemotherapeutic agents. *Developmental Neuropsychology, 5*, 17–24.

DuPaul, G. J., & Barkley, R. A. (1993). Behavioral contributions to pharmacotherapy: The utility of behavioral methodology in medication treatment of children with attention deficit hyperactivity disorder. *Behavior Therapy, 24*, 47–65.

DuPaul, G. J., & Kyle, K. E. (1995). Pediatric pharmacology and psychopharmacology. In M. C. Roberts (Ed.), *Handbook of pediatric psychology* (2nd ed., pp. 219–240). New York: Guilford Press.

Farwell, J. R., Lee, Y. J., Hirtz, D. G., Sulzbacher, S. I., Ellenberg, J. H., & Nelson, K. B. (1990). Phenobarbital for febrile seizures: Effects on intelligence and on seizure recurrence. *New England Journal of Medicine, 322*, 364–369.

Fletcher, J. M., & Copeland, D. R. (1988). Neurobehavioral effects of central nervous system prophylactic treatment of cancer in children. *Journal of Clinical and Experimental Neuropsychology, 4*, 495–538.

Forsythe, I., Butler, R., Berg, I., & McGuire, R. (1991). Cognitive impairment in new cases of epilepsy randomly assigned to carbamazepine, phenytoin and sodium valproate. *Developmental Medicine and Child Neurology, 33*, 524–534.

Furukawa, C. T., DuHamel, T., Weimer, L., Shapiro, G. G., Pierson, W. E., &

Bierman, C. W. (1988). Cognitive and behavioral findings in children taking theophylline. *Journal of Allergy and Clinical Immunology, 81,* 83–88.

Furukawa, C. T., Shapiro, G. G., Bierman, C. W., Kraemer, M. J., Ward, D. J., & Pierson, W. E. (1984). A double-blind study comparing the effectiveness of cromolyn sodium and sustained-release theophylline in childhood asthma. *Pediatrics, 74,* 453–459.

Furukawa, C. T., Shapiro, C. G., Kraemer, M. J., Pierson, W. E., Bierman, C. W. (1983). Theophylline vs. cromolyn sodium out-patient management of childhood asthma. *Journal of Allergy and Clinical Immunology, 71,* 130.

Gergen, P. J., Mullally, D. I., & Evans, R. (1988). National survey of prevalence of asthma among children in the United States, 1976 to 1987. *Pediatrics, 81,* 1–7.

Ghoneim, M. M., Hinrichs, J. V., & Mewaldt, S. P. (1984). Dose–response analysis of the behavioral effects of diazepam: I. Learning and memory. *Psychopharmacology (Berlin), 82,* 291–295.

Ghoneim, M. M., Mewaldt, S. P., Berie, J. L., & Hinrichs, J. V. (1981). Memory and performance effects of single and 3-week administration of diazapam. *Psychopharmacology, 73,* 147–151.

Gourley, R. (1990). Educational policies. *Epilepsia, 31*(Suppl. 4), S59–S60.

Gustadt, L. B., Gillette, J. W., Mrazek, D. A., Furukawa, J. T., LaBrecque, J. F., & Strunk, R. C. (1989). Determinants of school performance in children with chronic asthma. *American Journal of Diseases in Children, 143,* 471–475.

Herranz, J. L., Arteaga, R., & Armijo, J. A. (1988). Side effects of sodium valproate in monotherapy controlled by plasma levels: A study in 88 pediatric patients. *Epilepsia, 23,* 204–214.

Hill, M. R., & Szefler, S. J. (1992). Advances in the pharmacologic management of asthma. In S. J. Yaffe & J. V. Aranda (Eds.), *Pediatric pharmacology: Therapeutic principles in practice* (pp. 317–334). Philadelphia: Saunders.

Jenkins, C. R., & Woolcock, A. J. (1988). Effect of prednisone and beclomethasone dipropionate on airway responsiveness in asthma: A comparative study. *Thorax, 43,* 378–384.

Joad, J., Ahrens, R. C., Lindgren, S. D., & Weinberger, M. M. (1986). Extrapulmonary effects of maintenance therapy with theophylline and inhaled albuterol in patients with chronic asthma. *Journal of Allergy and Clinical Immunology, 78,* 1147–1153.

Kovacs, M., & Goldston, D. (1991). Cognitive and social cognitive development of depressed children and adolescents. *Journal of the American Academy of Child and Adolescent Psychiatry, 30,* 388–392.

Legarda, S. B., Booth, M. P., Fennell, E. B., & Maria, B. L. (1996). Altered cognitive functioning in children with idiopathic epilepsy receiving valproate monotherapy. *Journal of Child Neurology, 11,* 321–330.

Lindgren, S., Lokshin, B., Stromquist, A., Weinberger, M., Nassif, E., McCubbin, M., & Frasher, R. (1992). Does asthma or treatment with theophylline limit children's academic performance? *New England Journal of Medicine, 327,* 926–930.

Litt, I. F., & Cuskey, W. R. (1980). Compliance with medical regimens during adolescence. *Pediatric Clinics of North America, 27,* 1–15.

Mahapatra, S. (1990). Reading behavior in children with epilepsy. *Psychological Studies, 35,* 170–178.

Mazer, B., Figueroa-Rosario, W., & Bender, B. (1990). The effects of albuterol aerosol on fine-motor performance in children with chronic asthma. *Journal of Allergy and Clinical Immunology, 86,* 243–248.

Meltzer, E. O. (1990). Antihistamine- and decongestant-induced performance decrements. *Journal of Abnormal Child Psychology, 21,* 79–89.

Milavetz, G., Vaughn, L. M., Weinberger, M. M., & Hendeles, L. (1986). Evaluation of a scheme for establishing and maintaining dosage of theophylline in ambulatory patients with chronic asthma. *Journal of Pediatrics, 109,* 351–354.

Milgrom, H., & Bender, B. G. (1993). Psychological side effects of therapy with corticosteroids. *American Review of Respiratory Disease, 147,* 471–473.

Mitchell, W. G., Zhou, Y., Chavez, J. M., & Guzman, B. L. (1993). Effects of antiepileptic drugs on reaction time, attention, and impulsivity in children. *Pediatrics, 91,* 101–105.

Mulhern, R. K. (1994). Neuropsychological late effects. In D. J. Bearison, & R. K. Mulhern (Eds.), *Pediatric psychooncology: Psychological perspectives on children with cancer* (pp. 99–121). New York: Oxford University Press.

Mulhern, R. K., Wasserman, A. L., Fairclough, D., & Ochs, J. (1988). Memory function in disease-free survivors of childhood acute lymphocytic leukemia given CNS prophylaxis with or without 1,800 cGy cranial irradiation. *Journal of Clinical Oncology, 6,* 315–320.

Nitschke, R., Wilson, D., Bowman, M., Chaffin, M., Sexauer, C. (1990, September). *MRI detection of transient leukocephalopathy and neuropsychological findings in children treated for acute lymphocytic leukemia.* Paper presented at the third annual meeting of the American Society of Pediatric Hematology/Oncology, Chicago.

Nolte, R., Wetzel, B., Brugmann, G., & Brintzinger, I. (1980). Effects of phenytoin- and primidone-monotherapy on mental performance in children. In S. I. Johanessen (Ed.), *Antiepileptic therapy: Advances in drug monitoring* (pp. 81–90). New York: Raven Press.

Norman, P. S. (1985). Newer antihistaminic agents. *Journal of Allergy and Clinical Immunology, 76,* 366–368.

Ochs, J., Mulhern, R. K., Fairclough, D., Parvey, L., Whitaker, J., Ch'ien, L., Mauer, A., & Simone, J. (1991). Comparison of neuropsychological functioning and clinical indicators of neurotoxicity in long term survivors of childhood leukemia given cranial radiation or parental methotrexate: A prospective study. *Journal of Clinical Oncology, 9,* 145–151.

O'Dougherty, M., Wright, F. S., Cox, S., Walson, P. (1987). Carbamazepine plasma concentration. Relationship to cognitive impairment. *Archives of Neurology, 44,* 863–867.

Pegelow, C. H. (1992). Survey of pain management therapy provided for children with sickle cell disease. *Clinical Pediatrics, 31,* 211–214.

Powers, S. W., Vannatta, K., Noll, R. B., Cool, V. A., & Stehbens, J. A. (1995). Leukemia and other childhood cancers. In M. C. Roberts (Ed.), *Handbook of pediatric psychology* (2nd ed., pp. 310–326). New York: Guilford Press.

Rachelefsky, G. S., Wo, J., Adelson, J., Mickey, M. R., Spector, S. L., Katz, R. M., Siegel, S. C., & Rohr, A. S. (1986). Behavioral abnormalities and poor school performance due to oral theophylline use. *Pediatrics, 78,* 1133–1138.

Rappaport, L., Coffman, H., Guare, R., Fenton, T., DeGraw, C., & Twarog, F.

(1989). Effects of theophylline on behavior and learning in children with asthma. *American Journal of Diseases of Children, 143,* 368–372.

Riva, D., & Devoti, M. (1996). Discontinuation of phenobarbital in children: Effects on neurocognitive behavior. *Pediatric Neurology, 14,* 36–40.

Sachs, H. & Barrett, R. P. (1995). Seizure disorders: A review for school psychologists. *School Psychology Review, 24,* 131–145.

Schain, R. J., Ward, J. W., & Guthrie, D. (1977). Carbamazepine as an anticonvulsant in children. *Neurology, 27,* 1023–1028.

Schecter, N. L. (1985). Pain and pain control in children. *Current Problems in Pediatrics, 15,* 1–67.

Schlieper, A., Alcock, D., Beaudry, P., Feldman, W., & Leikin, L. (1991). Effects of therapeutic plasma concentrations of theophylline on behavior, cognitive processing, and affect in children with asthma. *Journal of Pediatrics, 118,* 449–455.

Sepp'al'a, T., & Visakorpi, R. (1983). Psychophysiological measurements of oral atropine in man. *Acta Pharmacologica Toxicologica, 52,* 68–74.

Seuss, W. M., Stump, N., Chai, H., & Kalisker, A. (1986). Mnemonic effects of asthma medication in children. *Journal of Asthma, 23,* 291–296.

Shanon, A., Feldman, W., Leikin, L., Ham Pong, A., Peterson, R., & Williams, V. (1993). Comparison of CNS asverse effects between astemizole and chlorpheniramine in children: A randomized, double-blind study. *Developmental Pharmacology Therapy, 20,* 239–246.

Shapiro, E. S. (1996). *Academic skills problems: Direct assessment and intervention* (2nd ed.). New York: Guilford Press.

Silverstein, F. S., Parrish, M. A., & Johnston, M. V. (1982). Adverse behavioral reactions in children treated with carbamazepine (Tegretol). *Journal of Pediatrics, 101,* 785–787.

Springer, C., Goldenberg, B., Ben Dov, I., & Godfrey, S. (1985). Clinical, physiological, and psychological comparison of treatment by cromolyn sodium or theophylline in childhood asthma. *Journal of Allergy and Clinical Immunology, 76,* 64–69.

Stein, M. A., & Lerner, C. A. (1993). Behavioral and cognitive effect of theophylline: A dose–response study. *Annals of Allergy, 70,* 135–140.

Stein, M. A., Krasowski, M., Leventhal, B. L., Phillips, W., & Bender, B. G. (1996). Behavioral and cognitive effects of methylxanthines: A meta-analysis of theophylline and caffeine. *Archives of Pediatric and Adolescent Medicine, 150,* 284–288.

Stores, G., & Hart, J. (1976). Reading skills of children with generalized or focal epilepsy attending ordinary school. *Developmental Medicine and Child Neurology, 18,* 705–716.

Thompson, P. J. (1987). Educational attainment in children and young people with epilepsy. In J. Okley & G. Stores (Eds.), *Epilepsy and education* (pp. 15–24). London: Medical Tribune Group.

Thorndike, R. L., Hagan, E. P., & Sattler, J. M. (1986). *Stanford–Binet Intelligence Scale* (4th ed.). Chicago: Riverside.

Trimble, M. R., & Cull, C. A. (1988). Children of school age: The influence of antiepileptic drugs on behavior and intellect. *Epilepsia, 29,* 15–19.

Vermeulen, J., & Aldenkamp, A. P. (1995). Cognitive side-effects of chronic antiepileptic drug treatment: A review of 25 years of research. *Epilepsy Research, 22,* 65–95.

Vining, E. P. G., Mellits, E. D., Dorsen, M. M., Cataldo, M. F., Quaskey, S. A., Spielberg, S. P., & Freeman, J. M. (1987). Psychological and behavioral effects of antiepileptic drugs on children: A double-blind comparison between phenobarbital and valproic acid. *Pediatrics, 80,* 165–174.

Vuurman, E. F., van Veggel, L., Uiterwijk, M. M., Leutner, D., & O'Hanlon, J. F. (1993). Seasonal allergic rhinitis and antihistamine effects on children's learning. *Annals of Allergy, 71,* 121–126.

Yaster, M., & Deshpande, J. K. (1988). Management of pediatric pain with opioid analgesics. *Journal of Pediatrics, 113,* 421–429.

Wechsler, D. (1974). *Wechsler Intelligence Scale for Children—Revised.* New York: Psychological Corporation.

Weldon, D. P., & McGeady, S. J. (1995). Theophylline effects on cognition, behavior, and learning. *Archives of Pediatric and Adolescent Medicine, 149,* 90–93.

CHAPTER SEVENTEEN

Summaries, Training, Ethics, and Direction

DEBORAH L. ANDERSON
RONALD T. BROWN
LAURA WILLIAMS

SUMMARIES

A variety of factors influence cognition in children and adolescents with chronic illness, and many of these affect the course and outcome of an illness. Consistent with the model provided by Garmezy (1981), we have highlighted the role of risk and protective factors that predict cognitive problems or, conversely, adaptation. In this chapter we describe demographics, disease parameters, individual differences, and family characteristics that affect cognition in chronically medically ill children.

Demographic Factors

Demographic factors include such variables as age of disease onset, gender of the child, and social resources of the family, including educational level of the parents and household income. The effect on cognitive capabilities of diseases such as cancer, congenital cardiac conditions, and insulin-dependent diabetes mellitus is related to both the age at which the child is diagnosed with the disease (Rovet & Fernandes, Chapter 7) and the timing of disease intervention (Armstrong & Mulhern, Chapter 4; Delamater, Brady, & Blumberg, Chapter 9). Age can thus be either a risk or a protective factor. For example, children diagnosed with insulin-dependent diabetes mellitus during the preschool years are more severely affected by the disease than children diagnosed at a later age (Rovet & Fernandes, Chapter 7). Alternatively, age can be a protective factor, such as the case of children with congenital heart defects, where earlier correction is associated with better learning outcomes (Delamater, Brady, & Blumberg, Chapter 9). Although gender has not been the focus of a great deal of research on cognitive outcome, recent data suggest that females who have received either central nervous system radiation or chemotherapy for leukemia are at significantly greater risk for cognitive neurotoxicities than are their male counterparts (Armstrong & Mulhern, Chapter 4; Brown et al., 1998). A wealth of data attests to the notion that social class is a significant predictor of cognition. Children from lower socioeconomic backgrounds have fewer economic and educational resources, and this negatively affects cognitive outcome. Some diseases, such as asthma and HIV/AIDS, have traditionally been associated with lower socioeconomic classes (Frank, Allison, & Cant, Chapter 8; Lemanek & Hood, Chapter 5; Wolters, Brouwers, & Perez, Chapter 6). With the additional financial burden associated with illness, a family's limited resources can be further depleted. Economic resources and education may help insulate the family and child from the devastating effects of a disease. Higher educational attainment may enable the family to access better medical care and to understand better the child's disease and treatment options. Alternatively, employment outside the home for caretakers poses an additional role that may result in stressors, which can directly affect the parents' coping skills and indirectly affect the child's adaptation to the disease.

Medical Parameters

Several disease-related variables, such as duration and severity of illness, clearly affect cognitive factors in the medically ill child or adolescent. As noted, age at onset is one aspect shown to influence outcome. Another important dimension related to time is length of illness. Specifically, children who have received longer periods of treatment typically have a greater number of school absences and may have received invasive and prolonged therapies associated with cognitive toxicities (Armstrong & Mulhern, Chapter 4; Handler & DuPaul, Chapter 16). Moreover, as periods of illness increase, opportunities to experience typical peer relationships are diminished and compromised. Cognitive adaptation in the chronically ill youngster may be detrimentally affected by social isolation from school, family, or peers (Schuman & La Greca, Chapter 13).

Severity of disease is another important factor in children with a chronic illness. Specific diseases and the degree of associated pathology place children at greater risk for such marked events as respiratory arrests that result in hypoxic events for children with asthma, cerebral vascular accidents (CVAs) for children with a more severe phenotypical expression of sickle cell disease, or a prolonged seizure event resulting in ischemia of brain tissue. Thus, the severity of disease per se may not necessarily be associated with poor cognitive outcome; rather, it is the specific event that is associated with more severe diseases that results in impaired cognition. The frequency of marked events also may be associated with adherence to various medical regimens. Adherence can serve as a protective factor in maintaining adequate cognitive functioning. For example, children with insulin-dependent diabetes mellitus who carefully adhere to a prescribed treatment regimen of strict dietary control, meticulous monitoring of blood glucose levels, and subsequent titration of insulin have been shown to demonstrate better cognitive adaptation than their less adherent diabetic peers.

Individual Differences

Characteristics of the individual play a role in the cognitive functioning of children and adolescents with chronic diseases. For children who have sustained traumatic brain injuries, premorbid adjustment has been an important ingredient in successful adaptation to the recovery process (Ewing-Cobbs & Bloom, Chapter 12). Good premorbid functioning is an important protective factor for children with chronic diseases, since it predicts positive adaptation to the illness and its associated stressors as well as cognitive functioning throughout and following the disease process. An adequate level of cognitive functioning is especially related to the child's and family's capacity to understand the disease and its management. Children with learning disorders are at greater risk for experiencing problems with compliance and having difficulties in effectively managing their disease. For example, for children and adolescents with insulin-dependent diabetes mellitus, the presence of learning disabilities is a significant risk factor and predicts poorer glycemic control because children may not possess the cognitive schemata necessary to follow a complex medical regimen successfully (Rovet & Fernandes, Chapter 7).

Another component of individual differences that affects disease management is coping style and perceptions associated with causality of disease, particularly given the significant role that these variables play in the learning environment (Kaslow, Rehm, & Siegel, 1984). Coping style and perceptual set are important in learning and cognition as a whole, and when coupled with medical illness may synergize to have substantial effect on cognitive adaptation in children with chronic diseases. For example, individuals characterized by more active coping styles have better disease adaptation. Moreover, those who have internal, stable, global attributions for positive events have better disease adaptation (Lemanek & Hood, Chapter 5; Schoenherr, Brown, Baldwin, & Kaslow, 1992). These latter constructs are particularly important in pediatric psychology because they are amenable to intervention and change, unlike other disease-related factors that may be difficult to control or alter because of their association with the pathophysiology of the disease.

Ecological Issues

Although one must bear in mind individual characteristics of the child, the specific characteristics of the environment also must be considered. Families, schools, and peers play an integral role in the child's environment. Over the past several years there has been increasing emphasis on the effect of the family system on a child's illness and, in turn, the effect of the disease on the family system (Barakat & Kazak, Chapter 15). Families not only provide the genetic hardware for children's mental abilities, but also shape the organizational process and environmental influences to help the child maximize that genetic potential. Families clearly can provide a great deal of support during diagnosis, treatment, and recovery. Peers and families are also important in providing the social support that enhances reintegration to school (Madan-Swain, Fredrick, & Wallander, Chapter 14) and negotiation of the stressors associated with academic performance and peer relationships (Schuman & La Greca, Chapter 13). Peers are especially important for normalizing the illness experience and assisting the chronically ill child or adolescent to become comfortable participating in routine daily activities. Finally, peers are critical in the school reintegration process as they play a unique role in assisting with reinvolvement in the more typical tasks of childhood and adolescence.

THE ROLE OF THE PSYCHOLOGIST IN THE HEALTH CARE SETTING

It is clear that the clinician must consider a myriad of factors when working with a chronically ill child, whether in the school system or the health care setting. The roles of psychologists are typically varied and include assessment, intervention, consultation, and liaison (American Psychological Association, 1998). These activities may be conceptualized as part of the health matrix model (see Figure 17.1). With the changes in the delivery of health care, psychology as a profession also has recognized the significance of timing of intervention. This is likely to assume greater importance during the next several years as the focus shifts to preventing disease and reducing the economic burden of health care costs. The health matrix model recognizes that service and prevention activities may be applied across the spectrum of diseases as psychology makes a contribution to health care. Moreover, the psychologist can make an important contribution to children's or adolescents' functioning through each of these services.

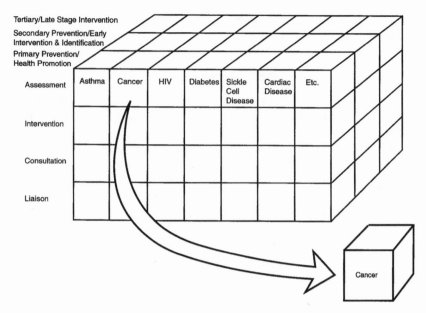

FIGURE 17.1. Health service matrix role. From American Psychological Association (1998).

Assessment

Psychologists may be asked to evaluate the emotional, behavioral, neuro-psychological, and academic functioning of children and adolescents being managed for a chronic illness who also have comorbidity of learning or emotional problems. For example, if a child is encountering difficulties in adhering to the prescribed medical regimen, a psychologist may wish to evaluate whether emotional factors such as anxiety and depressive symptoms are impeding compliance to the prescribed regimen or whether a learning disability or other cognitive factors, including developmental delays, are preventing successful adherence. Methods of assessment might include the administration of traditional psychological tests of mental abilities and academic achievement, as well as measures to assess attention and other cognitive factors that may affect the child's ability to follow through with health care providers' recommendations regarding treatment regimens. The astute pediatric psychologist gathers information with the goal of making a differential diagnosis and considers comorbidity of emotional factors that may accompany a learning disorder. There may be a complex intertwining of emotional and learning factors associated with cognitive adaptation to the disease and resulting adherence. Although some learning difficulties may be present prior to and separate from disease development, others may be the direct result of disease pathophysiology and/or treatment. Because of these complexities, the psychologist needs a firm understanding of the disease process and pathophysiology so the patient's needs may be best met.

Intervention

Intervention efforts for a child suspected of having some type of cognitive impairment or learning disability might include arranging for appropriate classroom placement, including special education services (Madan-Swain, Fredrick, & Wallander, Chapter 14), educating parents about the specific accommodations needed so that learning may be maximized, and working directly with the child to assist in issues of adjustment and adaptation to the disability. Intervention efforts also may include school visits in which students in the patient's classroom are taught about their peer's disease and its effect on the ability to function in class and participate in activities. The psychologist can be important in assisting the chronically ill child with successful reintegration into the classroom by minimizing peer misperceptions regarding the disease and maximizing successful adaptation to classroom routines. Peer education is key in promoting friendships and social support around the child's disease and possible cognitive limitations.

In addition, the pediatric psychologist devotes much effort in assisting the family to adapt to cognitive changes that may have occurred as the result of the disease and in providing support in negotiating the emotional impact and losses associated with the disease. Finally, children with a chronic illness will require support and assistance in adapting to the cognitive limitations that may be imposed by their disease. In this endeavor, the psychologist may provide intervention prior to the hospitalization, during the inpatient stay, and throughout the recovery period following discharge. The types of individual psychotherapies vary depending upon the developmental level of the child and the degree of cognitive impairment. For example, an adolescent receiving chemotherapy for cancer may benefit from cognitive behavioral therapy in coping with the loss of memory and physical changes that frequently accompany this treatment. On the other hand, the younger child whose linguistic skills may not be sufficiently developed to allow expression of emotions may benefit from play therapy, and the family may need additional support on a systems level (i.e., family psychotherapy).

Consultation

Psychologists frequently are called upon by their health care colleagues to provide consultation on the cognitive adaptation of the medically ill child.

Several styles of consultation are used by psychologists. The most traditional model has often been referred to as the independent functions approach. In this model, the psychologist receives a referral from the physician, contacts the family and conducts an assessment independently with the child, and communicates the findings to the referring physician by means of a report (Roberts & Wright, 1982). The primary goal of this model is to seek and apply expert knowledge to a specific problem in a specific patient. A clear drawback of the independent function model is that little information is shared directly among professionals, sacrificing both potential knowledge gain and important and perhaps helpful collegial relationships. In general, this model seems to work best for outpatient settings, allowing the consultant to communicate that the referral has been received and actions have been taken.

The indirect consultation approach involves little or no direct contact between the patient and the pediatric psychologist. This approach closely resembles the traditional notion of psychiatric liaison work. An example might be a psychologist who receives a description of a patient with a history of chronic school failure and then assists the physician in accessing psychological testing via the child's school psychologist. The primary emphasis lies in providing medical professionals with guidance and instruction so they can interact more effectively and conscientiously with children, adolescents, and their families (Kush & Campo, 1998; Roberts & Wright, 1982). Education and input are often provided during case conferences, staff development meetings, outpatient medical clinics, and through participation in medical rounds (Olson, Mullins, Chaney, & Gillman, 1994). A pediatric psychologist may assist pediatricians and other physicians through education on recognition of the signs of emotional and psychological distress, as well as on understanding the need for referral when behavior problems are reported. In addition, a consulting psychologist may work indirectly by providing medical professionals with disorder-specific treatment protocols and step-by-step intervention strategies for managing common behavior problems (Roberts & Lyman, 1990). An even broader role for the pediatric psychologist who chooses to work indirectly is to intervene at multiple system levels in a medical setting so that a child's and family's interactions with the health care system flows smoothly and meets their needs (Woolston, 1994).

Regarded as a "best practice," the collaborative approach uses direct patient contact provided by both the referring medical practitioner and the pediatric psychologist. Intervention generally occurs over four steps: (1) Referral is sought by the treating physician; (2) the psychologist speaks with the physician to gather background information about the patient and a description of the physician's concerns; (3) the psychologists completes the consultation with the patient and his family; and (4) the psychologist provides feedback to the referring physician about the patient's symptoms, diagnosis, and treatment options for follow-up. This model is typically considered the most desirable because it offers close collaboration and communication between medical staff and psychologists, including solid communication about treatment planning and intervention options (Roberts & Lyman, 1990). This type of consultation is particularly prevalent in outpatient specialty clinics like hematology/oncology, pediatric neurology, and endocrinology.

Finally, in the collaborative team model, the psychologist works within an interdisciplinary team of health care providers. Each of the individual team members provides information from the perspective of his or her area of expertise. The psychologist is then responsible for the development of the treatment program. Thus, for a child with a learning disability that may be comorbid with insulin-dependent diabetes mellitus, the psychologist can provide valuable information to team members regarding how to communicate with the child and family in a manner that maximizes adherence to treatment.

Liaison

Liaison activities involve educating the medical team and other professionals regarding the psychosocial aspects of the disease and services that are provided by psychologists. For example, it is important for the child's school to have an understanding of the medical needs required by the child during the course of the academic day (Madan-Swain, Fredrick, & Wallander, Chapter 14). If a program that addresses these needs can be developed before the child reenters school, subsequent disease adaptation is enhanced. Liaison activities also include work with health care professionals to assist in understanding the child's level of cognitive functioning and gearing communication regarding disease accordingly. Also, lectures to nursing staff on child development or management of pain, for example, and assisting the treatment team in dealing with losses associated with death and dying are activities for which pediatric psychologists are well trained.

Timing of Intervention

Intervention efforts may proceed in accordance with various disease states. Although diseases vary in their courses, typically interventions may be categorized as primary, secondary, or tertiary.

Primary Prevention

Primary prevention targets disease before it develops. An example includes research by Rodrigue (1996), who examined the effects of a program designed to promote healthy attitudes and behaviors related to sun exposure in mothers of children under the age of 10 years. Three groups were compared that included a comprehensive prevention program group, an information-only group, and a no-information control group. Findings revealed that although both the comprehensive prevention program and information-only groups demonstrated increased levels of knowledge about sun exposure, only the comprehensive prevention group demonstrated positive changes in sun-safe behaviors, attitudes, and beliefs that were maintained at 3 months following the intervention.

Secondary Prevention

Secondary prevention includes the assessment of early disease states and appropriate intervention so as to prevent exacerbation of symptomatology. Psychologists successfully have used secondary prevention efforts in their work with premature and low-birth-weight infants who are at increased risk for developmental disabilities. Although not all of these children are necessarily destined to evidence significant delays in development, the premise is that early identification allows for appropriate stimulation and remediation of the indicated areas of impairment so as to minimize the subsequent impact of the disease. Secondary prevention is important in pediatric psychology for some chronic illnesses and focuses on providing intervention programs for chronically ill children and adolescents who are at specific risk for later cognitive and developmental problems.

Tertiary Prevention

Tertiary preventions include interventions that psychologists might use with children and adolescents who are already suffering from a chronic illness (American Psychological Association, 1998). For psychologists working with the chronically ill child, tertiary prevention services may assist the child in adjusting to the diagnosis, coping with the treatment regimens, and securing interventions for educational late effects (Armstrong & Mulhern, Chapter 4). Currently, tertiary prevention encompasses the majority of clinical efforts by mental health personnel in general psychological practice. Because of the economic increases in the delivery of health care and as a result of the changes in its management and delivery, there has been an impetus to shift efforts from the tertiary arena to primary and secondary efforts. It is hoped that this strategy will not only reduce the costs of delivering health care but also minimize the sequelae of illness for children and their families.

CLASSIFICATION OF DISEASE

The previous chapters described various diseases, including cancer, asthma, HIV/AIDS, insulin-dependent diabetes mellitus, sickle cell disease, cardiac diseases, seizure disorders, and traumatic brain injuries. The chapters are summarized here.

Cancer

Most literature in pediatric oncology pertains to neurotoxicities associated with prophylactic chemotherapy and radiation and the effects of brain tumors on cognitive functioning (Armstrong & Mulhern, Chapter 4). Services in these areas have been aimed at providing assessments of mental abilities and academic skills and working with school programs to accommodate the special needs of these children (Madan-Swain, Fredrick, & Wallander, Chapter 14). To date, these services have been delivered primarily at the tertiary level, whereby children diagnosed with various malignancies are provided with the appropriate cognitive, emotional, and behavioral interventions. Future research should include the provision of secondary intervention efforts in which children at risk are identified and special programs are provided (e.g., Head Start) that minimize later cognitive deficits. Unfortunately, few studies are available that have evaluated the efficacy of primary prevention efforts directly aimed at reducing the rate of cancer in children and adolescents. Examples of primary prevention programs include those directed at reducing smoking in adolescents and decreasing skin cancer (e.g., Rodrigue, 1996).

Asthma

Consistent with research on other diseases, pediatric psychologists have directed their efforts primarily toward assessment when working with children who have asthma. Assessment efforts have not only addressed the cognitive impact of medications used in managing the disease and respiratory arrests associated with asthma but also have focused on cognitive style and attribution, which affect ongoing disease management and daily coping (Lemanek & Hood, Chapter 5). No studies could be located that address primary prevention efforts for children with asthma. Secondary prevention may include educating children and their families to both recognition of environmental stimuli that are likely to trigger an asthma attack and the identification of physiological cues that indicate an impending respiratory event. Tertiary efforts include teaching children strategies that minimize the length and severity of asthma attacks, as well as psychological testing that identifies possible cognitive toxicities associated with medication used to manage asthma. Additionally, psychologists can assist the family in developing contingencies for adhering to medication regimens. This is particularly important for children who are at risk for learning problems and who thus may have difficulty comprehending the importance of adherence and remembering the prescribed doses.

HIV

Psychologists have made significant contributions both to the prevention and intervention efforts in children and adolescents with HIV disease. Assessment has become a standard of care for this population, and psychologists are core members of treatment teams. Frequently, decrements in neurocognitive functioning are markers of disease progression and alert the team to possible exacerbation of disease (Wolters, Brouwers, & Perez, Chapter 6). Given the nature of disease transmission, intervention typically occurs at a family level and may include the caregiver, child, and other family members who struggle with the demands imposed by this catastrophic illness. A great deal of effort has been directed toward primary prevention of HIV by emphasizing the deleterious effect of unprotected sex and intravenous drug use. Secondary prevention efforts might include family planning services offered to adolescents already diagnosed with the disease. Once again, most services provided in clinics are comprised of tertiary intervention and include ongoing psychological testing that frequently is a core component of clinical trials with this population. Psychotherapy aimed at coping with the progressive effects of the disease and its affect on individuals, families, and peers is strongly indicated.

Insulin-Dependent Diabetes Mellitus

Insulin-dependent diabetes mellitus is another disease in which the psychologist plays an important role in terms of assessment and intervention. Significant contributions have been made in assessment that have resulted in increased physiological understanding of the disease (Rovet & Fernandes, Chapter 7). Intervention efforts often are directed at assisting patients and their families to manage the disease more effectively. Such efforts may include focusing on family dynamics that may impede the child's willingness or ability to comply with the treatment regimen. Although discussion is limited in the literature, secondary efforts might include identifying children recently diagnosed with insulin-dependent diabetes mellitus who are at risk for nonadherence because of specific learning disabilities or other comorbid psychiatric problems like depression or attention-deficit/hyperactivity disorder. Interventions have been almost exclusively at the tertiary level, which include assessment of learning disabilities that may be the result of early disease onset and addressing issues of poor glycemic control or difficulty with adaptation to the disease.

Sickle Cell Disease

Recent emphasis has focused on the role that psychologists play in assisting in the care of children and adolescents with sickle cell disease. Services are all encompassing and range from assessment, intervention, consultation with physicians in working difficult families, and liaison with the treatment team in managing pain (Frank, Allison, & Cant, Chapter 8). Primary prevention efforts include working with potential parents in genetic screening. An example of secondary prevention efforts is the model program used in the Children's Hospital at the Medical University of South Carolina. In this program, the medical personnel at the sickle cell center work collaboratively with the county school system to assure that school attendance is not interrupted by ongoing medical treatment, and provisions are made for assisting the child in maintaining academic progress and preventing any academic delays. Children and adolescents are monitored carefully so those at risk for academic difficulties are provided additional resources and assistance from school personnel and hospital staff. Tertiary intervention comprises most of the psychologists' work with this population and includes neuropsychological assessments, family psychotherapy, and pain management.

Cardiac Disease

Services for children with congenital cardiac disease include assessment of psychological problems that may have etiology in syncope, assisting mothers in negotiating the stressors of caring for an infant with a congenital heart defect, and helping the older child deal with the limitations imposed by the disease. Consultation and liaison activities include working with the medical staff in assisting families of children with cardiac anomalies and comorbid psychological adjustment difficulties. Unfortunately, there have been few investigations stressing primary prevention efforts, with the exception of the literature in the area of behavioral medicine that teaches children weight control, diet management, and the importance of exercise (Hopper et al., 1996). Secondary prevention efforts might involve a program of anxiety management for adolescents who, by family history, are at risk for cardiac conditions. Finally, the work of DeMaso and colleagues (1991) and Davis, Brown, Bakeman, and Campbell (1998) exemplify tertiary prevention efforts. These investigators have targeted families and children with congenital heart defects in the assessment and adaptation to their disease.

Seizure Disorders

Given the high frequency of comorbidities among children with seizure disorders and other neurological diseases (Anderson et al., in press), psychologists have an important role in the assessment and management of these children and adolescents. Assessment roles include the identification of comorbid psychiatric conditions and the iatrogenic effects of anticonvulsant medications and their effects on learning. Intervention efforts include assisting children and their families to adhere to medication regimens and to adjust to the illness. Consultation and liaison efforts may involve educating teachers and school personnel regarding the characteristics of a seizure disorder and how to manage an event in the classroom. Liaison activities involve a close working relationship with physicians in assisting them to recognize comorbid psychological conditions and adjustment problems. Intervention efforts have been limited to the tertiary arena, where psychologists provide assessment and monitoring of neurocognitive functioning for children who have been managed with anticonvulsant medication. Finally, therapeutic efforts might focus on seeking social support from peers, adherence to medical regimens, and assisting parents in negotiating the stressors of having a chronically ill child.

Traumatic Brain Injuries

Children and adolescents with traumatic brain injuries require psychological services at both an assessment and intervention level. Assessment is crucial in identifying areas of deficit (Ewing-Cobbs & Bloom, Chapter 12) to design an effective program of rehabilitation. Families and children also need ongoing assistance in dealing with the devastating effects of such a trauma during recovery and rehabilitation. Given the long-standing nature of the recovery and rehabilitation process, consultation and liaison is an ongoing component of treatment and involves sustained collaboration with the medical team and school personnel. Intervention efforts are most promising at the primary prevention level and include public service initiatives emphasizing the importance of wearing seat belts (Roberts & Turner, 1986) and bicycle safety helmets to prevent such injuries. Secondary prevention efforts might include providing education for children and adolescents at risk and their caregivers (i.e., children with attention-deficit/ hyperactivity disorder and learning disabilities) regarding safety issues in preventing injuries. Finally, tertiary prevention includes a wide array of psychological services.

TRAINING AND COMPETENCE

Medical professionals who provide services to children, adolescents, and their families often request assistance from their colleagues in pediatric psychology to help with assessment and diagnosis of emotional and behavioral problems and to contribute to treatment planning and intervention. Guidance and assistance are offered for a variety of presenting problems, including emergent psychiatric issues (e.g., suicide attempts, psychosis), malingering and somatic illnesses with spurious etiologies and symptoms, emotional distress associated with physical illnesses, and behavioral problems reported by parents during visits with physicians. In addition, psychologists are often asked to consult and provide assessments for children who are suspected of having learning disabilities, cognitive deficits associated with medical treatment, and multiple developmental problems (Kush & Campo, 1998). Clearly, the diversity of conditions as well as the numerous roles a consulting pediatric psychologist must fill make this position challenging and fulfilling.

Training programs in pediatric psychology originated during the 1960s at the University of Iowa and the University of Oklahoma Health Sciences Center (Davidson, 1988). In the years that followed, a number of pediatric psychology training opportunities emerged, primarily in response to growing concern about a lack of psychologists trained to work in medical settings providing care for the medical *and* mental needs of children, adolescents, and their families. Pediatric psychology is well designed to meet the need for this kind of specialized service because the discipline concentrates on health and illness behavior of children and adolescents and the unique experiences of children in the medical setting.

A number of graduate programs in clinical psychology offer specialized training in pediatric psychology in addition to expertise in clinical child psychology (for review, see Drotar, 1998). However, independent programs of pediatric psychology, with separate specialty and proficiency standards, do not currently exist. In fact, there has been a general lack of agreement about the necessary components of training and the sequencing of training required for specialization in pediatric psychology (Peterson & Harbeck, 1988). In general, most professionals agree that training in clinical child psychology, including expertise in severe psychopathology, is essential at the graduate level, followed by specialized training in chronic and acute childhood diseases, plus direct clinical experiences at the internship and postdoctoral levels. A generous breadth and depth in training experiences is essential.

BREADTH AND DEPTH

Issues of Pathophysiology

One of the most important ingredients for successful consultative work in the pediatric area is a solid knowledge of typical childhood diseases and their manifestations in various populations. A basic understanding of pathophysiology and disease process provides a necessary context for assisting children and families in both understanding and coping with serious illnesses. In conducting neuropsychological assessments with children and adolescents, knowledge of areas affected by specific diseases guides the choice of instruments, norms, and interpretations of results. For example, different cancer treatment regimens pose varying levels of neurotoxicities that may well affect memory and cognitive functioning. In addition, radiation and chemotherapy may have long-term negative sequelae. Thus, for psychologists with an interest in pediatric psychology, a critical area for training actually lies within the domain of health psychology. Health psychology as a discipline focuses on training graduate students in health care delivery systems as well as in knowledge of illness and disease management (Davidson, 1988).

Developmental Issues

Having a background and solid training in human growth and development is a crucial component for assessing and treating children who are medically ill and their families. The psychologist must adopt a systems paradigm that considers not only the child or adolescent but also the family and environment that affects the child's adaptation to the illness. A child's understanding of medical illness is determined by developmental level. Younger children will have a more concrete perspective of sickness and death, whereas an adolescent may understand more abstract issues related to his or her illness. The pediatric psychologist must be sensitive to these developmental differences in assessment and treatment planning.

Psychopathology

The pediatric psychologist will be called upon to assist the medically ill child or adolescent with emotional and behavioral issues. For this reason, thorough training in clinical child psychopathology is fundamental. Emotional and behavioral problems may not always be comorbid with the medical illness. In some cases, these difficulties are present before the diagnosis of a chronic illness, yet may affect the child's adaptation to the disease and adherence to the recommended treatment regimen. The psychologist's understanding of psychopathology also must extend into the adult realm of functioning, as services will also include assessment, treatment, and referral of the children's parents and other adult caregivers (Davidson, 1988). Ideally, the competent pediatric psychologist has experience using a variety of treatment modalities, including individual psychotherapy, family systems therapy, and group interventions.

Systems Issues

A working knowledge of how systems of care operate and interact within the medical setting is important for maximizing the effect of service to children who suffer from chronic illnesses. Systems of care include the family, medical team, school, and community. Intervention with the family may involve education about the disease and symptom management, referral for psychological services, and ongoing assistance in adaptation to the illness. Pediatric psychologists also work directly with the medical team to provide information about the patient's emotional and behavioral status and the psychologist's plans for intervention. The psychologist may play a unique role in facilitating communication among team members as well as between health care providers and the family. Schools provide an important source of information about the child's behavior and ability to function in an academic and social setting. In addition, the psychologist may work closely with the school to develop a reasonable plan to reintegrate the child to the classroom following an absence associated with medical illness and treatment.

ETHICAL ISSUES

Given the specialized needs of patients seen by psychologists, a unique set of ethical issues must be considered. Belar and Deardorff (1995) provide a thorough review of ethical guidelines pertinent to the practice of health psychology. They discuss five ethical principles as they apply to clinical health psychologists, and these principles are also appropriate for the pediatric psychologist. They include (1) competence, (2) integrity, (3) professional and scientific responsibility, (4) respect for people's rights and dignity, and (5) concern for others' welfare.

Competence

The principle of competence includes issues related to training, assessment, sensitivity to cultural differences of patients, and awareness of personal problems that may affect the psychologist's ability to care for patients. As discussed in the preceding section, the pediatric psychologist requires a breadth and depth of training in areas related to pathophysiology, developmental issues, clinical and emotional issues and how they affect chronic illness in children, and systems issues in the health care setting. Education consists of graduate-level course work as well as supervised clinical experience. It is not unusual for this level of expertise to be pursued by means of specialized postdoctoral training. Competency in training also entails an awareness of one's limits of expertise. The areas falling within the practice of pediatric psychology are extremely diverse, making it unlikely that any individual psychologist can claim proficiency in all related clinical tasks. The competent psychologist recognizes those cases outside his or her areas of expertise and seeks consultation or makes referrals accordingly. Because of the high level of research and clinical activity, psychologists must keep abreast of current literature. In terms of assessment, the competent psychologist understands that test results must be interpreted within the context of their use with medically ill children. This may entail using, when available, standardization data specifically for medical patients. Results should be discussed with both the patient and referring physician in a manner that promotes clear and accurate understanding. Another facet of competency involves sensitivity to differences in the cultural backgrounds of patients and their families. In particular, obtaining a good understanding of the patient's health belief model is a crucial component of assessment and is important in guiding intervention. Finally, although working with medically ill children and adolescents is certainly a rewarding experience, it is a stressful one. If the psychologist handles stress poorly, there will likely be a negative effect on clinical effectiveness. It is the responsibility of psychologists to monitor their own stress levels and seek assistance as necessary to avoid compromise of patient care.

Integrity

The principle of integrity within pediatric psychology includes advertisement of services, role clarification, awareness of duplication of services, and avoiding the imposition of one's own values on the patient. When advertising services or endorsing products, psychologists must ensure that all information is factual. Any claims about product effectiveness must necessarily be empirically based. It is particularly important for psychologists to clarify their role to children and families with whom they work. Given the variety of health care professionals that may be involved with any one patient, families may quickly become confused as to which individual delivers what services. Therefore, several explanations may be necessary before patients and families have a clear understanding of how the psychologist can assist them. Also, children and adolescents referred to pediatric psychologists may already be involved with a mental health professional. In this case, it is the ethical responsibility of the psychologist to obtain appropriate releases and discuss with the other professional the need for additional psychological treatment and how treatment focuses will be kept distinct. Finally, in working with chronically ill children and families, psychologists must be cognizant of their own health belief system and avoid insistence that the patient adopt these beliefs in the recovery process.

Professional and Scientific Responsibility

Professional and scientific responsibility includes standards of conduct and the role of consults and communication with other health professionals (American Psychological Association, 1992). Psychologists working with chronically ill children or adolescents are expected to maintain the same level of professional conduct as clinicians in general practice. Quality of care should be assured by periodic review of services. Pediatric psychologists often work in collaboration with a team of health care professionals. Regular communication with other involved professionals is imperative either through chart notes, team meetings, or direct communication. Psychologists should also understand the competencies of other team members so that professional relationships, consultations, and referrals are appropriate and enhanced.

Respecting Rights and Dignity

This fourth principle primarily involves issues of confidentiality. Psychologists providing services to the chronically ill child or adolescent face special challenges to confidentiality, including communicating information to the referral source, charting information in a generally circulated medical chart, and discussing the patient's status within the context of a multidisciplinary team or with family members. The ethical psychologist strives to maximize confidentiality within the limits of the law. For example, if information about psychological status is to be shared with a multidisciplinary team, the patient should be explicitly informed of this plan.

Concern for Others' Welfare

The principle of concern for others' welfare pertains to protecting the rights of the child, adolescent, or family being treated. The issue of informed consent is central to this ethical principle. Informed consent involves disclosure to the patient (or legal guardian if the identified patient is a minor) of the nature of the proposed treatment, associated risks and benefits, and alternative treatments available. It implies that the person has the capacity to consent, has been provided with adequate information, has not been coerced into consent, and that consent has been appropriately documented. Pediatric psychologists may be asked to evaluate the family's health beliefs concerning treatment, evaluate level of understanding, and clarify misconceptions about treatment. Often psychologists play an important role in communicating information to children or adolescents at appropriate developmental levels. Finally, psychologists may be called upon to assist patients and families cope with emotions that arise in response to learning about uncertainties of treatment through the process of informed consent.

Psychologists who work with chronically medically ill children are faced with a unique set of professional and ethical challenges. The task is to provide competent clinical care to children and their families within a multidisciplinary setting. This entails protecting patients' confidentiality while simultaneously communicating appropriate information to the health care team. Ensuring that communication between team, family, and patient is clear and occurs at a developmentally appropriate level and in a culturally relevant context is part of the psychologist's role. Recognizing the boundaries of one's expertise and seeking outside consultation when indicated is crucial.

FUTURE DIRECTIONS

Not only are the roles of pediatric psychologists diverse, but their responsibilities are widespread as well. Service delivery may be at many levels, including the level of the individual, the family, the multidisciplinary team within the clinic or hospital setting, and the health care community. Services may be provided within the context of an intervention model and can be primary, secondary, or tertiary in nature. Activities may include assessment, intervention, consultation, and liaison. In these endeavors, psychologists will likely be employed in clinical settings that serve children with a multitude of acute and chronic medical illnesses. To function as a competent pediatric psychologist, psychologists must be broadly trained in content areas encompassing pathophysiology, development, psychopathology, and various systems. Finally, the pediatric setting poses a unique set of ethical challenges to even the most competent and seasoned psychologist. Clearly, pediatric psychology is an exciting and richly rewarding field. We anticipate that this book will assist in the stimulation of clinical interests and research productivity for individuals already in the fields of clinical child, pediatric, and school psychology as well as those who are currently training. The contributions of each of the authors is very much appreciated, and it is anticipated that the clinical and research interests that emerge from this work will enhance our ability to care for children with chronic illnesses. We hope that the end result will enhance the quality of life of these children and their families.

REFERENCES

American Psychological Association (1992). Ethical principles of psychologists and code of conduct. *American Psychologist, 47,* 1597–1611.

American Psychological Association. (1998). *Final report to the Bureau of Professional Affairs on expanding the role of psychology in the health care delivery system.* Unpublished report.

Anderson, D. L., Spratt, E. G., Macias, M. M., Jellinek, M., Holden, K., Griesemer, D., & Barbosa, E. (in press). Use of the pediatric symptom checklist in a pediatric neurology population. *Journal of Pediatric Neurology.*

Belar, C. D., & Deardorff, W. W. (1995). *Clinical health psychology in medical settings: A practitioner's guidebook.* Washington, DC: American Psychological Association.

Brown, R. T., Madan-Swain, A., Walco, G. A., Cherrick, I., Ievers, C. E., Conte, P.

M., Vega, R., Bell, B., & Lauer, S. J. (1998). Cognitive and academic late effects among children previously treated for acute lymphocytic leukemia receiving chemotherapy as CNS prophylaxis. *Journal of Pediatric Psychology, 23*, 333–340.

Davidson, C. V. (1988). Training the pediatric psychologist and the developmental-behavioral pediatrician. In D. K. Routh (Ed.), *Handbook of pediatric psychology* (pp. 507–538). New York: Guilford Press.

Davis, C.S., Brown, R.T., Bakeman, R., & Campbell, R. (1998). Psychological adaptation and adjustment of mothers of children with congenital heart disease: Stress, coping, and family functioning. *Journal of Pediatric Psychology, 23*, 219–228.

DeMaso, D. R., Campis, L. K., Wypij, D., Bertram, S., Lipshitz, M., & Freed, M. (1991). The impact of maternal perceptions and medical severity of children with congenital heart disease. *Journal of Pediatric Psychology, 16*, 137–149.

Drotar, D. (1998). Training students for careers in medical settings: A graduate program in pediatric psychology. *Professional Psychology: Research and Practice, 29*, 402–404.

Garmezy, N. (1981). Children under stress: Perspectives on antecedents and correlates of vulnerability and resistance to psychopathology. In A. I. Rabin, J. Arnoff, A. M. Barclay, & R. A. Zucker (Eds.), *Further explorations in personality* (pp. 196–269). New York: Wiley.

Hopper, C. A., Munoz, K. D., Gruber, M. B., MacConnie, S., Schonfeldt, B., & Shunk, T. A. (1996). A school-based cardiovascular exercise and nutrition program with parent participation: An evaluation study. *Children's Health Care, 25*, 221–230.

Kaslow, N. J., Rehm, L. P., & Siegel, A. W. (1984). Social cognitive and cognitive correlates of depression in children. *Journal of Abnormal Child Psychology, 12*, 605–620.

Kush, S. A., & Campo, J. V. (1998). Consultation in the pediatric setting. In R. T. Ammerman & J. V. Campo (Eds.), *Handbook of pediatric psychology and psychiatry: Vol 1. Psychological and psychiatric issues in the pediatric setting* (pp. 23–40). Boston: Allyn & Bacon.

Olson, R. A., Mullins, L. L., Chaney, J. M., & Gillman, J. B. (1994). The role of the pediatric psychologist in a consultation liaison service. In R. A. Olson, L. L. Mullins, J. B. Gillman, & J. M. Chaney (Eds.), *The source book of pediatric psychology* (pp. 1–9). Boston: Allyn & Bacon.

Peterson, L., & Harbeck, C. (1988). *The pediatric psychologist: Issues in professional development and practice.* Champaign, IL: Research Press.

Roberts, M.C., & Lyman, R. D. (1990). The psychologist as a pediatric consultant. In A. M. Gross & R. S. Drabman (Eds.), *Handbook of clinical behavioral pediatrics* (pp. 11–28). New York: Plenum Press.

Roberts, M. C., & Turner, D. S. (1986). Rewarding parents for their children's use of safety seats. *Journal of Pediatric Psychology, 11*, 25–36.

Roberts, M. C., & Wright, L. (1982). Role of the pediatric psychologist as consultant to pediatricians. In J. Tuma (Ed.), *Handbook for the practice of pediatric psychology* (pp. 251–289). New York: Wiley-Interscience.

Rodrigue, J. (1996). Promoting healthier behaviors, attitudes, and beliefs toward sun exposure in parents of young children. *Journal of Consulting and Clinical Psychology, 64*, 1431–1436.

Schoenherr, S. J., Brown, R. T., Baldwin, K., & Kaslow, N. J. (1992). Attributional styles and psychopathology in pediatric chronic-illness groups. *Journal of Clinical Child Psychology, 21*, 380–388.

Woolston, J. L. (1994). General systems issues in child and adolescent consultation and liaison psychiatry. *Child and Adolescent Psychiatric Clinics of North America, 3*, 427–439.

Index